W9-CCO-133

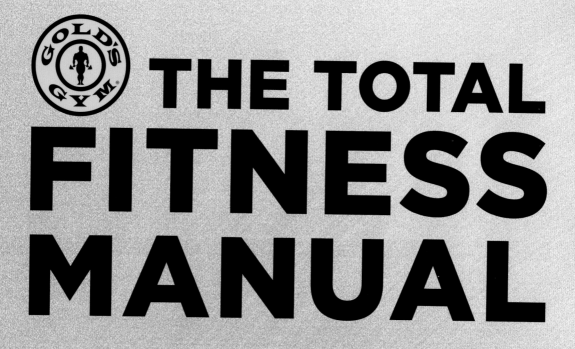

GOLD'S GYM THE TOTAL FITNESS MANUAL

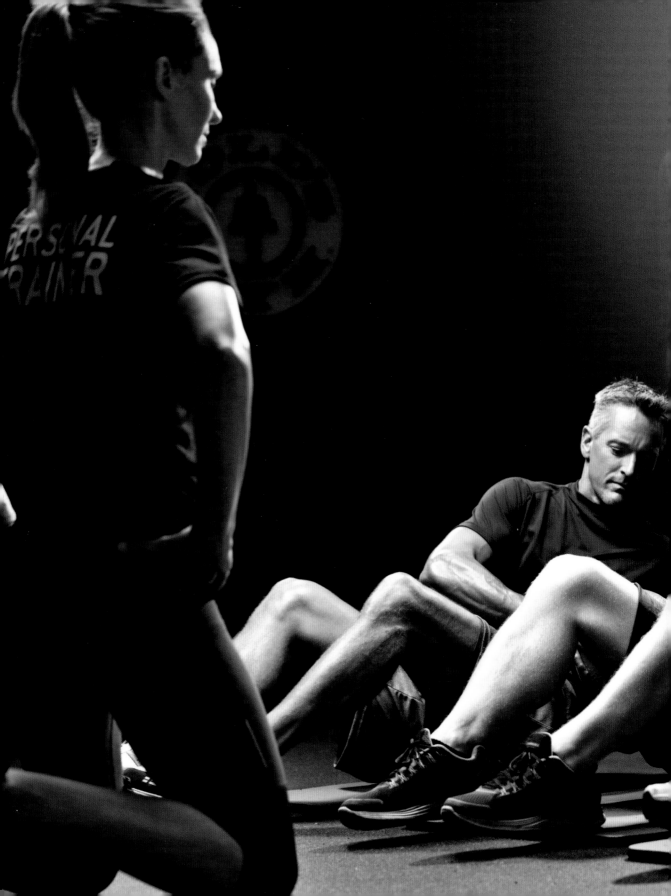

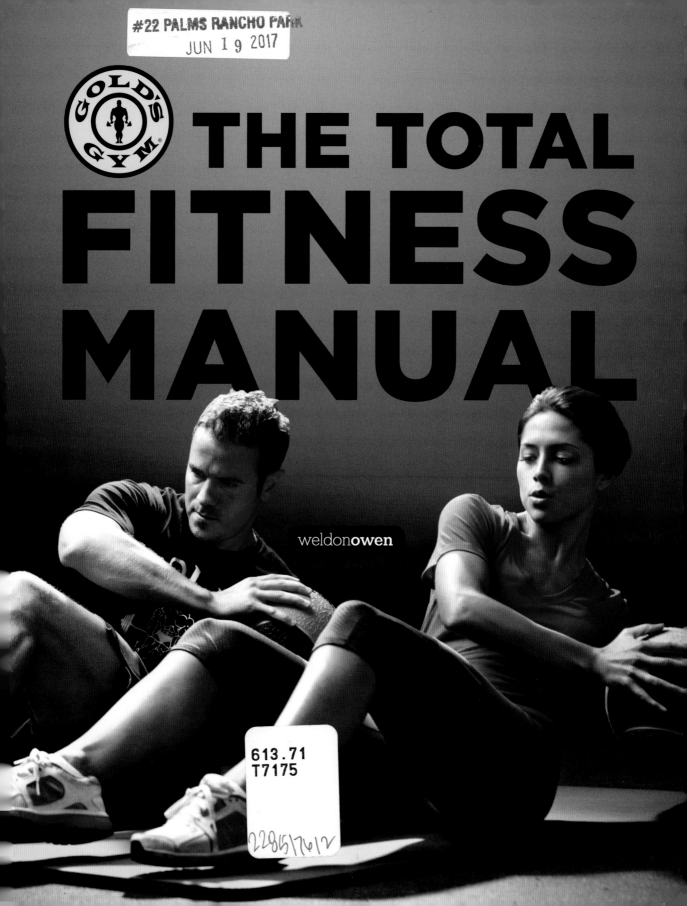

GOLD'S GYM

THE TOTAL FITNESS MANUAL

weldon**owen**

CONTENTS

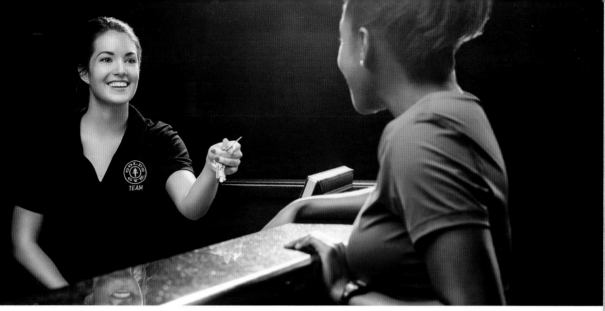

GET STRONG

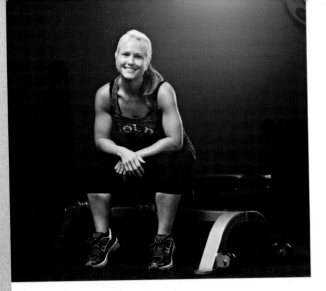

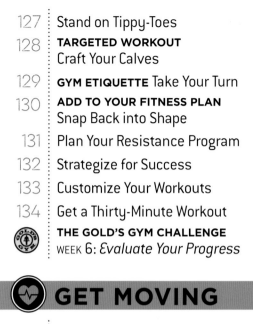
GET MOVING

STAY HEALTHY

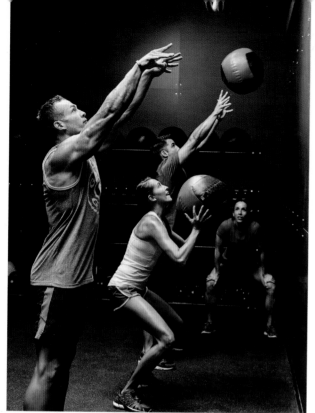

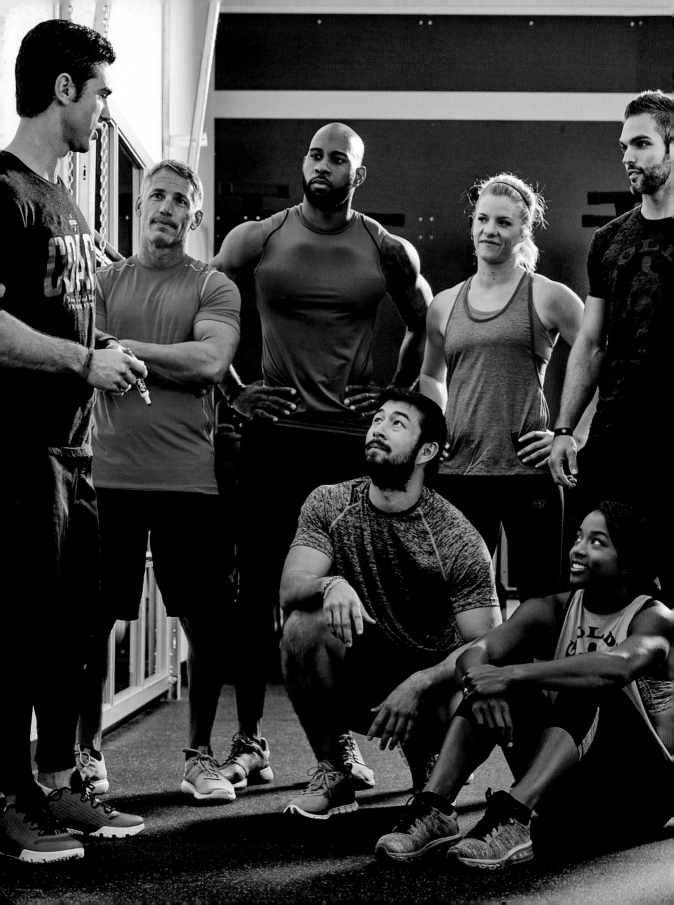

A TRADITION OF STRENGTH

In 1965, fitness enthusiast Joe Gold took the knowledge and expertise he'd gained while working out at the world-famous Muscle Beach and opened his first gym in Venice, California.

This first Gold's Gym featured homemade equipment and a can-do spirit that made it an instant hit with local bodybuilders. In 1977, the gym gained international renown when it was featured in the movie *Pumping Iron,* starring Lou Ferrigno and a Gold's Gym regular by the name of Arnold Schwarzenegger.

Joe Gold's passion for fitness was the driving force behind that original location's success. Today, that same passion can be found in the staff, trainers, and members at over 700 clubs across America and around the world in countries including Japan, Australia, Venezuela, Russia, India, the Philippines, and beyond.

Gold's Gym remains the go-to gym for celebrities and professional athletes—and anyone looking to get into the best shape of their life. No matter what your fitness goals may be, you'll find the latest and best equipment, classes, and services to suit your needs, whether that means getting ready for a beach vacation or looking to make major life changes.

But more importantly, at Gold's Gym you'll find a welcoming and supportive community. For more than 50 years, Gold's Gym has been showing people that strength comes in many forms. Joe Gold realized that every body has a unique path to achieving their health and fitness goals. Today, we're still dedicated to helping you set and attain those goals, in the gym and throughout your life.

TAKE THE GOLD'S GYM
CHALLENGE

Each year, Gold's Gym challenges its members to set personal fitness goals, and then meet with Gold's Gym's personal trainers to guide them on a 12-week journey. Thousands of people take the Challenge, with some spectacular results—and big cash prizes.

Winners in a number of age- and gender-based categories are chosen based on total body transformations including: the amount of weight lost, muscle tone, inches lost, percentage of body weight lost, personal testimonials, and before and after photos. Gold's Gym Challenge participants have lost over 188,000 pounds combined.

TRY IT AT HOME Taking the Gold's Gym Challenge gets you on the course to fitness, with expert advice, a supportive community both online and at the gym, and of course, the chance to win prizes. Can't wait to get started? This book also offers a home-based program you can do to get a feel for how the Gold's Gym Challenge works. Scattered throughout the chapters, you will find weekly Challenge pages, with each one taking you another step closer to achieving your goals.

GO FOR THE GOLD Once you've fully read up on the Gold's Gym Challenge in the pages that follow—and maybe tried the home-based program, it's time to get serious. Check out the Challenge rules and guidelines online at goldsgym.com or visit your local club for a personalized assessment. You really can transform your body in just 12 weeks. What are you waiting for?

HOW IT WORKS

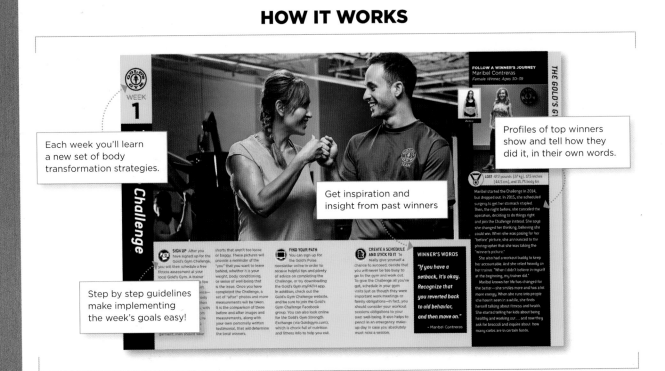

Each week you'll learn a new set of body transformation strategies.

Get inspiration and insight from past winners

Profiles of top winners show and tell how they did it, in their own words.

Step by step guidelines make implementing the week's goals easy!

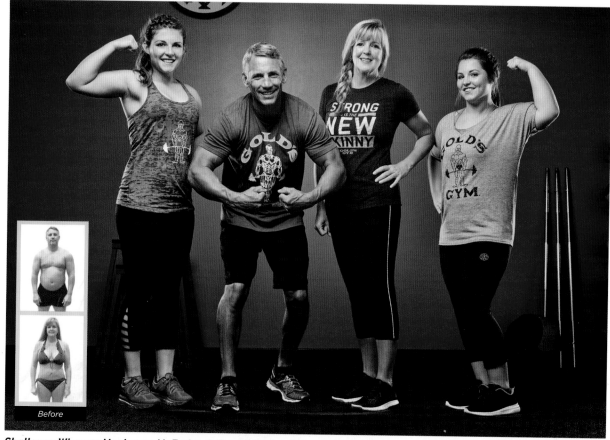

Before

Challenge Winners Mackenzy McFarland, Tom McFarland, Donna Dombrowski, and Sidney McFarland

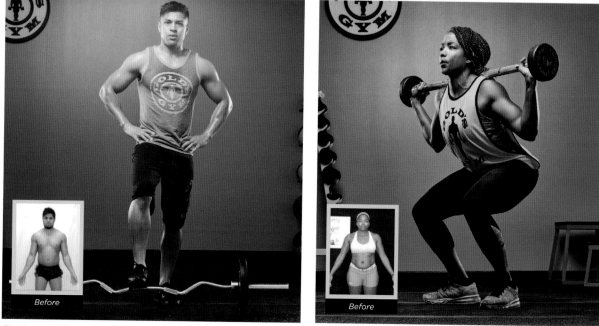

Before

Before

Challenge Winner Hedwin Lopez

Challenge Winner Ashley Friend

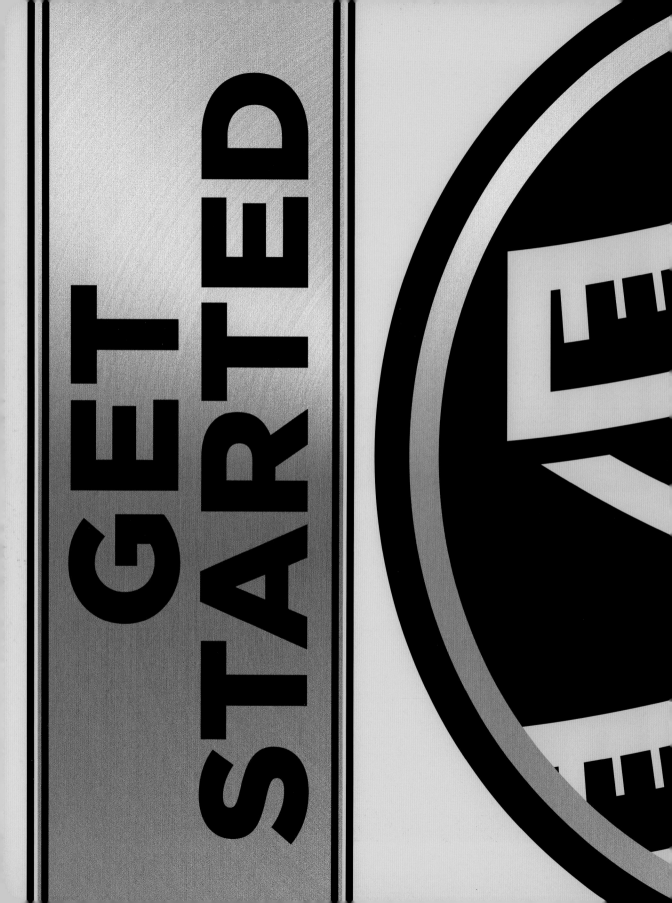

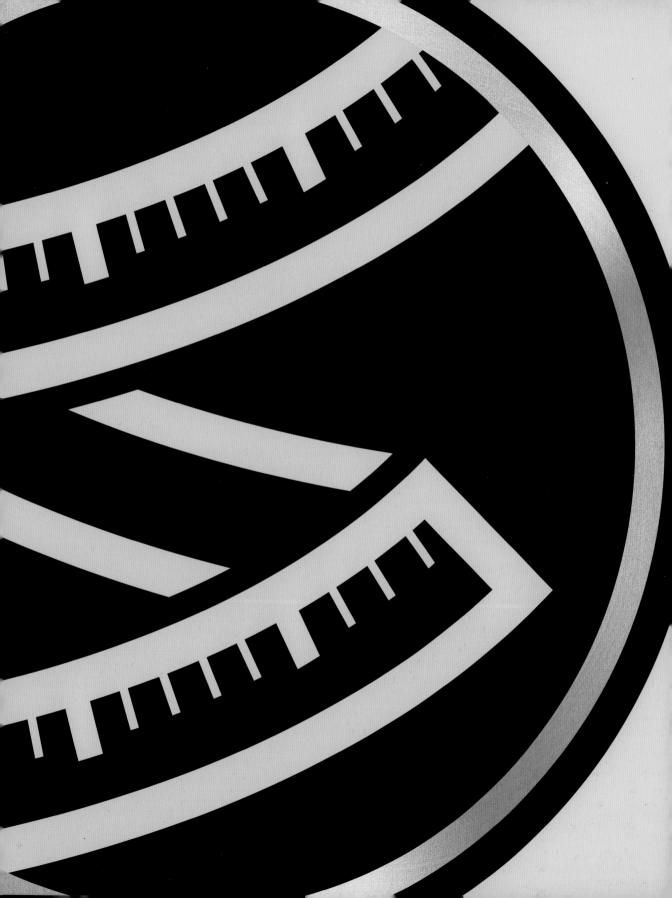

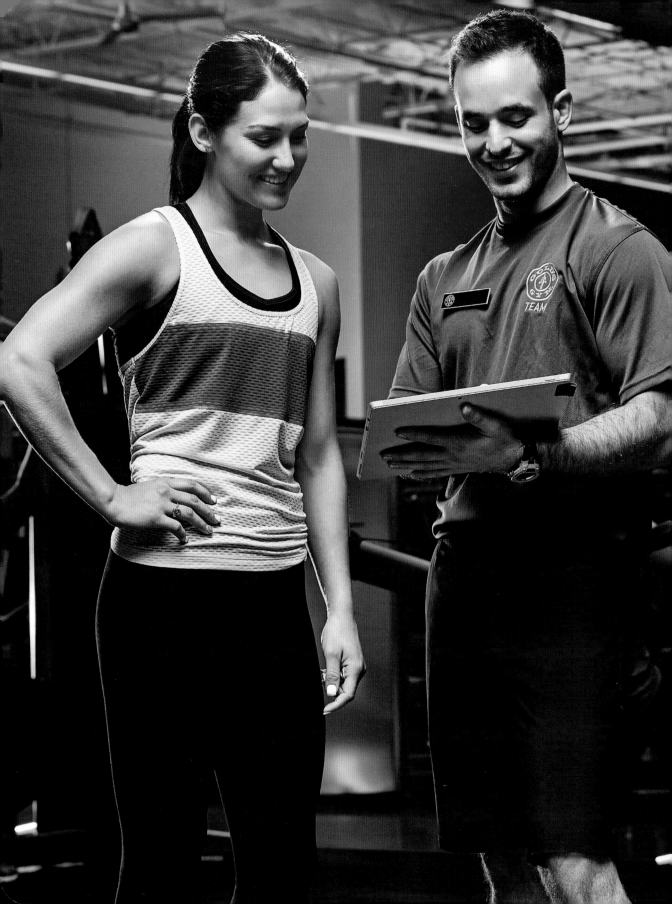

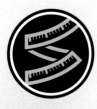 It might happen after a period of indulgence—the winter holidays or a summer vacation trip—or just come gradually, after too much time on the couch and at the fridge. You look in the mirror, and you barely recognize the person you see.

Have you gained some weight? Lost muscle tone? Is your posture drooping, or do you just appear a bit weary, even depressed? These are the signs, sure indicators that it's time to hit the gym and to start monitoring your diet. But what if you're unsure of how to prepare properly for this upcoming fitness renovation? Your first step, of course, is to check with your doctor before beginning any exercise program.

CHOOSE THE RIGHT GYM

Choosing the right gym is paramount. You need a fitness venue like Gold's Gym that caters to all levels of clients—remember, today's beginner will soon become tomorrow's intermediate. Trainers should be knowledgeable and supportive, and there should be a choice of several, so you can find the personality that meshes best with your own. All equipment must be up to date and the level of cleanliness high. It helps if you determine what type of gym you seek—one that focuses on resistance training, one that gives you lots of cardio options, one with dance and yoga classes, or a mix of all three. Don't get drawn in by glossy advertising alone. Instead, pay each of your potential choices a guest visit, and talk to the members about the quality and depth of service. Nothing beats first-hand input.

FOCUS ON DIET AND NUTRITION

Once you choose a gym and start your new fitness regimen, it's time to focus on diet and nutrition—what to eat, when to eat, how to eat. Learn the value of different macronutrients like carbs, proteins, and, yes, even fats. Begin to understand the process of hydration and how to give your body the necessary amounts of H_2O it requires to properly function.

OUTFIT YOURSELF APPROPRIATELY

You will also need to outfit yourself in the right clothing and footwear—like tops and bottoms that wick moisture away and athletic shoes that have the right support—and stock a gym bag with toiletries, towels, water, and snacks. From there on, it's up to you to stick to your program, work toward your fitness goals, and maintain a positive attitude.

001 PICK YOUR HEALTH GOALS

Before starting any fitness regimen, you naturally need to determine your goals. Do you want to improve your looks, boost your sports performance, raise your endurance, or improve your overall health? Do you simply want to lose weight or also tone up and gain muscle mass?

Gold's Gym's GOLD'S PATH™ program breaks fitness goals into the four most popular categories so that you can more easily find your starting point.

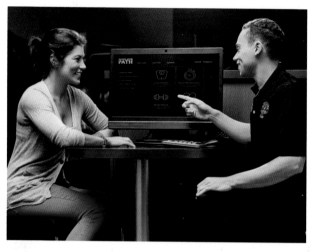

 LOSE WEIGHT Get lean, lose inches, reduce body fat percentage, and keep it off.

 BOOST PERFORMANCE Increase endurance, gain functional strength,and improve sport performance.

BUILD MUSCLE Gain strength, increase lean mass, or increase body definition.

IMPROVE OVERALL HEALTH Get fit, reduce stress, move better, feel better, and live better.

Your workouts will vary based on each of these goals, so it's a good idea to consult a trainer at first to customize your regimen with these specific outcomes in mind. Once you start actively training, it helps to post an upcoming athletic event on your calendar—whether it's a 5K charity walk or a 50-mile bike-a-thon—to give you something concrete to work toward.

002 FIND THE RIGHT PLAN FOR YOU

The challenge to creating a fitness program is avoiding the latest here-and-gone fads and finding a plan that makes you feel great—and then sticking with it. The Gold's Gym Challenge is a 12-week full body transformation contest exclusively available to Gold's Gym Members. Not a member? Visit your local Gold's Gym where a personal trainer can customize a 12 week transformation plan to jumpstart your fitness journey.

Exercise is a proven way to get in shape, stay fit, and improve your outlook. And the best part? There is a range of fitness options and workout tools to choose from. You might want to experiment with free weights, cardio training, dance classes, Pilates, yoga, running, swimming, martial arts, and biking, until you find the right combination.

Once you have a plan, stay realistic about your progress. Heightened expectations can sabotage any fitness plan—if you want too much too fast, you're likely to be disappointed. If you want to obtain results faster, talk with a trainer. He or she can point out the level of improvement you should be seeing and ease any concerns. A trainer can also help you tweak or expand your current program. So don't lose sight of your goals, and remember that, as with many disciplines, the slow way is ultimately the fast way.

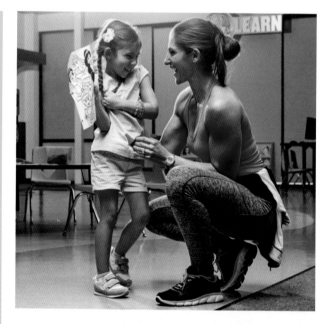

THINK about it

If you're tied down with the kids, many gyms offer a "kid's club" or "mommy and me" program. You can also offer to watch a friend's or neighbor's kids in exchange for them watching yours.

003 EVALUATE YOUR LIFESTYLE

While formulating your plan, imagine your day-to-day life, and consider how your new regimen can benefit it. If you have a sedentary desk job, an exercise program could compensate for all that inactivity. If you have a more physical job, exercise will help you keep up with on-the-job demands, especially as you grow older. And even if you participate in any sporting activities during the week or on the weekends, working out will help you achieve that high level of fitness your sport requires. A successful exercise plan will even allow you to spend a few hours crashed in front of the TV—without feeling guilty.

To avoid falling prey to these typical excuses for resisting a visit to the gym, try these motivational tricks.

I FEEL TOO TIRED AFTER WORK. Schedule a morning workout or a lunchtime session with a buddy.

MY DAY IS TOO BUSY. Pencil an hour workout into your planner as if it were an important meeting.

I FEEL SORE AFTER A WORKOUT. Simply vary the body part you concentrate on during your next session.

I HAD TO MISS MY END OF WEEK SESSION. No regrets … just reschedule it. Don't fall into the common trap of giving up after one disappointment.

004 FIND YOUR STARTING POINT

Every fitness program should start with establishing a baseline to evaluate future improvements. Start with the Gold's Gym fit test. The 10- to 15-minute test includes five exercises—crunches, push-ups, a pull-up for men or a bent-arm hang for women, squats, and a bench step test. Your results will generate a Fit Score, which you can use to track your health the way you use your body-fat index and cholesterol levels to help you track wellness issues. Your score indicates your level of fitness compared to Americans your age, and the test is free.

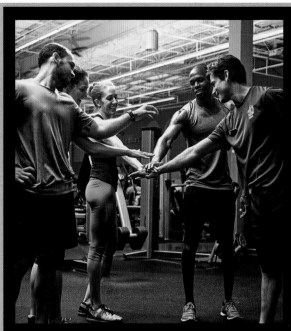

Ask the EXPERT

HOW DO I STICK TO A FITNESS PLAN?

Looking for ways to stick to your program? Here are some smart, stick-to-it strategies provided by the experts at the Gold's Gym Fitness Institute.

TELL FRIENDS Share your health and fitness goals with friends, family, or online; it helps to have a support group from the get-go.

TAKE A PIC Display an unflattering photo of yourself in plain sight to remind you of the cost of slipping.

TRASH THE BAD Purge your home of unhealthy, tempting foods. Make it easy on yourself, and stock up on healthy choices.

CAN THE EXCUSES Create a no-excuse mind-set—stash workout clothes in the office or in your car's trunk.

TRICK YOURSELF Tell yourself you only need to do a half hour of work—then stay for an hour.

CHANGE UP YOUR MUSIC Experiment with a variety of music mixes to keep yourself engaged and upbeat while you work out. Switch it up when it becomes routine.

PUSH HARDER Push yourself to go the extra distance when you are tiring during a run or workout routine; just think how good you'll feel if you finish. Plus, you'll have momentum for the next time.

MAKE FRIENDS Make gym buddies who will expect to see you there for workouts or classes.

005 STEP ABOARD

Monitoring your progress is a regular part of any fitness program, so your weight losses or gains should be checked and recorded every week or so. The best way to do this is with a quality scale that is as accurate as possible. There are three basic types to choose from.

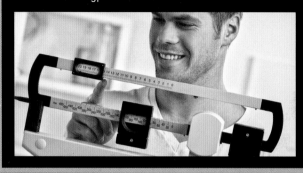

BALANCE SCALE This is the upright scale with adjustable weights that is found in your doctor's office or at the gym. Balance scales are quite accurate, but expensive.

DIGITAL SCALE Electronic digital scales with lit displays are accurate and easily portable. They operate on batteries or even on solar power. If the batteries are low, readings may be inaccurate. Some digital scales also offer additional features, like readouts with information about weight-related topics such as your percentage of body fat.

SPRING SCALE With these traditional scales, you step onto a platform, your weight compresses a spring, and a needle points to your weight. They are fairly reliable and can be recalibrated to zero with a knob or button; they cannot take much rough jostling, however.

006 MEASURE BODY FAT

These days, there are also several types of devices that measure the percentage of fat in your body. Although there is not a lot of research yet on just how this number relates to your general health, it may be an indicator of your chances of a weight-related ailment.

BODY FAT SCALES There are home body fat scales that use bioelectrical impedance (BIA) to gauge mass, water, and fat by sending an electrical current through your body and timing how long it takes. At present they are considered unreliable—drinking a lot of water can change readings by 10 percent.

HANDHELD BIA DEVICES These easy-to-use devices are often used in gyms, but they suffer the same reliability issues as body fat scales, and are often costly.

CALIPERS Caliper gauging, also known as the "pinch test," measures skin thickness at different places in your body. The resulting numbers are then plugged into a formula that estimates body-fat percentage based on age and gender. The pinch test is fairly accurate, but it can't be done properly without assistance, and it only measures subcutaneous fat.

HYDROSTATIC WEIGHING The most accurate readings of body fat come from hydrostatic weighing—which means you sit on a special stool underwater and expel as much air as possible while the machine weighs you. Check with a local university to find a facility that offers it. New high-tech machines that are nearly as accurate as hydrostatic weighing (that allow you to stay dry) are now offered at some gyms.

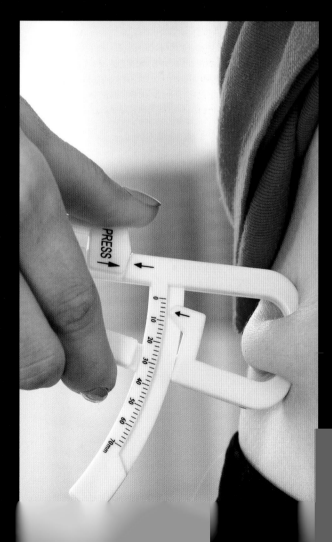

007 TAPE YOUR PROGRESS

Keeping track of your body measurements is essential. To start, go to your local Gold's Gym and get a full fitness assessment (all good gyms should provide this for free).

GET MEASURED Whether you are joining the 12-Week Challenge or just starting up a general fitness program, schedule a visit to a Gold's Gym to get your vitals down on paper. Be sure you bring along shorts (men) or a bathing suit (women) for your "before" photo. It will help inspire you to get in shape and keep the momentum going. A trainer will note the following:

- Weight
- Waist
- Thigh
- Hip
- % Body fat

To make the most of this data, you can also measure yourself weekly at home. Rather than just weighing yourself, taking measurements is the most accurate way to tell if you are shaping up. You might see a loss of an inch or more, even if your weight isn't budging. That's an indication that you're making progress—losing fat and gaining muscle. Measure at the same time of day (and be sure to keep the tape parallel to the floor). Measuring also allows you to calculate your hip-to-waist ratio, which helps determine health risks. Record these numbers in your fitness journal from week to week.

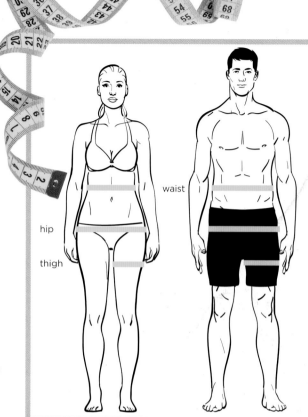

waist

hip

thigh

008 SNAP SOME SELFIES

Scales and body-fat percentages may give you important numbers, but don't get stuck on those figures as your only measures of progress. It is actually your own figure that will give you a true sense of how far you've come on your fitness program. And the best way to judge this is to snap some photos of yourself before you even start your plan.

STRIP DOWN Strip down to just your skivvies or a swimsuit, and take or have someone take pictures of you from all four sides. Seeing yourself from all angles may be pretty disheartening, but don't try for flattering shots: in these "before" photos you want to see the real state of your body.

STICK 'EM UP Stick the photos in a spot you can't miss them, and then every few weeks, snap a new set to see just how far you've come. Eventually, there will come a day when you know for sure you are snapping a set of true "after" pics. These before and after photos are better than any scale for telling the story of your own transformation.

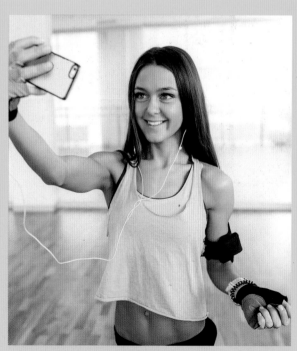

009 FIND THE RIGHT GYM FOR YOU

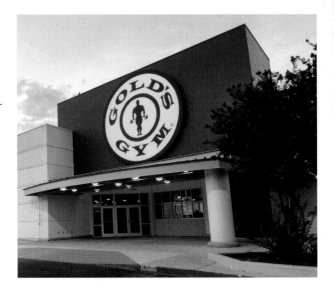

We may like to believe that we can become workout kings or queens at home, but sometimes it takes repeat visits to a dedicated space—a gym, health club, or athletic organization—for us to initially achieve real change. And the value of input or customized workouts from a professional trainer cannot be overstated. This is not to say a home gym won't offer you benefits, but many people find that first familiarizing themselves with all the equipment available at a commercial gym helps them determine how to best furnish a home gym.

There are certain steps you should take before purchasing a gym membership, including heeding these suggestions.

CREATE A MUST-HAVE LIST Draw up a list of must-haves—features or classes you would find in your ideal gym based on your established fitness goals. These could include a spacious free weight area, a variety of cardio machines, or a range of yoga classes. Even fitness newbies want to know their options.

RESEARCH ONLINE Avoid buying into hyped-up advertising or inflated fitness promises offered by competing facilities, and perform your own online research. Also, check online for feedback from satisfied or unhappy clients. Whatever gym you join should have an app so that you can link to the community and see class schedules, gym hours, and the like.

TAKE ADVANTAGE OF DEALS Look for introductory offers or coupon deals that allow you to try out gyms before signing up.

SCOUT THE LOCATION Location matters—Look for a gym near work if you plan on lunchtime workouts, or one near your home for early morning or evening sessions. A bonus would be if it's close enough to walk or bike to, for added cardio benefits.

CHECK OUT CLASS SIZES You don't want to feel packed into an overbooked class. Check out studio services, such as GOLD'SFIT® and GOLD'SCYCLE™.

MAKE SURE IT'S CLEAN Cleanliness should be an important factor, especially in the locker room and shower areas.

FEEL THE VIBE Ambience can affect attitude, so make sure the lights are not too bright, the décor too bold, or the music too loud. And always put substance above glitz or glamour. You'll do better in a supportive environment with a friendly community.

THINK *about it* Some deals on gym memberships or personal training may be offered in January or September, but don't focus on joining a gym only then. Any time is a great time to get in better shape!

010 ASK THE RIGHT QUESTIONS

Suppose you've finally found what seems to be the gym of your dreams. But don't get the membership just yet. You might want to take a moment to look over the following checklist of questions and make sure everything is in order before you sign any of the paperwork.

HOURS Does your location offer a discount membership if you visit during off-peak hours?

EQUIPMENT What is the age of the equipment, and how often does it get replaced?

INSTRUCTION Are you shown how to use the equipment as part of the service, or is there a fee?

STAFF Is the staff certified? Are they trained to handle medical emergencies? Are there qualified personal trainers available?

AMENITIES What amenities or extras does the locker room provide, such as towels, shampoo, body wash, hair dryers, and Wi-Fi?

CHILDCARE If you're a parent, does your choice offer childcare? Are there kids' classes?

FEES Are all services included in your membership, or are there extra charges for certain classes or for the use of special equipment?

EXTRAS Do members get discounts on massage therapy or other extras?

CANCELATION What do you need to do in order to cancel? Are there penalty fees?

011 LEARN THE LINGO

Like any sport or athletic pursuit, the fitness world has developed its own language. Your trainer may use words or phrases that are unfamiliar to you, or other members may use slang expressions you don't understand. Not to worry. Just look over the following list of terms, and pretty soon you will be speaking fluent "gym" with all the other exercise buffs.

REP Repetitions; how many times you complete a single exercise in a row: "I did 12 reps of a bench press."

1RM (ONE-REP MAXIMUM) The maximum amount of weight you can lift in a single repetition.

SET A group of repetitions done without stopping.

SUPERSET A combination of complementary exercises done back to back in one "superset" with little to no rest.

FAILURE The point at which you cannot do one more rep. Reaching failure is believed to encourage muscle growth.

SPOT When someone assists another person with an exercise.

RESISTANCE TRAINING Any exercise using resistance, like weights, machines, medicine balls, or elastic bands.

SELECTORIZED MACHINES Also known as universal machines, refers to weight machines upon which poundage is selected by inserting a pin into the weight stack.

FREE WEIGHTS Typically refers to dumbbells and barbells.

BAR A long straight bar that holds plate weights.

EZ CURL BAR A curved weight bar often used for bicep curls.

COLLAR The attachment that secures the plate weights to a barbell or curl bar.

NEGATIVES Negative training is when the muscle lengthens during an exercise, called an eccentric contraction.

CIRCUIT A series of different exercises performed back to back with little or no rest.

PYRAMIDING Performing sets of downward or upward scaling reps or weight, such as 4 sets by 12-10-8-6 or 6-8-10-12

INTERVALS Training at a low intensity for a period of time, followed by a high-intensity period.

HIIT (HIGH-INTENSITY INTERVAL TRAINING) This interval strategy alternates periods of short, intense exercise with less intense recovery periods. Also known as Tabata™ training.

RECOVERY Refers to rest taken between exercises. Short recovery is best for fat burn and conditioning, long recovery is best for powerlifting and bulking.

DOMS (DELAYED-ONSET MUSCLE SORENESS) The pain and stiffness felt in muscles several hours to days after unaccustomed or strenuous exercise.

MAXIMUM HEART RATE Calculated by subtracting your age from 220. It is used when determining your training zone.

TARGET HEART RATE A good target heart rate for vigorous training is 70 to 85 percent of your maximum heart rate.

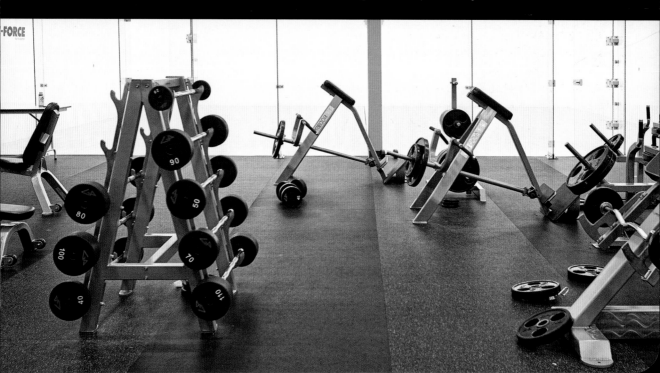

012 DISCOVER YOUR WORKOUT PROFILE

Before you commit to a fitness program and begin to create an exercise regimen that will truly work for you, it's helpful to understand what type of gym-goer you are. Just seven questions—crafted by Gold's Gym Fitness experts—can help you zero in on your workout profile.

Are you the grinder, who's allowed your workout to get a little stale? Or maybe you're a little too laid-back, showing up at the gym, but not really putting in the effort. You might be a real workout warrior, who makes fitness a priority; a fledgling who has a lot to learn; or the butterfly who uses the gym as just another social venue. Once you know your fitness personality, you can calculate how to get the most from your gym time and how to mix up your routine for a better workout.

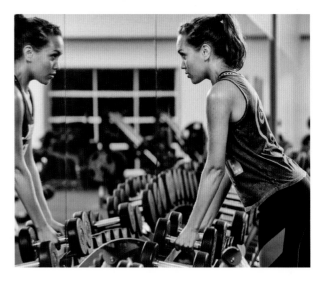

HOW WOULD YOU DESCRIBE YOUR PERSONALITY IN GENERAL?

☐ A. Dependable, organized, and steady

☐ B. Agreeable, fun-loving, and pretty mellow

☐ C. Intense (at times), motivated, and definitely adventurous

☐ D. Shy with strangers, but warm and generous with friends and family

☐ E. Outgoing, easy to be around, and loyal

WHY DID YOU JOIN A GYM?

☐ A. I missed the routine of daily practice, having played a lot of team sports when I was young.

☐ B. Just seemed like the thing a healthy adult should do.

☐ C. I couldn't afford to build a home gym.

☐ D. I wanted to start doing more than just long walks.

☐ E. My friends joined.

OUTSIDE OF THE GYM, HOW DO YOU STAY ACTIVE?

☐ A. I'm always up for a pickup game.

☐ B. I don't really stay active—that's why I go to the gym.

☐ C. I do triathlons, 10K races—you know, all that fun stuff.

☐ D. Maybe I'll take an afternoon walk or go for an easy bike ride.

☐ E. I love to do charity walks with groups, or fun runs with my family.

WHAT IS THE EXTENT OF YOUR GYM KNOW-HOW?

☐ A. I can pretty much jump on any cardio or weight machine in the joint.

☐ B. I know what I need to know.

☐ C. I know the next big fitness trend before anyone else.

☐ D. It's passable. I've mastered a few machines and the treadmill.

☐ E. Pretty good. And if I need help, I just ask one of the trainers.

HOW FAR IN ADVANCE DO YOU PLAN YOUR WORKOUT?

- [ ] A. No need to plan—I've got my routine down pat.
- [ ] B. I don't. I just let my mood decide.
- [ ] C. Weeks in advance. Doesn't everyone?
- [ ] D. I wait to see what cardio and weight machines are available.
- [ ] E. I usually check in with friends to find out what their workout plans are before I start to plan mine.

WHAT DO YOU DO BETWEEN SETS OR CARDIO SESSIONS?

- [ ] A. Towel down, grab a drink of water, and then keep going.
- [ ] B. Send a text or check my e-mail.
- [ ] C. Check my heart rate, and then get right back to work.
- [ ] D. Look for a free machine that I already know how to use.
- [ ] E. Stop to chat with a gym buddy.

WHAT ARE YOUR LISTENING/VIEWING HABITS AT THE GYM?

- [ ] A. I plug in my headphones, turn on the music, and get to work.
- [ ] B. I take TV over music—if I control the remote.
- [ ] C. I spend free time carefully crafting workout playlists.
- [ ] D. Sometimes I read books, sometimes I watch television. It's a toss-up.
- [ ] E. I don't like wearing headphones—I feel like I'm tuning out the people around me.

MOSTLY As – DAILY GRINDER

You grew up playing sports and started at the gym early, but now you've settled into a routine that lacks variety and is so dull that you might even quit. Try new things, like biking to work or running to the gym to add some scenery. You can also take classes—boot camp or mixed martial arts work many muscle groups and also deliver mucho cardio. Or join a training group that simulates a sports league … anything to break out of your routine rut and restore your love of fitness.

MOSTLY Bs – LAID-BACK LIFTER

You visit the gym because you know you should, but your heart isn't in it—plus you aren't pushing yourself toward any fitness goals. But going to the gym is half the battle, so try taking a group workout class that incorporates weights and weight-room exercises like squats and curls to get more out of your gym time. Hire a trainer for a session or two, and create a road map for your fitness future. The key is seeing the gym as an ongoing commitment to your body, not as a daily duty.

MOSTLY Cs – WORKOUT WARRIOR

Fitness rules your life. Being active and healthy is one of your priorities, and you enjoy it. You don't need much workout advice, but you should slow down at times to let your body rest and enjoy a little variety. You're a high achiever with a regimented workout, but adding variety makes you stronger and works more muscle groups. Try a yoga class to give your muscles a good stretch, a Zumba® class for a fun twist, or a mixed martial arts class to punch up your routine.

MOSTLY Ds – FITNESS FLEDGLING

You're a recent recruit (even after a few years at the gym) who's still working to get in shape, so you're wary of trying unfamiliar machines or new classes. Yet discovery is really enjoyable. The problem is you get in a rut because you do only what you know— you're stuck in a safety net. Ask for a free physical assessment (most gyms offer them) to gauge your fitness level. Then consult a trainer on how to use a given machine properly, or approach a teacher if you're nervous about a certain class.

MOSTLY Es – GYM BUTTERFLY

Being social is half the reason you hit the gym. Working out while catching up with friends keeps you going back. You just need to ensure that between conversations, you really are burning calories. If your routine isn't showing results, cut back on the chitchat, and try circuit training. Cross-train on the bike and then the elliptical—and minimize your rest period. Get your workout done faster; you'll then have more time to socialize. Also consider recruiting your friends for a boot camp or cycling class.

013 CHOOSE A TRAINER

A trainer is one of the most vital and helpful tools in your fitness toolbox. A good one will motivate and stimulate you, ensuring that your physique continues to improve.

Choosing the right one for you is essential and also sets you at ease while doing so. A good trainer will literally have your back and wants optimum results for you.

CHECK THEIR EXPERIENCE It's a good idea for you to interview different trainers to get a handle on their individual areas of expertise and what modalities they are most qualified to teach—especially if you should have certain limitations. Perhaps you suffer from tennis elbow or experience recurring lower-back pain. You will naturally be looking for a qualified trainer who is equipped to work effectively in such situations, one who will not in any way worsen your condition.

CHECK THEIR PRIORITIES The qualifications of trainers may vary, but bear in mind that your safety and personal goals should always remain their top priority.

CHECK THEIR STYLE It's important to get a sense that a trainer is not going to push you beyond your realistic capabilities, especially in the beginning. There's a fine line between challenging clients and intimidating them—the best trainers know how to walk it.

CHECK THEIR PERSONALITY Perhaps you have engaged a highly qualified trainer to work with based on his or her knowledge and experience, but you soon discover your personalities just aren't meshing. He may be too humorless; she may be too critical. Finding someone simpatico—who is truly on your wavelength—allows you to feel confident while achieving real results.

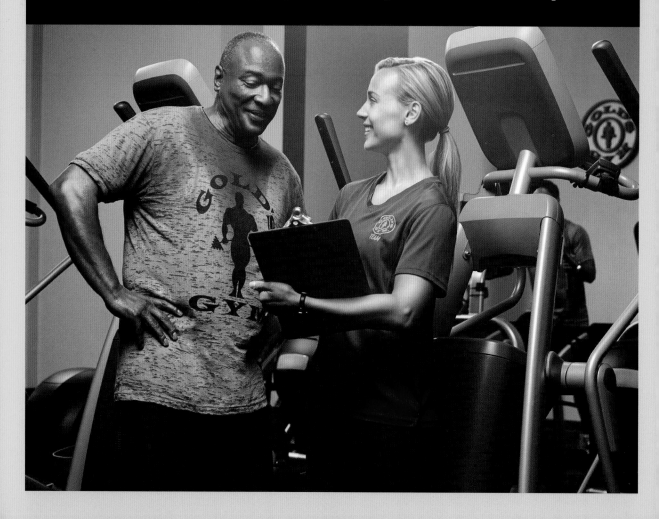

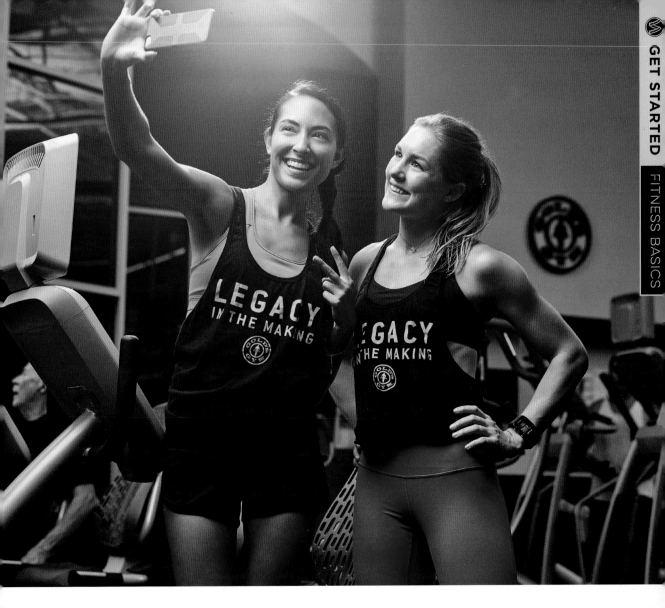

014 BUDDY UP!

Working with a trainer can help you achieve your goals, but sometimes, when motivation starts to lag, choosing to buddy up with a friend or partner can be very productive.

COOPERATION This is a cooperative partnership: one party counts on the other, and vice versa.

COMPETITION Friendly competition is a great motivator. If one of you is stronger than the other, don't make your competitions about who can lift the most weight or perform the most reps. See which one can first top a personal best.

ACCOUNTABILITY Knowing that someone is waiting at the gym for you at a certain time will encourage you to keep to your workout schedule.

015 POST YOUR SUCCESS!

One helpful way to stay motivated during the sometimes frustrating fitness process is to post your success or progression on social media or an Internet site —Facebook, Instagram, Twitter, or your own blog, for instance.

Set aside your vanity for a bit, and post several of those not-so-flattering "before" pictures you've taken (see #008). Then, after you have maintained that gym-going lifestyle over the course of several weeks or months, begin to post your "after" progress pictures. This sharing of your fitness evolution will be the means of both patting yourself on the back for a job well done and helping to motivate others to begin their own fitness programs.

016 WORK OUT AT HOME

Once you have familiarized yourself with the equipment at your gym and feel that you are staying on a regular schedule, it might be time to consider creating another workout center at home. This gives you some backup if you can't get to the gym, and lets you share workouts with a spouse, child, or friend. A home workout center can't often compete with the range and versatility of a commercial gym, it does offer one valuable benefit—convenience. For simple but effective home workouts, try using some of the following low-tech equipment, which take up little room.

FREE WEIGHTS Weight-training tools, which help to increase strength and bone density, are a must for your home gym. Handheld dumbbells and small hand weights have multiple uses, including isolation exercises. Also consider a set of barbells and a basic bench or a floor mat.

RESISTANCE BANDS These giant rubber bands come in various levels of resistance, and are lightweight and portable. There are flat bands or tubular varieties, which you can attach to handles for easier gripping.

JUMP ROPES Very little can beat these schoolyard favorites for offering low-tech but highly effective cardio workouts. Gold's Gym offers a variety, including the 3-IN-1 Jump Rope that offers adjustable weight, length, and speed.

MEDICINE BALL These weighted balls are great for high-speed, high-intensity resistance training.

STABILITY BALL This large inflatable ball can be used for a host of exercises, and can also be utilized like a bench for support. Gold's Gym offers the StayBall, which is weighted with sand for greater stability.

017 COVER YOUR BASES

To cover a lot of fitness bases, little beats the one-stop workout station called the home gym. This versatile machine allows you to focus on multiple areas such as chest (press and fly), shoulders (press and raises), arms (biceps and triceps), legs (extensions and curls), back (lat pull-down and rows), and abs (resisted crunches). Features to look for include adjustable seats and legwork components, variable bench positions, and effective levels of resistance—at least 150 pounds (68 kg) worth. You can try out the Olympic-width Gold's Gym Rack and Bench (shown below) with adjustable uprights and safety spotters; weight plate storage; a squat rack; independent utility bench; flat, incline, and decline bench positions; six foam leg developers with Olympic sleeve; a rolled preacher pad; removable curl yoke; and exercise chart.

When factoring price, ask yourself how much you intend you use the machine. Portability is another factor: does it fold up, or do its size and weight make it impossible to move out of the way? Certain models can equal the footprint of a love seat.

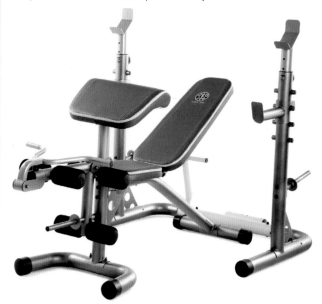

018 USE A STAND-IN

You'd be surprised at how many items already in your home can be substituted for gym equipment. Try using canned goods for hand weights, a full laundry detergent jug in place of a kettlebell, a chair back as a support during leg raises, an ottoman or picnic table seat for bench dips, or a filled duffel bag for lifts and curls. Or fashion a length of cotton clothesline into a jump rope. For some people, kitchen counters are the perfect height for doing triceps push-ups or impromptu barre work.

STAYBALL
by GOLD'S GYM

019 SELECT YOUR HOME MACHINE

The following exercise machines, which focus on different goals and supply varying levels of impact, are all popular choices for home workout centers. Look for models with electronic displays that show heart rate, calories burned, speed, and incline or resistance levels and that also allow you to program customized workouts. **Note:** Make sure to keep young children away from any equipment with moving parts, even if it is not in use.

ELLIPTICAL MACHINE

With its circular up-and-down motion—a cross between a treadmill and a stair-stepper—this machine offers cardio benefits and also helps strengthen legs, hips, and glutes because you are able to increase resistance—or work out in reverse! Because it is nearly impact free, this machine is good for those with joint problems or weight issues. Gold's Gym has numerous models of ellipticals, such as the Stride Trainer 550i.

TREADMILL

The treadmill, a time-honored weapon in the home gym arsenal, makes up more than half the fitness equipment market. The running/rapid walking motion specifically affects cardio-respiratory health. Look for models that feature a flexible surface, speed and grade adjustments, and an emergency stop device, such as the space-saving Gold's Gym Trainer 520 that comes with 16 preset workout apps.

STATIONARY BIKE

There are two types of workout bikes—the flywheel models and the air or bike models (such as the Gold's Gym Air Cycle). An upright flywheel bike (like the Gold's Gym Cycle Trainer 300 Ci) resembles a normal bicycle, while the recumbent (like the Gold's Gym Cycle Trainer 400 Ri shown here) has an upright seat that offers back support. The cardio benefits are similar for both positions. Some deluxe models offer a choice of moving scenery and allow you to participate in group classes—remotely.

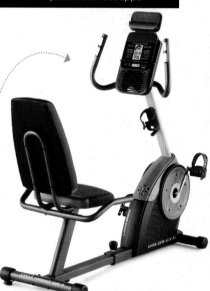

020 KEEP THESE MACHINES IN MIND

There a range of other popular home exercise machines available. Here are a few more to consider.

ROWING MACHINES A low-impact rower exercises all major muscle groups at once, fairly close to a total-body workout. Sleek new models feature digital readouts and use piston/hydraulic, flywheel, wind, or magnetic resistance. These machines have a long footprint; if this is an issue, look for models that fold up for easy storage.

CROSS-COUNTRY SKI MACHINES This machine, which simulates the striding, sliding motion of a cross-country skier, exercises both arms and legs, but remains easy on the knees. Look for a wide foot-bed for stability.

STAIR STEPPERS This machine, which simulates climbing stairs, is considered low impact, but some people find the strenuous action hard on the knees. Some machines offer hand grips to also work the arms.

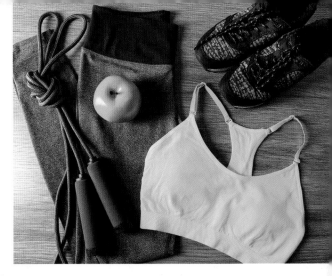

021 GEAR UP FOR PERFORMANCE

Gym-centric fashion has been with us since the 1980s, and we now see entire clothing lines dedicated to the "athleisure" movement, even some with celebrity branding. Yet, the basic uniform of the serious gym-goer has not changed much over the decades—a tank top or T-shirt, and shorts or leggings. Comfort and performance are the current watchwords. Hi-tech fabrics have even turned the T-shirt and shorts look into a perfect combination of functionality and old-school style.

Specialty shops and online vendors devoted to workout gear, as well as department and sporting goods stores, offer lots of workout clothing, with elite brands, budget options, and all the choices in between, along with various fitness trackers. Check your branch for a Gold's Gym Pro Shop with classic and modern Gold's Gym apparel. Also check out goldsgear.com.

022 KEEP IT WITH YOU

Extras like handy pockets further amp up the functionality of today's gear—do you really want to juggle your smartphone and keys while you're running on the treadmill? If you haven't stashed everything in a locker at Gold's Gym, look for clothing with hidden pockets—on the side, at the back, front, or in the waist—and you'll want them zippered to keep your things put.

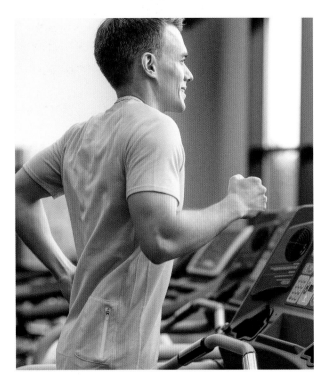

023 HANDLE WITH CARE

Even your gym clothes regularly get a workout—when you exercise, you are not only sweating, you are also shedding dead skin cells and body oils, so you need to remove both odors and grime when cleaning them. Yet proper laundering can pose some problems. Most exercise clothing is made of delicate synthetic stretch fabrics that need special handling—for one thing, they are not tolerant of strong detergents or fabric softeners. Always read the care labels carefully, especially for high-end brands.

Here are some pointers for getting the most life out of your hard-working gym duds:

RINSE OUT SWEAT Rinse out sweaty clothes while still at the gym, and place them in a zip-lock bag.

PRESOAK GARMENTS Remove sour odors by presoaking soiled clothing in a basin of cold water with 1 cup (237 ml) of white vinegar for 15 minutes. You can also add a cup of white vinegar to the rinse cycle.

AVOID SOFTENERS Avoid using fabric softeners on synthetics; they leave behind a coating that can lock in odors and damage delicate elastic fibers.

HOLD THE BLEACH Never use chlorine bleach.

TURN EVERYTHING INSIDE OUT Before you throw your workout clothes into the wash cycle, turn them inside out to protect colors and expose the most soiled areas.

MEASURE SPARINGLY Use slightly less detergent than recommended, and wash your load in cold water. Or look for detergents that are made specifically for workout clothing.

KEEP IT COOL Air-dry clothing or machine dry at the lowest setting. High heat can cause synthetic and stretch fabrics to shrink and lose flexibility.

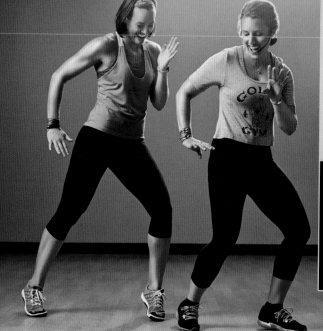

024 WICK IT AWAY

No one wants to feel like a sweaty mess during a workout. Technology comes to the rescue with sportswear fabrics that have the ability to wick moisture away from the body. Here are some possible stay-dry options:

POLYESTER This is a popular, breathable synthetic, but it does retain odors and has a high "stink factor."

COTTON Natural cotton doesn't retain odors, but it tends to hold moisture, so use it for low-sweat activities.

NYLON This fabric is lightweight, silky, mildew-resistant, and wicks moisture to the surface of the fabric.

BAMBOO Eco-friendly fabrics made from bamboo pulp are lightweight, naturally wicking, odor-repellent, and also protect your skin from ultraviolet rays.

POLYPROPYLENE This synthetic is water-resistant, making it ideal for wet weather activities. Its fibers force body moisture to the surface, where it can evaporate.

ELASTIC FIBER Fabric blended with elastic fibers, like Lycra or Spandex, lend them both super stretch and support. These stretch yarns are breathable, wick moisture, and dry quickly.

Ask the EXPERT

SHOULD I GO FOR COMPRESSION?

A recent boon for dedicated gym-goers is the advent of compression clothing. These super tight-fitting elastic garments are usually found as tops and bottoms, with a choice of short or long sleeves or compression leggings versus pants. There are also plenty of accessory pieces for arms and forearms, legs, and the knee and elbow regions.

Compression clothing is worn during and after strenuous or explosive workouts and are reportedly effective at easing soreness and speeding up muscle recovery. It is believed that they reduce inflammation—and the build-up of fluid and pressure—and increase blood flow to the affected areas, which removes the pain-inducing enzyme creatine kinase. Compression also helps speed blood to your heart after it has oxygenated your muscles—thus allowing you to train harder and do so for longer.

025 START OFF ON THE RIGHT FOOT

The modern athletic shoe is a marvel of engineering, with dozens of sporting applications. For your basic gym workout experience, look for a cross trainer that offers stability, style, shock absorption, traction, and a wicking footbed. And look for a proper fit—a workout shoe should feel comfortable right away. If you are involved in activities like kick-boxing or dance classes, discuss specialized footwear with your instructor. The following are some things to look for when buying workout shoes.

FLEXIBLE UPPER A flexible, lightweight upper will keep you agile and light on your feet.

STABLE BASE A stable base will support your foot, especially during lifting movements.

REINFORCED TOE A reinforced toe supports your foot during moves like push-ups.

NONSLIP SOLE A nonslip sole gives you safe support during kicks, lateral movements, and jumps.

THINK about it If you're making regular trips to the gym, be sure your sneakers can handle the heavy demands you're placing on them. Most workout shoes need to be replaced after approximately 100 hours of use.

026 STOCK YOUR GYM BAG

Don't get caught in the locker room with an oversized duffel filled with excess workout gear. Just stock your tote with these must-have items. These smart essentials will help you maximize your time at the gym.

WATER BOTTLE

Purchasing a high-quality, reusable bottle makes sense both financially (no overpriced bottled water) and environmentally (no plastic waste). Plus, insulated bottles will keep water or sports drinks cold and heated beverages hot. Look for models like the Gold's Gym Hydration Bottle with an easy-open snap lid.

BATTERY-POWERED IPOD CHARGER

What's worse than climbing onto the elliptical only to realize your iPod is kaput? By tossing a portable charger into your bag, you'll always have extra juice available to keep your music playing so that you can pace yourself during a cardio workout. Many of these chargers also work for cell phones and handhelds.

CHAMOIS TOWEL

These lightweight towels have been used by swimmers and divers for more than 20 years. A chamois towel is made of a highly absorbent hi-tech PVA material designed to dry your body more quickly than traditional, bulky cotton towels. Small microfiber towels are also effective during and after a workout.

RESEALABLE PLASTIC BAG

If you regularly squeeze in a morning workout at the gym before heading to the office, you don't want your dirty, sweaty gym clothes smelling up your tote—and all the other accessories inside it. Keep odors at bay by placing the gym clothes and socks you've worn in large, resealable plastic bags. These are available at most supermarkets and discount stores.

WEIGHT-LIFTING GLOVES

While you're weight lifting (or working out with other hands-on equipment) you'd probably rather obsess about your form, not blisters and calluses. Look for machine-washable fingerless gloves that are made of soft, durable leather or vinyl. Check your local Gold's Gym Pro Shop for a variety of styles, like the stretch mesh Tacky Training Glove—it comes in multiple colors for both men and women.

SHAMPOO AND BODY WASH

These multitasking products, which often feature a scent that is perfect for both men and women, save you from packing two separate bottles in your gym bag. Or look for travel-size bottles that don't take up room in your gym bag, and place them in resealable bags.

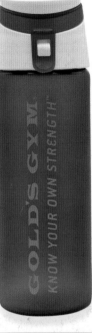

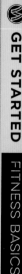

RECOVERY DRINK

It's important to repair your muscles with loads of protein and anti-inflammatory nutrients within 30 minutes of exercising. Take advantage of your gym's health bar or pro shop offerings, or bring drinks from home. Try Vanilla Créme Muscle Milk (select Gold's Gym Pro Shops) or shake up your own in a Gold's Gym Fusion Mixer or Basic Shaker Cup.

CLEAN T-SHIRT

There's nothing better than knowing a clean, dry T-shirt is waiting for you after a tough workout and a shower. Consider packing a pair of leggings or clean sweatpants, too. After all, do you really want to put your sweaty workout clothes back on? Check out the many styles for both men and women at your local Gold's Gym Pro Shop.

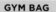

WORKOUT JOURNAL

You know it's important to keep track of your fitness goals—and, better yet, your progress. With a journal devoted to both exercise and general diet information, you'll be able to record the decisions you make and your victories, as well as jot down questions for trainers. Try the Gold's Gym Workout Journal, or, if you carry a tablet to the gym, you can plot your activities electronically.

GYM BAG

You, of course, need a gym bag to carry all your gear. Check your local Gold's Gym Pro Shop for a wide selection of carriers, including classic duffel bags, backpacks, and tote bags.

RUBBER FLIP-FLOPS

You'll want to protect your feet on damp changing-room floors and when you hop into the shower or visit the sauna or steam room. Plus, it's nice to have something clean and dry to slip into after a hard workout. Make sure to keep your flip-flops clean with soap, water, and a spritz of disinfectant spray.

027 PACE YOURSELF

Perhaps the hardest quality to cultivate during a long-term fitness plan is patience. In the results-based gym culture, you might push yourself to prove all that hard work is paying off, or you may want to demonstrate that you have the grit and determination to finish each exercise rotation quickly. This is especially true in a group environment, in which competition with others can override prudence. Yet, whether you are involved in high-intensity training or simply doing basic circuits, there are no gold stars for rushing to complete your reps. In fact, if you do rush, chances are you might finish only half of your intended goal. Not to mention, if you overdo it and get hurt, you won't be back on the machines for days.

028 WORK WITH A TEMPO

To get the most from your workouts, use tempo to guide you. With an appropriate amount of weight for your strength level, you should be able to count two seconds on raising, then lowering, the weight. This lets you focus on the muscles being used and maintain good form throughout the set. If you have to take time off from the gym, gradually working back up in the amount of weight you use will also help you avoid overtraining or injury.

To build up your endurance and stamina in the gym, it's crucial to include cardiovascular exercise as part of your regimen. Cardio includes any movements or activities that increase your heart rate for an extended period of time. Long duration, sustained cardiovascular training, or intervals of cardio with short rests between should both be used to get the best results, and should be completed multiple times per week. Nutrition also plays a large role in your endurance during exercise, so pay close attention to nutritional recommendations (see items 031–033 for more details).

029 WARM UP

Warming up is a frequently neglected (or even altogether forgotten) aspect of working out. Yet, it is important to have your muscles both warm and pliable for the often heavy workloads that will follow. A warm-up can be as simple as light dynamic stretching or a few minutes on a stationary bike in order to slightly elevate your heart rate and get those muscles and joints moving.

The tendency to dive right into an intense workout can result in injury due to the often excessive strain put on muscles and tendons at the sudden onset of explosive exercise. Taking a few minutes prior to your workout to properly warm up will not only help prevent injury, it will also properly prepare you for the work to follow. It's instinctive for a jungle predator to stretch out before pursuing its prey—and humans should learn from this behavior.

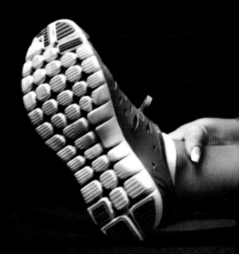

030 **COOL DOWN**

In the same way that warming up is vital to your gym longevity, cooling down is important as well . . . and for the same reasons. At the end of your workout, your muscles are pumped and filled with lactic acid—waste that has built up. Stretching at this time promotes the elongation of the muscle tissue, which helps transport vital nutrients more efficiently to your muscles, while aiding in the removal of the waste. Stretching will also help to keep you progressing and injury free.

Your greatest insurance in the gym is the care you give to your body by listening to it and offering it what it needs. Warming up and cooling down, though they may not seem glamorous, will keep you in this game for the long haul, and a few minutes before and after each session is a small price to pay for a lifetime of successful workouts.

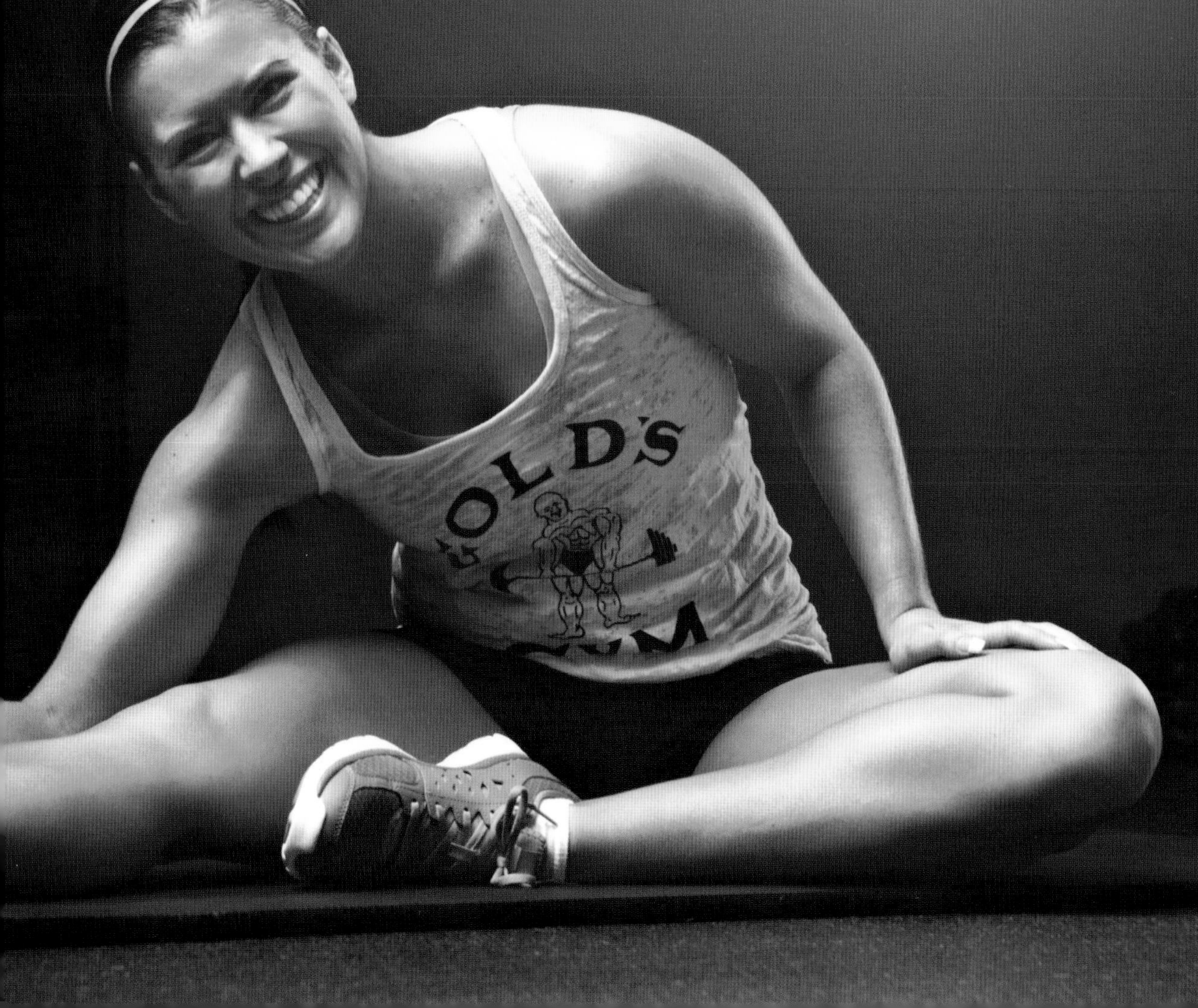

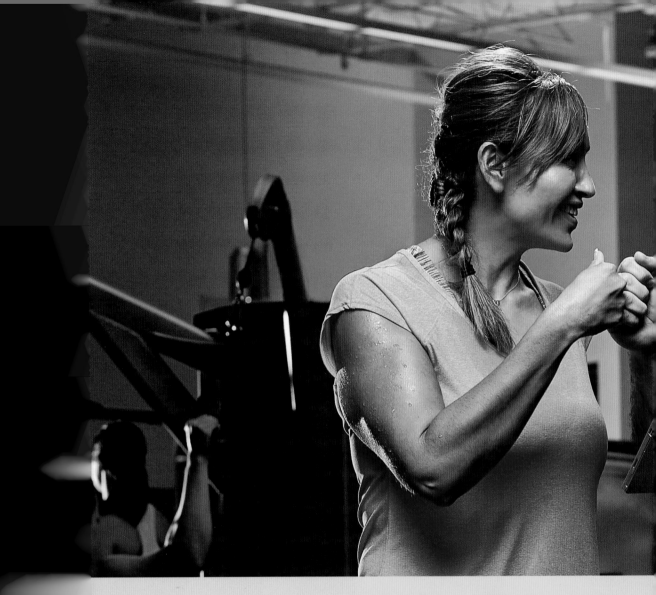

 SIGN UP After you have signed up for the Gold's Gym Challenge, you will then schedule a free fitness assessment at your local Gold's Gym. A trainer will weigh you and take a few measurements—your waist, hip, and thigh circumference— and also calculate your body fat percentage. You will then pose for "before" photos, with full-body images shot from the front and back. If you're a woman, wear a bathing suit or other form-fitting garment; men should wear shorts that aren't too loose or baggy. These pictures will provide a reminder of the "you" that you want to leave behind, whether it is your weight, body conditioning, or sense of well-being that is the focus. Once you have completed the Challenge, a set of "after" photos and more measurements will be taken. It is the comparison of these before and after images and measurements, along with your own personally written testimonial, that will determine the local winners.

 FIND YOUR PATH You can sign up for the Gold's Gym Pulse newsletter online in order to receive helpful tips and plenty of advice on completing the Challenge, or try downloading the Gold's Gym myPATH app. In addition, check out the Gold's Gym Challenge website, and be sure to join the Gold's Gym Challenge Facebook group. You can also look online for the Gold's Gym Strength Exchange (via Goldsgym.com), which is chock-full of nutrition and fitness info to help you out.

FOLLOW A WINNER'S JOURNEY
Maribel Contreras
Female Winner, Ages 30–39

Before

LOST 47.2 pounds (27 kg), 17.5 inches (44.5 cm), and 15.7% body fat

Maribel started the Challenge in 2014, but dropped out. In 2015, she scheduled surgery to get her stomach stapled. Then, the night before, she canceled the operation, deciding to do things right and join the Challenge instead. She says she changed her thinking, believing she could win. When she was posing for her "before" picture, she informed her photographer that she was taking the "winner's picture."

She also had a workout buddy who helped to keep her accountable. And she relied heavily on her trainer. "When I didn't believe in myself at the beginning, my trainer did."

Maribel knows her life has changed for the better—she smiles more and has a lot more energy. When she runs into people she hasn't seen in a while, she finds herself talking about fitness and health. She started telling her kids about being healthy and working out … and now they ask for broccoli and inquire about how many carbs are in certain foods.

CREATE A SCHEDULE AND STICK TO IT To really give yourself a chance to succeed, decide that you will never be too busy to go to your gym and work out. To give the Challenge all you've got, schedule in your gym visits just as though they were important work meetings or family obligations—in fact, you should consider your workout sessions obligations to your own well-being. It also helps to pencil in an emergency make-up day just in case you absolutely must miss a session.

WINNER'S WORDS

"If you have a setback, it's okay. Recognize that you reverted back to old behavior, and then move on."

~ Maribel Contreras

031 GET AN INTRODUCTION TO PROPER NUTRITION

Nutritional science studies and interprets the interactions of nutrients, and other substances in food, in relation to their effect on the maintenance, growth, reproduction, health, and disease of an organism. Nutrition is a key element in fitness, health, and in exercise—you can't out-train a bad diet.

Food is made up of macronutrients—carbohydrates, fats, proteins, and water—that are required in large quantities, along with micronutrients—minerals, vitamins, antioxidants, phytochemicals, and intestinal flora—that are needed in smaller quantities. A balanced human diet is composed of these different nutrients in the right proportions. The wrong ratios—or critical omissions—can affect both physical and mental health.

Exercise may be a big part of fitness, but up to 75 percent of your gains in the gym are also going to be based in your intake of macronutrients and micronutrients. If you need solid advice, a nutritionist can help—and many gyms out there, including Gold's Gym, have trained nutritionists on staff to assist you.

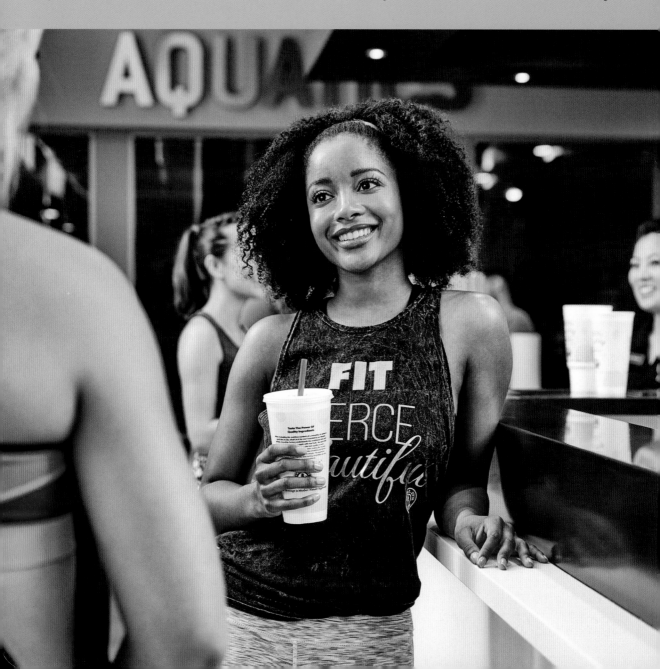

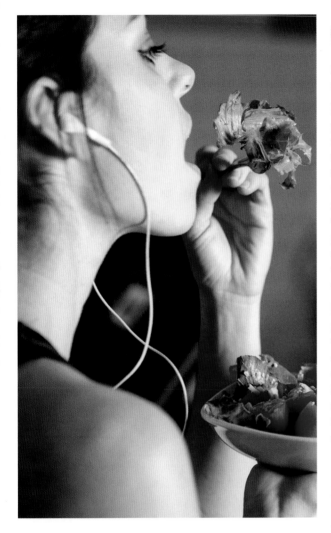

033 MAKE SOME SIMPLE CHANGES

It only takes three simple ideas to change the way you think about eating—planning, fueling, and recharging.

PLAN AHEAD When you are involved in a weekly fitness program, you not only want to keep hunger at bay, you also need to keep energy levels steady. Nutritionists recommend three meals, plus two snacks, in the course of a day. Balancing the right proportions of dietary macronutrients will allow you to maintain both your weight and energy levels. Try to create menus that are heavy on the vegetables, fruits, and healthy, whole-grain carbohydrates, with considered amounts of lean protein and polyunsaturated or monounsaturated fats. Also be sure to drink plenty of water, because a healthy diet combined with proper hydration will positively affect your workouts— and your daily life.

FUEL UP Always eat before you exercise. This helps to prevent low blood-sugar levels and hunger pangs during a workout, as well as provide energy to your muscles. Three or four hours before your workout, prepare a small meal of complex carbs—a whole-wheat waffle with yogurt and blueberries, whole-grain cereal with low-fat milk and banana slices, or a parfait of kiwi and orange slices over low-fat vanilla yogurt topped with low-fat granola. You can also have a light snack one to two hours before your workout.

RECHARGE Any intense workout that lasts longer than an hour will deplete your body of carbs and fluids. A small meal eaten soon after will remedy this, as well as help aid in muscle repair and recovery—muscles are most receptive to replacing glycogen within the first two hours after hard exercise. indulge in a protein drink at the gym bar, and follow that with a full, balanced meal two hours later. Try a baked sweet potato topped with chili, white-meat turkey in a whole-wheat wrap, pasta with chicken and veggies, or eggs scrambled with peppers, onions, and spinach.

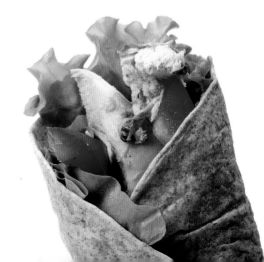

032 RETHINK YOUR EATING HABITS

Your workout plan should focus on two factors—eating smart and getting fit, in that order. Before achieving a better external physique through exercise, you need to start building up your body from the inside. This requires an awareness of the types of foods you should eat, those you need to avoid, and the supplements you may require.

Smart nutrition also means rethinking the ways you eat, the times and places you eat, and your attitude toward food in general. As your fitness regimen advances, you will likely find that many of your cravings have altered. You'll be less likely to indulge in salty or fatty snacks and become more concerned about the nutritional value of meals rather than simply the levels of satisfaction. Food will eventually become the ally rather than opposition.

034 MAKE SENSE OF MACRONUTRIENTS

Most nutritional guidelines indicate an approximate percentage of macronutrients—carbohydrates, proteins, and fat—humans require for optimal health, but their ratios are widely debated. Following a workout plan also affects these numbers.

In general, to maintain a healthy weight, women need 1,600 to 2,400 calories per day, and men need 2,000 to 3,000 calories. Age, sex, and level of activity, along with diet and fitness goals are among the factors that determine how those calories are portioned among the macronutrients. A nutritionist can answer a variety of questions for you on suggested intake amounts based on your goals, whether you're working toward weight loss, body building, or general fitness. Whatever breakdown of nutrients you follow, focus on variety, nutrient density, and healthy amounts of all food groups. Limit calories from sugars and saturated fats, and reduce sodium intake.

This chart below gives you sample recommended ranges of percentages of daily calories for varying goals, whether you want to build muscle, lose fat, or maintain the shape you're in.

NUTRIENT	MUSCLE BUILDING	FAT LOSS	MAINTENANCE
CARBOHYDRATES (4 calories per gram)	40 to 60 percent	10 to 30 percent	45 to 65 percent
PROTEIN (4 calories per gram)	25 to 35 percent	40 to 50 percent	10 to 35 percent
FAT (9 calories per gram)	15 to 25 percent	30 to 40 percent	10 to 35 percent

035 CHOOSE YOUR CARBS

Carbs are one of the main nutrients in our diets, and the most important one for those who are following a workout regimen—they are not only the top food source for energy, but they are also a source of recuperation. The digestive system turns carbs—most commonly sugars, starches, and fiber—into glucose (blood sugar), which the body then converts to energy that supports bodily functions and physical activity. When choosing carbs, remember, the more complex the better.

SIMPLE CARBS Simple carbs, such as white bread, white rice, or refined sugars, interfere with fat metabolism, may contribute to fat gain, decrease the body's energy needed for prolonged activity, increase hypertension (leading to high blood pressure) and can create an energy roller coaster as blood glucose levels fluctuate.

COMPLEX CARBS These carbs, found in natural, high-fiber foods like whole grains, fruits, vegetables, and beans, are far better for you than refined foods because they get absorbed more slowly into the system, avoiding spikes in blood sugar and offering sustained energy. They also make you feel more satiated after a meal and less likely to snack.

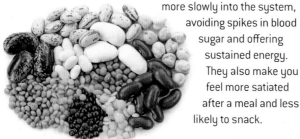

036 PICK YOUR PROTEINS

Proteins are organic molecules made up of amino acids—the building blocks of life— that produce the enzymes, hormones, neurotransmitters, and antibodies that enable the human body to function. Proteins also aid in growth of muscle tissue. As food is digested, proteins break down in the bloodstream into individual amino acids that trade with other amino acids already located in our cells. This provides a supply of frequently replenished amino acids that are ready when needed. Some fitness buffs believe that if you beef up on protein—which contains 4 calories per gram—you will gain muscle. Although it's true that proteins rebuild and repair muscles, your body can only handle a certain amount; the rest turns to waste. So limit your intake to six to seven ounces of protein daily—even if you are an athlete.

COMPLETE PROTEINS These generally come from animal sources and include beef, poultry, fish, milk, eggs, cheese, and yogurt. Plant-based soy is also a complete protein.

INCOMPLETE PROTEINS This group is made up of vegetable sources that don't contain all nine essential amino acids, or don't have sufficient quantities of them. They include nuts, seeds, beans, and grains. They should, ideally, be combined with each other to complete the essential amino acid profile—for example, you can pair rice with beans, toss some almond slivers over a leafy spinach salad, or spread peanut butter on whole-grain toast.

037 OPT FOR VEGAN PROTEIN

If you're a vegetarian or vegan, there's no need to become protein-deprived. There are plenty of plant-based foods that supply the necessary protein needed for a healthy diet.

LOWER-CALORIE SOURCES Foods made from soybeans offer some of the highest amounts of protein: tempeh and tofu contain 15 and 20 grams per half cup, respectively. Actual soybeans, known as edamame, are also a rich source. Legumes, like peas, beans, and lentils, make an excellent meat substitute. Peas contain 7.9 grams of protein per 8 ounces, about the same as a cup of milk. Although grains contain a relatively small amount of protein, quinoa (which is actually a seed) offers more than 8 grams per cup, as well as all nine essential amino acids. Not surprisingly, this little seed is often called the "perfect protein."

HIGHER-CALORIE SOURCES Nuts, which provide healthy fats and proteins, are invaluable in a plant-based diet. They can be high in calories—roasted almonds, cashews, and pistachios contain 160 calories per ounce along with their 5 to 6 grams of protein—so choose varieties that are raw or dry roasted. Nuts and seeds make an ideal protein-based snack for those times at work when you skipped lunch or when you're heading to the gym and need a nosh. Sesame, sunflower, poppy, chia, hemp, and flax are especially good choices because they also contain fiber, minerals, vitamin E, and omega-3 fatty acids. With all those calories, however, stick to recommended portions.

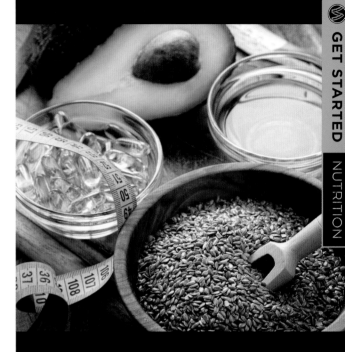

NUTRITION AND DIET APPS

 Tracking your nutrition can be time-consuming, but some people love to calculate all of their macros. Even if you're not the type to do so, the good news is that there are great apps that can make tracking almost effortless. Some will help you make sense of nutrition labels, which can steer you to better choices at the grocery store; others can help you track your calorie intake. Some even will send you reminders and motivational messages.

- *Calorie Counter Pro*
- *Carb Master Free Daily Burn*
- *DietHero*
- *Diet Point Weight Loss*
- *Diet Watchers Diary*
- *FatSecret*
- *Fooducate*
- *My Diet Coach*
- *MyFitnessPal*
- *Nutrino*
- *PRO MyNetDiary*
- *Shopwell*
- *SparkPeople Calorie Counter and Diet Tracker*
- *Thryve*

038 DON'T FEAR THE FAT

Fat often gets a bad rap as the culprit behind unwanted weight gain. However, a balanced diet requires this macronutrient: fat supports some body functions and helps to dissolve certain vitamins. As with carbs, there are different types—and it is important to know which of fats are beneficial and which are the ones to avoid.

THE BAD Saturated fat comes from animal sources, like red meat, poultry, and dairy products, and has been linked to higher levels of cholesterol and high-density lipoprotein (LDL), which can increase the risk of cardiovascular disease. Trans fats occur naturally in many foods, but most are made from oils using a process called partial hydrogenation. Trans fats also increase LDL levels and lower beneficial high-density lipoprotein (HDL). They are typically solid or semi-solid at room temperature.

THE GOOD There are healthier fat options, including monounsaturated fat (MUFA), which improves cholesterol levels, and polyunsaturated fat (PUFA), found mostly in plants or oils. Healthy fats, like olive, safflower, peanut, and corn oil, remain a liquid at room temperature.

THE VERY GOOD Heart-healthy omega-3 fatty acid is a PUFA that can actually decrease the risk of coronary artery disease. Sources include oily fish like salmon, tuna, sardines, and herring, as well as avocados, flaxseed, canola (rapeseed) oil, nuts, and many spices.

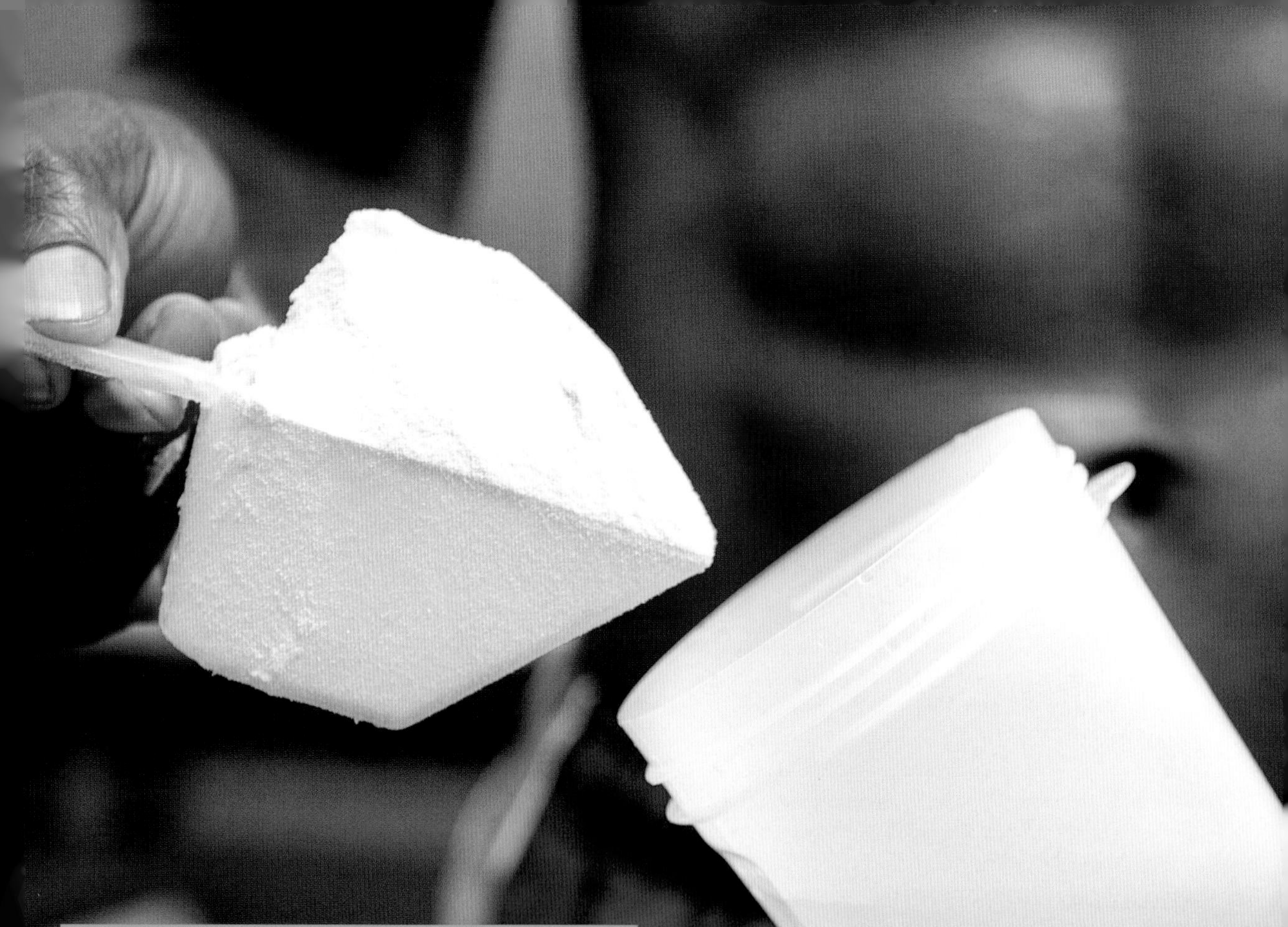

039 SUPPLEMENT SAFELY

Sports supplementation has become "big business"—and for good reason. Supplements do work in many cases. Products like protein powders, fish oil, or branched chain amino acids can fill in small deficiencies and increase performance, depending on the individual. Weight loss supplements or performance enhancers, on the other hand, contain powerful drugs that can be risky to ingest. And detoxes (diuretics) and laxatives offer only short-term results. In most cases, a healthy diet provides all the nutrients you require; sports supplements are meant to augment this balanced diet, not replace it.

When it comes to the micronutrients, although there are a mind-numbing number of vitamins available on the shelves of your pharmacy or health food store, most people find that taking a high-quality multi-vitamin serves them just fine. Unless you are diagnosed with a specific deficiency, your over-the-counter multi offers you the optimum amounts of your daily requirements in a single convenient tablet or capsule. Look for special customized products for men, women, and seniors.

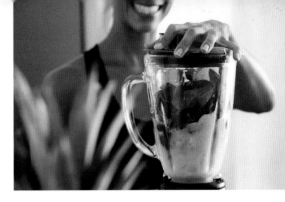

040 POWER UP WITH PROTEIN POWDER

Commercial protein powders allow you to prepare health shakes whether you need a satisfying snack or a meal replacement. These powders are typically made from high-quality sources like egg albumin, milk (whey and casein), and soy, plus they tend to contain all the essential amino acids that our bodies can't make, but which need to be part of our diets.

EGG ALBUMIN These protein powders, made from egg whites, are a high-quality source of protein. These kinds of powders were the original standard for body builders.

MILK PROTEINS Casein and whey protein powders are made from cow's milk—casein from the curds and whey from the liquid portion. The powders tend to have a slow rate of digestion.

SOY These powders offer a nutritious plant-based source of complete protein.

041 UP YOUR INTAKE

Although our diets should ideally supply our daily protein requirements, there are times when gym-goers might need the extra protein offered by these powders.

WHEN STILL GROWING Teens tend to need more protein as they work out or take part in sports.

WHEN BEGINNING AN EXERCISE PROGRAM If you're just starting to build muscle, your body will need extra protein.

WHEN INCREASING WORKOUT INTENSITY If you're amping up at the gym or prepping for a race, consider increasing protein intake.

WHEN RECOVERING FROM INJURY Consuming more protein can help you heal more quickly.

Signs of low protein intake include weakness during weight workouts, fatigue, and injuries that are slow to heal. Just bear in mind that 10 to 14 additional grams of protein a day will usually do the trick, yet some powders contain 80 grams per serving. That's simply too much, and breaking it down can be hard on the liver and kidneys.

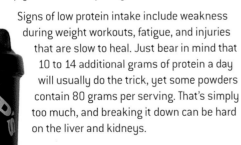

042 SHAKE IT UP

There are endless ways to make refreshing, healthy drinks from a basic protein shake recipe: two cups of liquid, fresh or frozen fruit and vegetables, nuts or seeds, and your choice of protein powder. The liquid can be water, milk—soy, almond, rice, or low-fat dairy—or yogurt. Seasonal fruits (such as pumpkins or peaches) or exotic types (like papaya, kiwi, or mango) are good additions. Parents wary of adding spinach or kale to kids' shakes can include a flavorful fruit. The taste of berries is particularly effective for masking the greens.

If you're among the super health conscious, add flaxseed or oats for fiber and micronutrients, banana for electrolytes, low-fat Greek yogurt for probiotics, chopped or slivered nuts for fiber and unsaturated fats, and cinnamon or cardamom for high levels of antioxidants. Simply combine your chosen ingredients with a handful of ice in a bullet processor or juicer for a perfect frothy mixture. Or you can use a countertop blender to combine fresh fruit or purées with cold water or a creamy option like soy or almond milk. Just avoid anything too hard or granular.

Even if you don't have time to make your own, Gold's Gym has a smoothie bar to help you power up before your workout, or get extra nutrition after!

SMOOTHIE RECIPE APPS

If you need some inspiration to help you devise delicious pre- and post-workout smoothies, great recipes for super-healthy shakes will be at your fingertips when you search the following apps. Many give recipe-specific nutritional info and also allow you to share your favorite ones with family and friends.

Also check online on the Gold's Gym Strength Exchange for delicious and healthful recipes.

- *Green Smoothies*
- *Instasmooth*
- *Pocket Smoothie Recipes*
- *Primal Smoothies*
- *Protein Pow*
- *Protein Shake Recipes*
- *Superfood HD*
- *Whole Living Smoothies*

043 BUILD BONE

No matter your age, working out places a lot of demands on your body. To help compensate for this, muscles require a solid, supportive framework—which means a healthy, functional, and strong skeletal system.

Exercise can help you maintain your bones—weight-bearing physical activity can cause new bone tissue to form and allow you to achieve greater peak bone mass. It also allows you to improve muscle strength, coordination, and balance, which in turn helps prevent falls and related fractures. But first you shoulder make sure you are doing the utmost nutritionally to sustain your skeleton. The two chief nutrients required for this are calcium, which builds strong teeth and bones, and vitamin D, which improves calcium absorption and bone growth. They can both be found in these following food sources, among others.

MILK

Dairy products are high in calcium, and the calcium they contain is extremely well absorbed. So have a glass of milk—just 1 cup (237 ml) of moo juice supplies 30 percent of the daily requirement.

HOW MUCH CALCIUM?
306 mg in 8 ounces (237 ml)

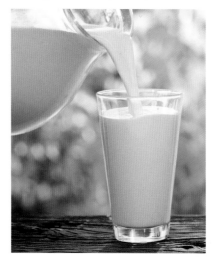

CHEESE

No need to binge on it or slather melted cheese over everything you eat—just one portion of cheddar cheese the size of a pair of dice, for example, supplies 30 percent of your daily calcium needs.

HOW MUCH CALCIUM?
195 to 205 mg in 1 ounce (28 g)

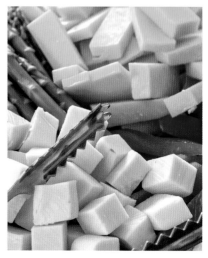

PLAIN YOGURT

With only about 160 calories, 1 cup (237 ml) of this creamy favorite can supply 42 percent of the recommended daily amount of calcium and 20 percent of vitamin D daily.

HOW MUCH CALCIUM?
415 mg in 8 ounces (237 ml)

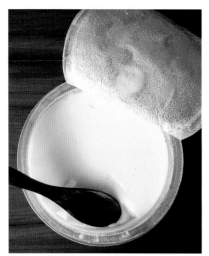

SARDINES

These small, canned fish, when packed with the bones, have surprisingly high levels of both vitamin D and calcium. They are also high in B12, B3, and B2. Serve in a pasta sauce or in salads.

HOW MUCH CALCIUM?
5 mg in 3 ounces (85 g)

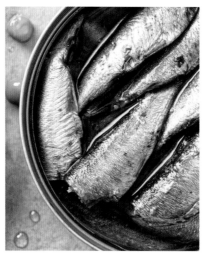

SALMON

This delicious pink fish not only contains heart-healthy omega-3 fatty acids, a mere 3 ounces (85 g) of sockeye also supplies more than 100 percent of your daily vitamin D.

HOW MUCH CALCIUM?
20 mg in 5.5 ounces (154 g)

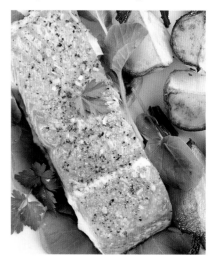

FORTIFIED CEREAL

Many of us love to start our day with a bowl of cereal. So, read the front of the box or the ingredient list to discover which healthy, whole-grain cereals offer you 25 percent of your daily vitamin D.

HOW MUCH CALCIUM?
100 to 1,000 mg in 8 ounces (226 g)

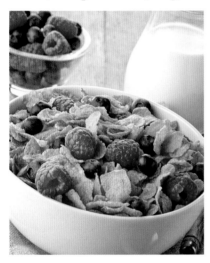

CABBAGES

Look to members of the cabbage family, like broccoli, kale, bok choy, cabbage, mustard, and turnip greens, for leafy sources of calcium. They also help build strong bones with folate and vitamin K.

HOW MUCH CALCIUM?
60 to 300 mg in 8 ounces (226 g)

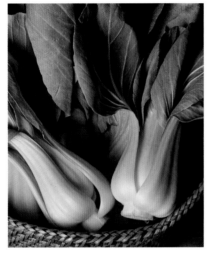

DANDELION

Look no further that your front lawn for a fresh source of calcium. Dandelion is high in this mineral—ounce for ounce more than milk—and it's packed with other nutrients. Use the greens in salad.

HOW MUCH CALCIUM?
52 mg in 1 ounce (28 g)

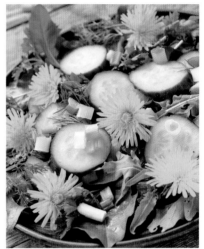

ORANGES

Whole oranges are potent sources of calcium, and their ascorbic acid may also aid in calcium absorption. If your prefer this morning staple in a glass, look for varieties with added vitamin D or calcium.

HOW MUCH CALCIUM?
60 mg in 1 average orange

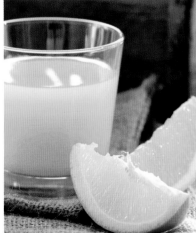

ALMONDS

These tasty nuts have a lot to offer. A ½ (118 ml) cup supplies you with 18 percent of the calcium you need each day. And they will also promote weight loss, colon health, and heart health.

HOW MUCH CALCIUM?
183 mg in 4 ounces (114 g)

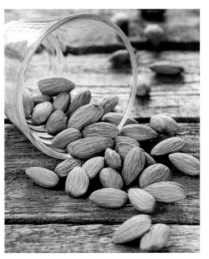

SESAME SEEDS

If you want to get the calcium you need without eating animal products, try out these tiny seeds. Sesame also supplies other nutrients and minerals—including copper, manganese, and iron—and fiber.

HOW MUCH CALCIUM?
88 mg in 1 tablespoon (14 g)

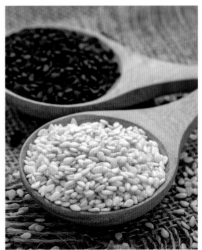

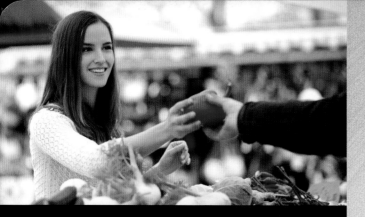

044 EAT RIGHT ON A BUDGET

We are all familiar with supermarket sticker shock: a few basic food items like eggs, milk, bread, lettuce, and cheese leaves your wallet distinctly lighter. Food costs will keep escalating, so it's important to shop wisely.

USE APPS Check out the many smartphone and tablet apps—some are even free—that let you plan menus, watch your calorie intake, and find alternative food options.

CLIP COUPONS Sign up online for one of several services that offer you customized coupons for the healthy foods you prefer—low-calorie frozen meals, gluten-free products, or organic foods, for instance.

GO ORGANIC Many organic farmers or ranchers don't bother with the expense and red tape required to earn "certified organic" labels. So simply make sure the product packaging says organically grown, and you will pay about 50 percent less than for certified foods.

MAKE SOUP There are many ways to augment low-sodium soup and turn it into a nutritious meal: add seasoning, spices, vegetables, meat, pasta, or even scrambled eggs. Studies show that dieters are less likely to overindulge when starting a meal with low-fat soup.

BUY FROZEN VEGGIES Slash the high price of fresh vegetables (and fruits) by opting to buy frozen in bulk. Flash-frozen produce works well in soups, casseroles, quiches, pasta, and health shakes.

AVOID WASTE Think before you discard any leftovers. Bones or meat scraps can be used in making soup stock. Vegetables can be added to an omelette or processed with your morning smoothie. Consider buying storage bags or disks that slow spoilage.

045 DISCOVER SUPERFOODS

They may not actually be miracle cures, but so-called superfoods are nutrient-rich powerhouses that offer large doses of antioxidants, polyphenols, vitamins, and minerals. They may reduce the risk of chronic diseases and prolong life. People who consume superfoods tend to be healthier and thinner than those who don't. Superfoods are also easy to fit into your diet if they aren't there already.

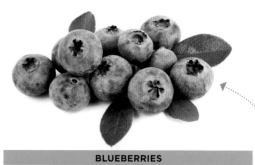

BLUEBERRIES

These berries are full of phytonutrients that neutralize free radicals (agents that cause aging and cell damage). Their antioxidants may also protect against cancer and reduce effects of age-related conditions, such as Alzheimer's disease. Try sprinkling blueberries in your yogurt or granola, or add them to your morning health drink.

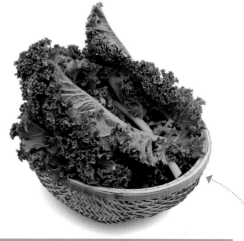

KALE

Phytonutrients found in kale appear to lessen the occurrence of a wide variety of cancers, including breast and ovarian. Scientists believe they trigger the liver to produce enzymes that neutralize potentially cancer-causing substances. Kale can be sautéed with olive oil and garlic or added to a vegetable smoothie.

BROCCOLI

Cruciferous vegetables like broccoli contain phytonutrients that may suppress the growth of tumors and reduce cancer risk. One cup (226 g) will supply you with your daily dose of immunity-boosting vitamin C and a large percentage of folic acid. Broccoli is a stir-fry star, but also try it as a salad ingredient.

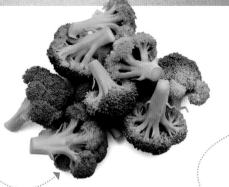

OATS

Oats are a rich source of magnesium, potassium, and phytonutrients. They contain a special type of fiber that helps lower cholesterol and prevent heart disease. Magnesium works to regulate blood-sugar levels, and research suggests that eating whole-grain oats may reduce the risk of type 2 diabetes. Oats can be used as a breakfast cereal, in baking, or mixed into meatloaf.

BLACK BEANS

A cup (226 g) of black beans packs 15 grams of protein, with none of the artery-clogging saturated fat found in meat. Plus, they're full of heart-healthy fiber, antioxidants, and energy-boosting iron. They make an excellent low-calorie soup or a piquant veggie dip.

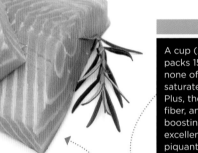

SALMON

Salmon contains omega-3 fatty acids, that the human body cannot produce by itself. Omega-3s reduce inflammation, improve circulation, increase the ratio of good to bad cholesterol, and may even slash cancer risk. Salmon is also a rich source of selenium, which helps prevent cell damage, and several B vitamins. Try an apple-and-horseradish glaze on baked salmon.

TOMATOES

These popular fruits contain lycopene, an antioxidant rarely found in other foods. Studies suggest that it could protect the skin against harmful UV rays, prevent certain cancers, and lower cholesterol. Plus, tomatoes contain plenty of potassium, fiber, and vitamin C. Try them in a tasty avocado, lettuce, and tomato sandwich, which contains another superfood—avocado!

AVOCADO

With its bad rep as too fattening, the avocado is so often overlooked. Yet along with its deliciously creamy taste, this superfood is filled with healthy fats and essential nutrients: oleic acid, lutein, folate, vitamin E, and glutathione to name just a few, that can help protect your body against heart disease, cancer, and eye and brain diseases. Toss a few chunks into a smoothie or eat it as a side with egg dishes in place of potatoes.

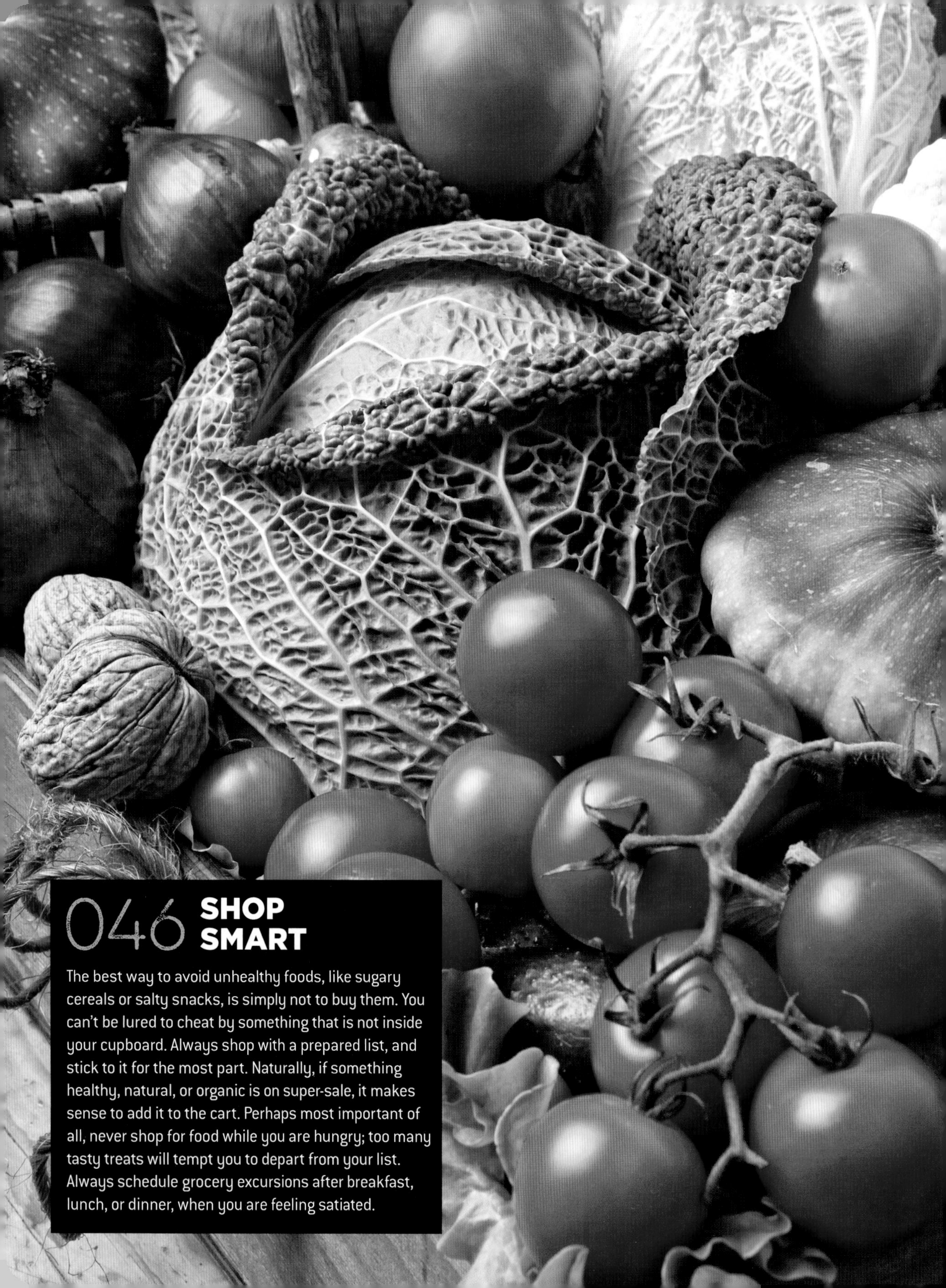

046 SHOP SMART

The best way to avoid unhealthy foods, like sugary cereals or salty snacks, is simply not to buy them. You can't be lured to cheat by something that is not inside your cupboard. Always shop with a prepared list, and stick to it for the most part. Naturally, if something healthy, natural, or organic is on super-sale, it makes sense to add it to the cart. Perhaps most important of all, never shop for food while you are hungry; too many tasty treats will tempt you to depart from your list. Always schedule grocery excursions after breakfast, lunch, or dinner, when you are feeling satiated.

047 AVOID GROCERY GOOFS

Many food items that shoppers believe are healthy choices have high—or hidden—calories as well as excess amounts of sugar, salt, or preservatives.

ENERGY BARS Don't let the advertising fool you—these are not legitimate alternatives to a healthy snack. Even if they do contain vitamins, minerals, and fiber, they are sweet treats, not health food. At least opt for varieties that offer whole grains, nuts, or dried fruit, and not those with chocolate or caramel.

GRANOLA Manufacturers insist this dense, whole-grain cereal is a healthy breakfast alternative, but they often add honey, sugar, and oil. A quarter-cup serving can have 150 calories—before you even add milk. Instead, try using granola as a topping lightly sprinkled on yogurt, health muffins, or oatmeal. And if the package lists three or more types of sugars in the ingredients (honey, brown sugar, and molasses, for instance), give it a pass; health food stores usually stock less-sugary alternatives.

TRAIL MIX Also known as GORP ("good old raisins and peanuts"), this snack is popular with both kids and adults. Yet, it was originally meant for hikers undertaking rigorous activity, not TV-tray noshers. The calorie-dense nuts and dried fruits are not meant to be gobbled by the handful, so watch portion control.

FRUIT YOGURT Yogurts that feature fruit at the bottom also contain extra sugar and preservatives. Stick with plain or vanilla varieties for your probiotic protein boost, and try adding fresh fruit, nuts, or flaxseeds.

PITA CHIPS Watch out, consumers—these so-called healthy snack chips can have as much fat and sodium as a bag of name-brand corn chips. Look for baked and seasoned varieties rather than fried, salty ones.

LO-CAL FROZEN MEALS Most of us love the convenience of popping a low-calorie dinner into a microwave. But not only do many frozen meals contain high levels of sodium, they also short-change diners on greens, with their small portions of limp, waterlogged veggies. Consider augmenting your meal with a salad or a serving of vegetables or fruit.

PACKAGED SANDWICH MEAT Some of these sliced meats have fewer calories than their deli-counter counterparts because they are packed with water, but they can also be very salty, especially those with smoky or peppery flavorings. Plain turkey or chicken are your best options.

FRUIT JUICE When it comes to increasing your intake of vegetables and fruits, as recommended, drinking fruit juice is one convenient solution. Unfortunately, many juices contain only marginal amounts of real fruit juice, if any, and most 100 percent fruit juices have had the beneficial fiber removed.

LO-CAL SALAD DRESSING Any foods with low-fat or fat-free labels are holdovers from days when saturated fat was falsely vilified. Manufacturers found that removing fat also removed flavor, which they made up by adding copious amounts of sugar. Simply use smaller portions of dressing or sour cream, rather than "diet" varieties.

CANNED SOUP This is "old news" in the nutrition world—canned soup may be good, but it is also loaded with salt. Try buying low-sodium soup and seasoning it with a little salt and the savory flavors of black or red pepper and spices, like basil, oregano, cilantro, cumin, or dill.

BROWN RICE Whole-grain brown rice offers more health benefits than white rice and is more filling, but it's not high on taste. Try combining whole grains with rice or regular pasta, and season the mix with herbs and spices.

049 PLAN AHEAD

One way to help ensure the effectiveness of a fitness program is to prepare a weekly diet plan. Take your pick of diet plan templates on the internet; many offer food and portion suggestions along with easy-to-prepare recipes. Once you have selected a plan, create a shopping list. If some recipes can be made ahead and frozen, get them ready before you start the plan. In addition to breakfast, lunch, and dinner, be sure the plan includes a few between-meal snacks for "grazing." Many nutritionists concur that consuming multiple small meals a day is healthier than the traditional three large meals. If the plan is still not satisfying you after two weeks, or you aren't getting the results you hoped for, try another plan, perhaps one with more emphasis on vegetables or juicing. And, of course, before embarking on any serious weight-loss regimen, always consult with a doctor first.

048 SIT DOWN!

We all do it—standing over the sink as we spoon up our oatmeal or grabbing a health bar for lunch as we rush to a meeting or gazing into the open refrigerator as we spoon down the ice cream. But, dining on our feet or on the run is not conducive to proper digestion. It is also makes it too easy to indulge in poor dietary habits. Mealtimes need to be acknowledged with a proper setting along with the proper amount of time allotted for you to slowly consume—and chew—your food.

So set the table, dim the lights, and put on relaxing music—even if it's only a date with yourself! And if you must eat on the run, invest in a bullet blender, and make healthy fruit and veggie smoothies to sip as you drive.

050 SHAVE PORTIONS

Reducing your calorie intake by about 20 percent is part of a good initial fitness routine. Here are a number of tricks that can help you eat less and resist going back for seconds.

FILL UP Drink a 16-ounce (480 ml) glass of water before mealtime. A full belly makes you less likely to overindulge.

ADJUST RATIOS Add nutrient-rich veggies and fruits to your recipes to make up for reduced portions of protein, fat, and carbs. Add spinach to pasta, extra green beans to stir fries, apple slices to cereal, or switch mushrooms for half the meat in ground-meat recipes.

CONTROL PORTIONS Never snack on foods right out of the bag or box— it's impossible to control intake, and studies say you can eat 50 percent more than you intended. If a snack package contains six servings, then divide it up into six zip bags.

FOOL THE EYE Use a smaller dinner plate than normal to fool your eyes into thinking your portion size has not shrunk. Put mixed drinks or cocktails in tall, thin glasses with extra ice to make them appear more substantial— and limit yourself to one.

CIRCLE THE BUFFET Look over the buffet offerings before deciding on what to choose to put on your plate. In studies, diners often put the first three things they saw on their plates, regardless of calories.

CONTRAST COLORS You are more likely to take bigger servings when the food color is similar to the color of the plate—white Alfredo pasta on white plates, for instance. So if you serve red meat, opt for pale plates, and with chicken or fish, use your darkest stoneware.

START WITH SOUP Research shows that when diners begin a meal with a brothlike soup, such as a consommé, they tend to consume less food overall.

SATISFY CRAVINGS Satisfy your craving for dessert at the end of a meal with a flavorful decaf tea like peppermint, chocolate, or raspberry peach.

STAY BUTTONED UP Fitted, more rigid clothing such as blue jeans, dress pants, or a tailored jacket will feel increasingly tighter as you continue to eat and warn you when to put down the fork. Don't just unbutton for comfort—stop eating!

PAY ATTENTION Concentrate on your meals. Don't watch TV or play computer games while you eat—you are likely to end up consuming more food while feeling less satisfied.

THINK *about it*

Differentiate between cravings and hunger. If you can comprehend the difference between wanting to eat and actually needing to eat, you can more easily eliminate unnecessary calories.

051 CARRY YOUR OWN SNACKS

The healthiest option when you're traveling is to bring your own snacks. Try these tasty treats, which are inexpensive and easy to tote along wherever you go.

PACK DRIED SNACKS Prepare individual servings of dried fruit; be sure to follow the serving size on the package label.

KEEP YOUR COOL For car travel, bring a small cooler with fresh fruit, such as apples, oranges, bananas, or grapes.

BRING THE GREENS Cut up raw veggies and carry them in a snap-lid bowl; they provide fiber and a nice crunch.

CHILL OUT Freeze individual cartons of low-fat yogurt ahead of time for a refreshing, gut-healthy treat.

BAG YOUR BREAKFAST Pour single servings of your favorite high-fiber cereal into sealable sandwich bags.

TAKE A CUP WITH YOU Invest in an insulated travel mug so you can indulge in homemade smoothies while you are on the go.

PACK A LUNCH Assemble a complete, healthy meal, including snacks, in storage containers, and store them in an insulated lunch box or cooler that you can toss in your back seat. Just be sure to pull over when you want to enjoy it!

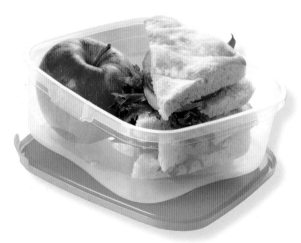

THINK *about it* Don't forget to hit the gym if your travel plans allow it. You can find Gold's Gyms throughout the U.S. and in many countries internationally. And many hotels have their own gyms or fitness centers.

052 ORDER WISELY

When dining out, it isn't always easy to make smart, healthful choices, especially when you're looking over a multi-page menu full of tempting items. The following guidelines could help you to stay on-plan.

GET IN THE CLEAR Begin with a clear, vegetable-based soup or side salad to reduce your appetite.

ASK FOR IT ON THE SIDE Always ask for salad dressing on the side, so that you can control how much you use.

LIMIT THE BREAD If the bread basket calls your name, eat one small piece with a drizzle of olive oil instead of butter.

LOSE THE FAT Avoid anything called crispy: that means "fried."

CHOOSE THE COOKING METHOD Opt for meats that are grilled, baked, broiled, roasted, or braised.

OPT FOR LEAN Order lean cuts of beef, like T-bone, sirloin, flank or strip steak, and pot roast. Or choose poultry or seafood.

DON'T GIVE IN TO TRENDS Don't cave in to "fad" foods of processed or fatty meat, like pork belly or short ribs; they are not worth the caloric beating you will take.

ORDER À LA CARTE Consider ordering salad and soup à la carte and then sharing a main course with a companion.

KNOW THE FACTS If you're dining at a chain restaurant, look up the menu online beforehand to get the nutritional info you need to make informed choices.

EAT LIKE A KID Remember that in many places, adults can order off the kid's menu. Sometimes that's just enough comfort food to satisfy you without trouncing your diet.

Ask the EXPERT

DO I HAVE TO SKIP DESSERT?

There's not much good to say about sugary foods—when following a fitness plan, avoid or limit processed foods and sugar. These empty calories offer nothing in the way of nutrition.

We all know that sticking to a fitness and nutrition regimen isn't easy. If you've been vigilant and eating clean, a little reward for all that hard work will probably do you more good than harm. You can go ahead and order that dessert, but be sure you partake in this kind of indulgence no more than once a week. You can even schedule in a regular cheat meal—just anticipating your weekly splurge can help ease the stress of sticking with the program.

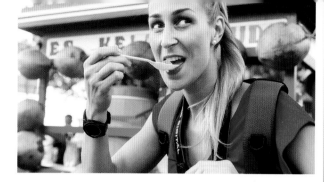

053 EAT SMART ON THE GO

So you've been exercising hard and watching your diet—and results are beginning to show. But once holiday or summer travel season shows up, you may find your good habits are at risk. Here are some safe bets for eating healthy on the go and what to steer clear of in a few common travel situations.

HOW TO ...	SAFE BET	STEER CLEAR
SNACK SMART WHILE YOU WAIT	When your only choice for a snack is a terminal or train station newsstand, opt for trail mix or a low-fat, high-protein energy bar. But follow the serving size on trail mix—it's typically about a cup (57 g) or a palmful—and pass on what's left to a neighbor to avoid calorie overload.	If an upscale coffee shop is an option, beware of added calorie traps that come with drinks. Whole milk, flavored syrups, and whipped cream can add 300 or more calories to your beverage. Instead choose bottled water to stay hydrated while traveling.
CONTROL CALORIES ON A FLIGHT	Some airlines offer economy passengers a snack box that contains tuna, hummus, baked pita chips, raisins, and organic crackers—all adding up to around 600 calories. Consider sharing it—and the calories—with a travel companion. Other airlines offer a turkey sandwich with light mayo that comes with a bag of baby carrots and a small candy bar. Or you might order an energy bar that's high in protein, but only contains 200 calories. Check your airline's website to see what sort of healthful options they have for fitness-conscious travelers.	Avoid salty snacks, which dehydrate you in the already dry cabin air. Also beware of high-sugar, high-fat treats that pack the equivalent calories of a meal but leave you feeling unsatisfied. Go easy on the alcohol, too, which could leave you feeling both dehydrated and logy after your flight.
EAT RIGHT ON THE ROAD	For a quick bite, stop at a mini mart, and head to the refrigerator section for low-fat string cheese, fat-free yogurt, or fresh fruit. For a meal, look for fast food restaurants that offer salads with grilled—not fried—chicken and low-fat or fat-free dressing. A baked potato topped with chili is a good way to get 15 percent of your daily serving of fiber. Pair it with water and lemon or unsweetened iced tea. Compared to a 20-ounce (290 ml) regular soda, this option will save more than 200 calories.	Avoid anything that's extra meaty, extra-crispy, slathered in gravy or melted cheese, super-sized, fried, or sugary.
TAILOR YOUR RESTAURANT MEALS	When dining in unfamiliar surroundings, check the menu for baked or broiled chicken or fish and steamed veggies. Don't be afraid to ask questions: "How is that prepared?" "What's the vegetable of the day?" or "Can I get a baked potato instead of fries?"	Avoid consuming oversized portions: split a large entrée with your travel companion—otherwise, high-fat, high-calorie items will leave you feeling guilty, sluggish, and sleepy for the rest of your trip.
KEEP IT HEALTHY AT THE BEACH	You are on vacation to relax, unwind, and enjoy, not to stress out or feel guilty after making bad food choices. Start the day off with a filling breakfast—an egg-white omelet with fruit and whole-wheat toast—to avoid making a bad decision at the beachside café. Stay hydrated with water and fresh-fruit smoothies.	Sure, the oceanside scenery may seem better with a drink in your hand, but splurging on sugary, mixed "umbrella" concoctions like piña coladas, margaritas, rum runners, and the like, will cost you two to four times the calories of a glass of beer or wine. And be careful of poolside snacks—you'll want to save those excess calories for a satisfying dinner.

054 STAY HYDRATED

Water is critical to human life, flushing our tissues and aiding metabolism. Some sports medicine specialists believe that half the population is mildly dehydrated at any given time. Sadly, these people don't even know they are dehydrated, having so rarely felt the benefits of true hydration. During workouts, when your body loses fluids through sweat, it's even more important to take frequent breaks with the water bottle.

Dehydration, especially if caused by intense physical activity like exercise, can decrease strength, endurance, and performance or skill levels in sports. Every cell and organ system in your body has to work harder, and because there is less blood volume, the cardiovascular system raises your heart rate to compensate. A properly hydrated individual, on the other hand, displays better decision-making skills, higher levels of concentration, elevated mood, and increased coordination. The following guidelines will help keep you hydrated during your normal busy days, as well as on your workout days.

EVERY DAY Drink eight 8-ounce (240 ml) glasses of water every day.

BEFORE AND AFTER WORKOUTS Drink 12 to 24 ounces (355–710 ml) of water before and after a workout.

DURING WORKOUTS Drink 8 ounces (240 ml) of water every 20 minutes during a workout.

DURING EXTENDED WORKOUTS For extended workouts lasting more than an hour, combine water with low-calorie sports drinks that replace lost electrolytes and provide sugar for energy.

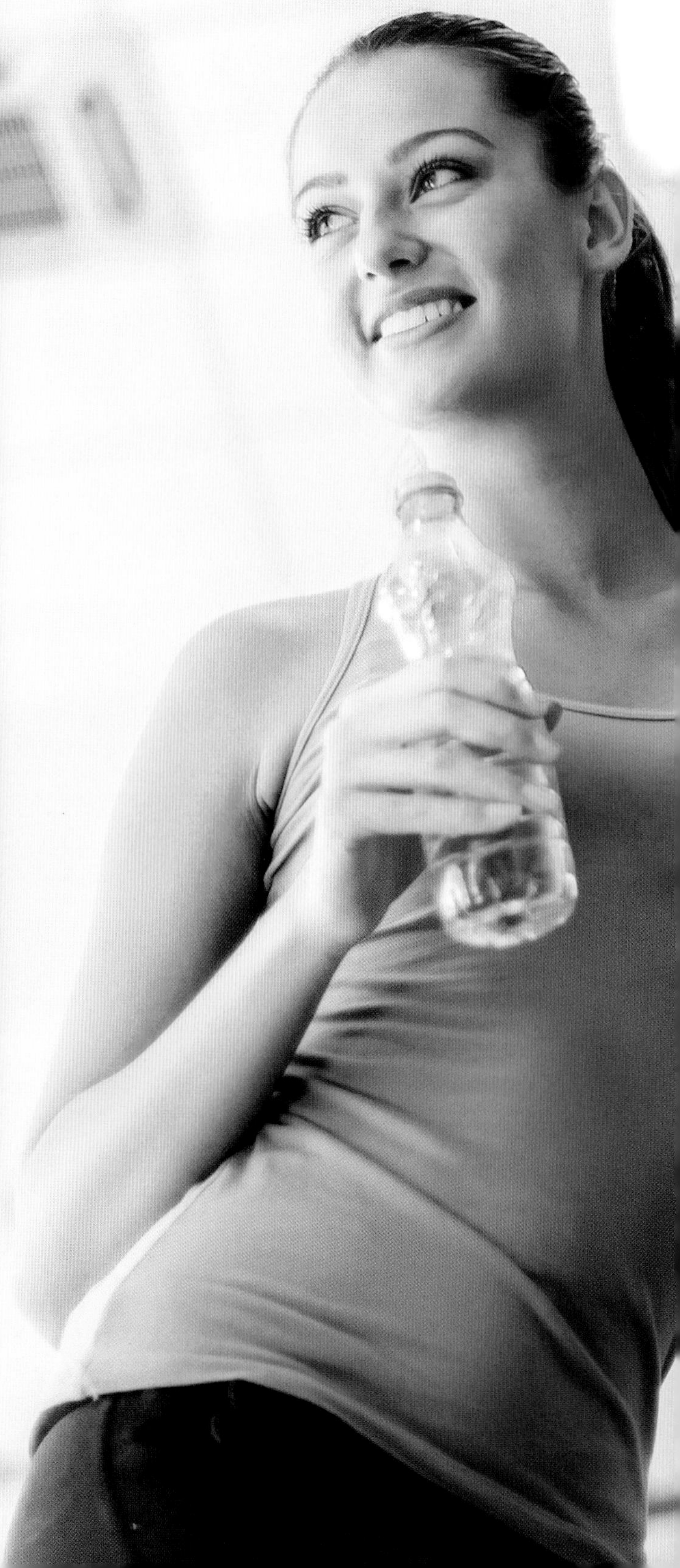

055 CURB THE CAFFEINE

Drinking coffee or black tea does not count as part of your daily water requirement—the caffeine in these beverages acts as a diuretic, flushing water from your body. The famous "caffeine rush" may give you a false sense of energy when you are feeling tired or fatigued, but caffeine is a stimulant that will ultimately leave you feeling even more run-down after it peaks.

A small amount can ease headaches, but too much can actually trigger them. If you want to limit caffeine, cut back gradually until you indulge only two days a week. If you must use caffeine to boost your metabolism—studies show that coffee and green tea do have this effect—be aware that coffee has a half-life of 6.5 hours. If you plan to turn in by 10:00 p.m., stop drinking coffee by 2:30 p.m., so that you have at least an hour with no caffeine in your system.

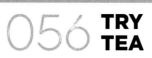

056 TRY TEA

Want a hot beverage that won't produce all the side effects of caffeinated drinks? Try herbal teas. These can come in a multitude of tasty varieties, including blackberry, ginger, rose hip, hibiscus flower, peppermint, chamomile, lemon balm, and more. There are herbal teas to wake you up, those to calm you before bedtime, and even those to serve as dessert. Many herbal teas contain vitamin C and antioxidants, and some can aid digestion and respiration.

When served plain, herbal teas add zero calories to your diet. That makes them excellent "craving quenchers" to sip while you watch TV, work on the computer, or cook dinner. And don't forget to try them iced for summertime refreshment before, during, or after a workout.

Commercial herbal teas can be purchased in most supermarkets … or check out a health food shop for more unusual or healthful varieties.

057 GO GREEN

When you crave a caffeinated beverage, it's definitely smart to go green … as in green tea, one of the healthiest drinks around. Its chock-full of antioxidants and nutrients that have powerfully beneficial effects on your body.

Among the many claims made for this tea: it can improve brain function, promote fat loss, and boost the metabolism. Just remember, however, that like other caffeinated beverages, green tea can act as a diuretic.

Whatever the claims, green tea is delicious either hot or cold. Just be sure to buy quality organic green tea or order it at restaurants that brew it fresh. Beware of canned and bottled varieties with added flavors—often those flavors also add sugars and calories.

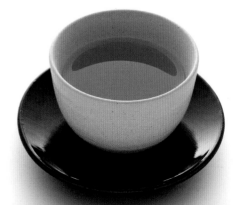

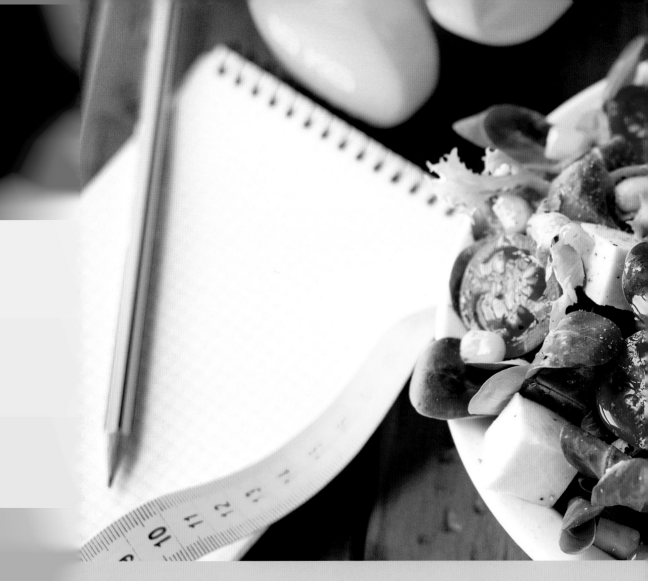

 START WITH A JOURNAL During the 12 weeks of the Challenge, it is a good idea to carefully monitor your food intake. You might think you are fully aware of everything you eat daily—but then you write it all down. Suddenly, all those impulse noshes, late-night snacks, car-trip indulgences, and other dietary lapses will glare up at you from the written page or your smartphone screen. So start keeping a journal (in an old-fashioned book or in digital form) to record everything that you eat. *Everything.* Once you discover all the "hidden" calories that you consume each day—that bagel and cream cheese you glommed down in the office break room, those fries you got from your friend's plate, or those cookies you mindlessly gobbled in front of the TV—you will start becoming a more conscious eater. You will be more likely to nix unnecessary snacks and make healthier choices. Remember, following a balanced diet will help you evolve into that fit and toned person you wish to become.

FIND AN ALTERNATIVE Your food journal will reveal your diet weaknesses—salty potato chips, ice cream double-dips, or ballpark franks, for instance—giving you a better chance of eliminating those foods. It's important to forego empty calories during the Challenge, but you can supply yourself with some smart, satisfying alternatives: air-popped popcorn instead of potato chips, frozen coconut milk instead of ice cream, or smoked salmon in a whole-wheat pita instead of a hot dog.

FOLLOW A WINNER'S JOURNEY
Matt Morrissey
Male Winner, Ages 40–49

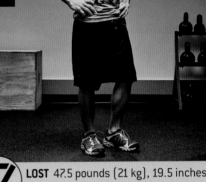

Before

LOST 47.5 pounds (21 kg), 19.5 inches (49.5cm), and 10.3% body fat

Matt realized he had to make a change when he saw photos of himself at a family wedding. "I knew it was time to do something about my weight," he says. "My body was sore constantly, and I would injure myself doing simple things like playing on my coed volleyball team. I was hurting and out of shape."

His game plan for the Challenge included either steady-state cardio in the mornings—30 minutes of constant activity like walking uphill on a machine—or high-intensity interval training (HIIT), a form of cardio that really burns calories. At night, he and his daughter followed a series of bodybuilding videos for the first two months. He eventually grew bold enough to try new machines to see what muscles they worked on. "It was a learning experience. I was trying to teach myself."

Matt still goes to the gym almost every night. He has upped his caloric intake and increased the protein percentage in his diet to try to add some mass.

PLAN A WEEKLY MENU There's a saying among fitness experts: "You can't out-train a bad diet." That is why it is so important to plan weekly menus—seven days of meals and snacks—and then shop for all your grocery items at the same time so you can avoid impulse shopping. Gold's Gym and many other fitness websites offer an almost infinite number of healthy menu options. You can also take cell phone shots of healthy meals you've prepared and show them to a trainer or nutritionist to see if you are on the right track.

WINNER'S WORDS

"One of the biggest things for me is my family. [They] motivated me, and I think that's a huge part of my success.

~ Matt Morrissey

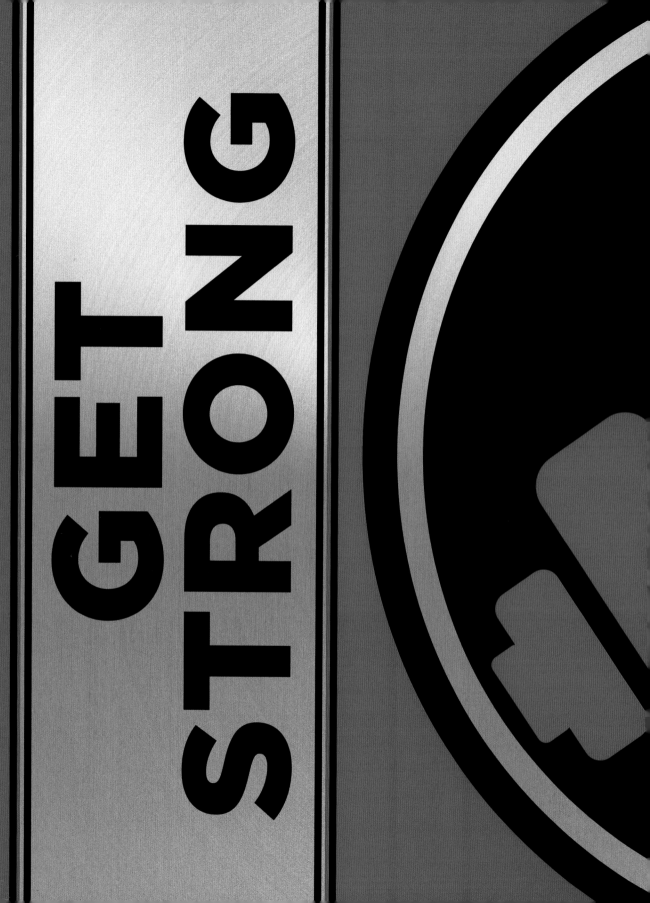

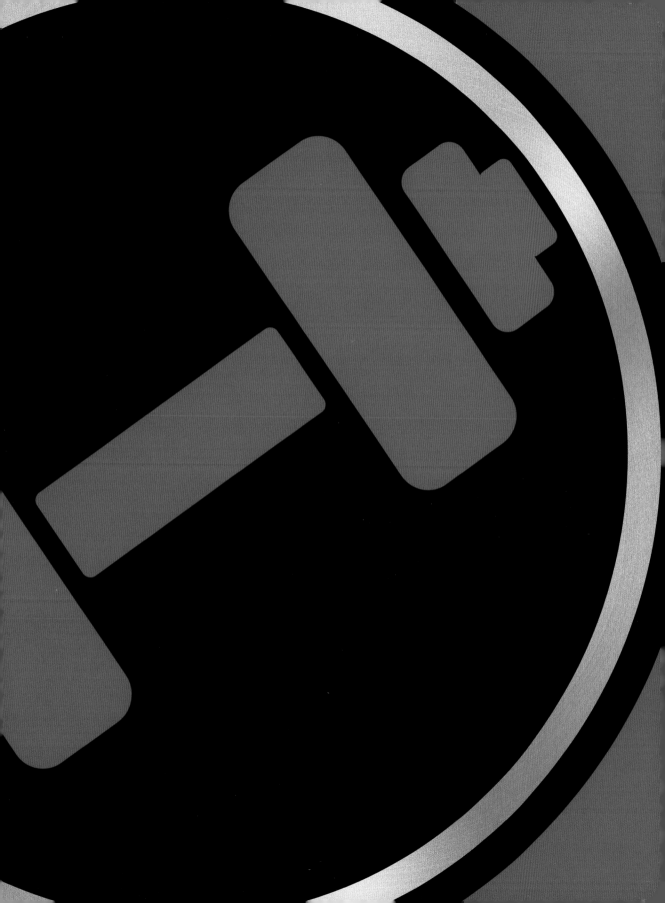

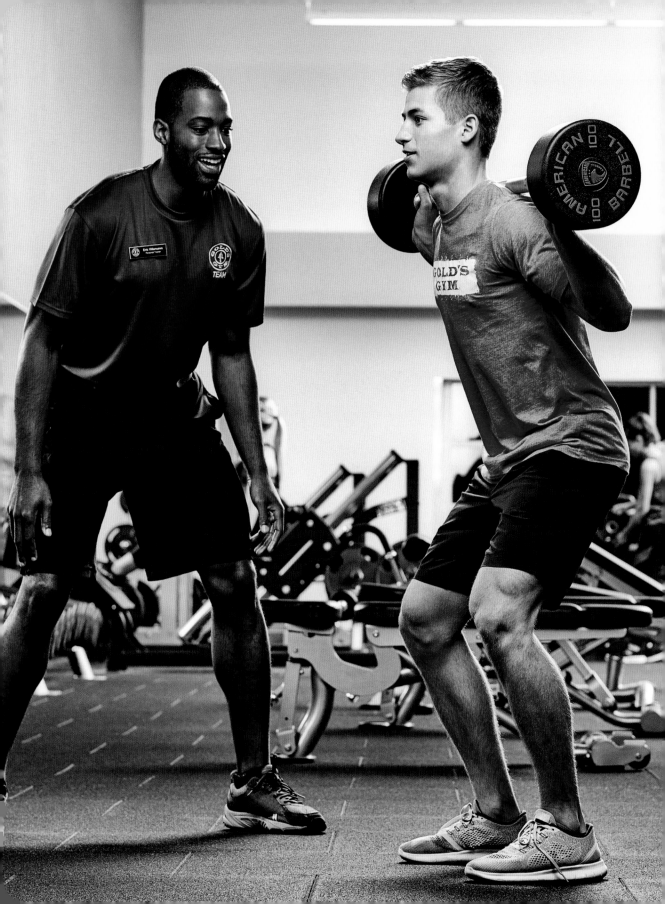

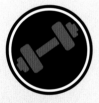 Resistance training is a key part of any fitness regimen. It not only increases strength, power, and endurance, it also tones muscles and can make them larger. Making resistance training a part of your regimen has other benefits, too.

APPRECIATE THE BENEFITS

A resistance workout acts as a major metabolism booster because the body continues to burn far more calories after a strength session than after aerobic exercise. When training is done through a full range of motion, it will improve flexibility, renew fluidity, and reduce the risk of injuries, muscle pulls, and back pain. It also improves posture, aids balance and coordination, and can prevent loss of muscle mass. Its results also work wonders on your self-image and state of mind. There are indications resistance training can even enhance cognitive function. Healthwise, resistance training can reduce resting blood pressure, help control blood sugar, and improve cholesterol levels. Studies indicate that resistance training can positively affect insulin sensitivity, resting metabolic rate, body fat, glucose metabolism, blood pressure, and gastrointestinal transit time, and reduce risk factors for diabetes, heart disease, and cancer.

CHOOSE THE METHOD

At Gold's Gym, you'll find a wide range of strength-building tools—resistance-based machines such as the leg press or the pec deck, or hand-held free weights like barbells, dumbbells, and medicine balls. You can even exercise without implements or tools, using your own body weight to create resistance. Depending on whether your goal is to increase muscle size or build strength, your training volume—the number of reps per set—will differ. To gain size, you need to stress the muscle by upping the volume of reps per set, while maintaining an optimum amount of weight. If you want to focus on strength, your volume of reps per set will be less, but you will work with increased weight.

FOLLOW THE PROGRAM

When augmented by a healthy diet and a cardiovascular exercise program, resistance training can benefit your life every single day. Whether it's carrying grocery bags from the car, keeping up with your kids, engaging in your favorite recreational sports, or simply fighting off the encroachments of aging, a regular strength regimen that burns fat, builds muscle, and stabilizes your skeletal system will leave you feeling fit, energized, and confident.

058 START RESISTANCE TRAINING

Many of us who are new to the gym experience, or who simply want to get fit, may ask a trainer, "Why get involved in weight training or bodybuilding?" A wise pro will be quick to point out the numerous benefits of resistance work, or "pumping iron," as enthusiasts call free-weight exercise. The advantages include increasing one's bone density, enhancing the shape of the body, and improving posture and functionality. Weights are also the key to giving yourself a customized workout by augmenting your own natural shape and musculature—resistance training allows you to pinpoint each muscle group with precise, controlled movements. This can result in better muscle definition and, with dedication and time, a truly sculpted physique. In fact, there is such an extensive list of positive attributes that not investigating resistance training in some capacity is like having a sporty car but no fuel.

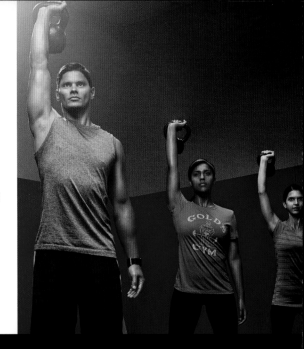

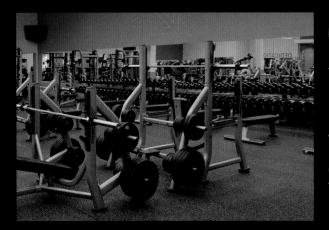

059 COMPARE YOUR OPTIONS

The three main tools of resistance training are free weights, resistance machines, and your own body weight. Resistance machines are the weight machines, like the leg press or lat pull-down, that target specific areas of the body. Hand-held free weights, such as barbells, dumbbells, kettlebells, and medicine balls, allow for a wide range of motion. Exercises that use your own body weight for resistance, a practice sometimes referred to as calisthenics, are aid free. Each method has its advocates, but there are also certain drawbacks. This table explains some of the pros and cons.

MODALITY	PROS	CONS
RESISTANCE MACHINE	Ideal for beginners	Restricts range of motion
	Encourages proper form	Does not work ancillary muscles
	Follows predetermined resistance path	Popular machines may be in heavy rotation
FREE WEIGHT	Allows full range of motion	May require a spotter
	Develops ancillary muscles	Dismounts can be risky
	Easily utilized at home	Users need to work up to compound lifts
BODY WEIGHT	No equipment needed	No way to increase resistance
	Exercise anywhere, any time	Isolating certain muscles is tricky
	Builds strength, flexibility, and mobility	Less ability to build mass, especially in legs

060 CALCULATE THE NUMBERS

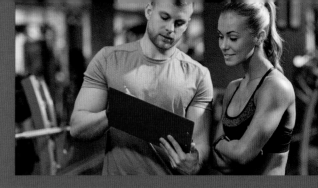

If you are a novice heading for the resistance machines or the weight room, the first thing you probably think is, "How much weight should I aim for?" and then, "How many reps and sets should I perform?" Although there is no one formula for determining the ideal weight or perfect number of reps and sets for a given machine or exercise, there are some useful guidelines. Getting close to the right numbers could be the difference between a successful session with great results and wasted time on the gym floor.

When you begin, choose weights that are light enough so that you can do 12 to 17 reps over two to three sets—but only do 10 to 12 reps initially. Those extra reps are "in the tank"—meaning you could do them, but don't want to push your muscles yet. You don't want to shock your brain or nervous

system with a searing workout, not until they figure out how to properly coordinate the movements the exercise requires. In order to concentrate on your form, start with two sets of 12 reps or three sets of 10 reps. Your nervous system will soon learn which muscle fibers to contract and which to relax. Your muscles themselves will adapt to the workload. At about two weeks, speak to a trainer about increasing your weight load, performing fewer reps, but adding more sets.

061 LEARN THE WORKOUT BASICS

There are varying levels of definition—the visible development of muscles—that gym-goers hope to achieve, from simple toning to competitive bodybuilding. If you want to gain bulk along with body conditioning, consider a combination of speed lifting, interval training, and supersets. This is especially true if you want to achieve that "ripped" look of extreme muscle definition. If you seek to improve strength but not size, try short rep workouts using extra-heavy lifts. The logic behind this is that the less amount of time a muscle is stressed, the less likely it will be to expand in size.

To utilize resistance training properly, there are a number of factors you need to understand.

WARM-UP AND COOL-DOWN Whether you choose cardio or stretches before or after resistance training, leave time for properly warming up and cooling down.

TYPE OF LIFT Tailor your workouts to focus on specific body areas, especially the ones that might be problematic.

PROGRESSIVE OVERLOAD By gradually increasing your weights, your muscles will grow larger and stronger.

INTENSITY The weight as a percent of your one-rep max.

FREQUENCY The ideal frequency of workouts varies depending on each individual, but most people see the best results with three to four resistance-training sessions per week, never working the same muscle group two days in a row.

VOLUME This usually refers to the total number of sets and reps completed within a specified time period. Can be categorized by muscle groups or areas of the body.

VARIETY Switching the order of exercises (or the exercises themselves), rep schemes, or training volumes challenges your muscles, which will adapt by increasing their strength and size.

REST How long you rest between sets affects your results: 30-second to 60-second breaks increase muscle size and endurance; rests of two to four minutes result in strength alone.

RECOVERY Muscles need time to repair and grow after a workout. Try to allow 48 hours of recovery before re-working the same group.

WORKOUT APPS

Various fitness apps help you set and track your goals, join fitness groups, share ideas, and get advice. Others show exercises or guide you through various routines with step-by-step instructions, features to function as a personal trainer. Gold's Gym myPATH works with most fitness trackers, recording calories burned, workout duration, reps, and more, all in real time.

- Gold's Gym myPATH
- CARROT Fit
- Daily Burn
- Fitocracy
- FitStar
- Jefit Workout
- The Johnson & Johnson Official 7 Minute Workout
- Pocket Yoga
- Progression
- Sworkit
- Touchfit: GSP
- Workout Trainer

062 KNOW YOUR MUSCLES

Before you begin a resistance-training program, it's a good idea to familiarize yourself with the basics of your musculature. These illustrations provide a quick visual guide to the major muscle groups that you will be targeting during workouts. For more detailed information on their functions, see the individual tips indicated after the muscle names.

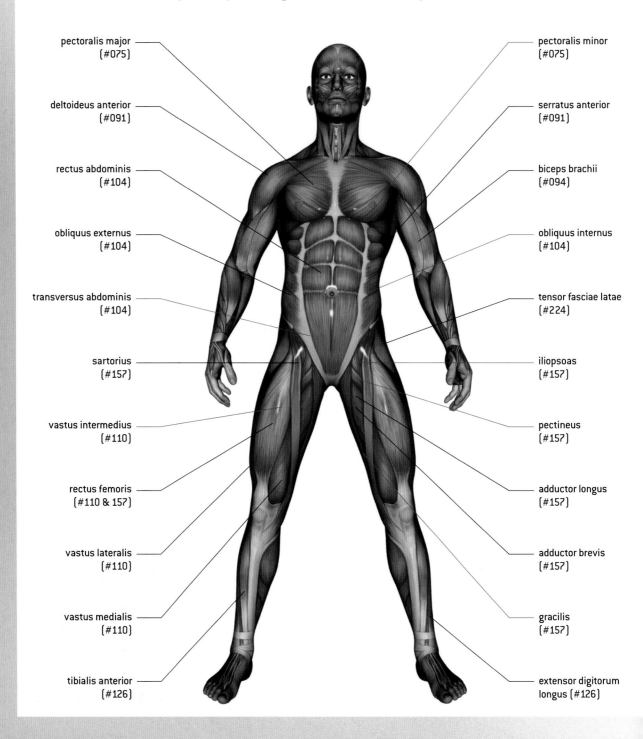

pectoralis major (#075)

deltoideus anterior (#091)

rectus abdominis (#104)

obliquus externus (#104)

transversus abdominis (#104)

sartorius (#157)

vastus intermedius (#110)

rectus femoris (#110 & 157)

vastus lateralis (#110)

vastus medialis (#110)

tibialis anterior (#126)

pectoralis minor (#075)

serratus anterior (#091)

biceps brachii (#094)

obliquus internus (#104)

tensor fasciae latae (#224)

iliopsoas (#157)

pectineus (#157)

adductor longus (#157)

adductor brevis (#157)

gracilis (#157)

extensor digitorum longus (#126)

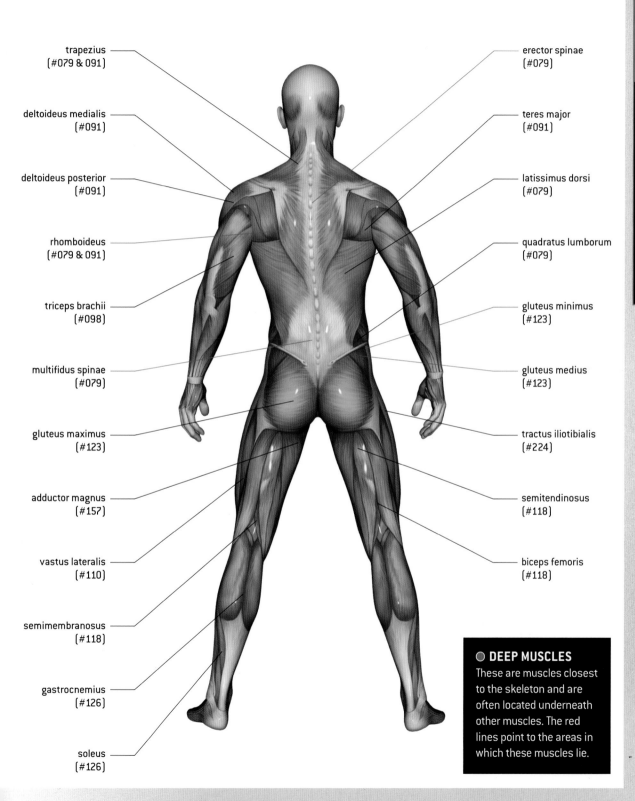

trapezius
(#079 & 091)

deltoideus medialis
(#091)

deltoideus posterior
(#091)

rhomboideus
(#079 & 091)

triceps brachii
(#098)

multifidus spinae
(#079)

gluteus maximus
(#123)

adductor magnus
(#157)

vastus lateralis
(#110)

semimembranosus
(#118)

gastrocnemius
(#126)

soleus
(#126)

erector spinae
(#079)

teres major
(#091)

latissimus dorsi
(#079)

quadratus lumborum
(#079)

gluteus minimus
(#123)

gluteus medius
(#123)

tractus iliotibialis
(#224)

semitendinosus
(#118)

biceps femoris
(#118)

⬤ DEEP MUSCLES
These are muscles closest
to the skeleton and are
often located underneath
other muscles. The red
lines point to the areas in
which these muscles lie.

HOW DO MUSCLES GROW?

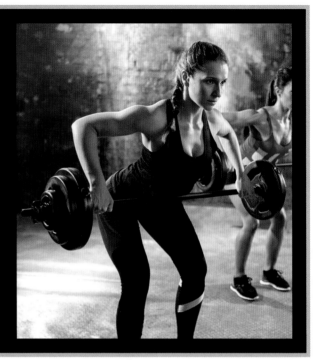

Muscle hypertrophy, or increased size of skeletal muscle, is the body's adaptive stance when increased resistance or force is placed upon the body. The number of muscle cells does not increase, but rather their size does. Resistance training generally results in two types of growth: sarcoplasmic hypertrophy and myofibrillar hypertrophy. The former focuses more on increased muscle glycogen storage and is found in professional bodybuilders and endurance athletes. The latter, which focuses more on increased myofibril (the rodlike unit of a muscle cell) size, is seen in powerlifters, Olympic lifters, and strength athletes. These two factors do not occur in isolation, with the result that both bodybuilders and strength competitors differ little in strength and muscle size. For the average gym-goer, a consistent progressive overload, whereby you increase the resistance and/or repetitions, will aid in muscle hypertrophy.

063 MASTER MUSCLE CONTROL

When learning to perform an exercise, you'll often hear the instruction to engage a particular muscle or muscle group—a task that sounds easier than it is. This is muscle control, or the ability to voluntarily flex or relax specific muscles. This calls for a deep connection between your mind and body.

During an exercise, you contract certain muscles in groups or in isolation, which causes the weight to move. Learning to target the correct muscles takes practice, however. For example, when executing a biceps curl, a neophyte will pick up a dumbbell, curl upward, and feel some sensation in the biceps , but also in the forearms and even the anterior deltoids because these muscles are all programmed to get the weight up. To practice control, forget about the lift and instead focus your mind on the contraction and relaxation of particular muscles. Beginners will be sure to feel other muscles come into play. For example, try to isolate the contraction of your latissimus dorsi (the large muscle on either side of your back). You'll probably feel your chest and shoulders muscles also contract.

To learn true muscle control, you must master two important actions: relaxation and contraction.

FULL-BODY RELAXATION Learning to engage a muscle also means learning to relax it. To practice this skill, stand tall and consciously look for tension in any muscle, and then relax it. With time and practice, you'll eventually be able to consciously relax a muscle without contracting those nearby.

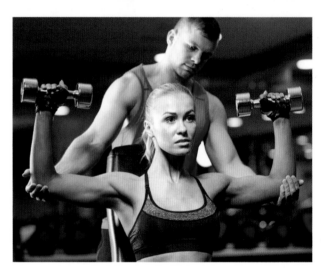

FULL-BODY CONTRACTION After practicing relaxation, try for full-body contraction. Again stand tall, but now try to contract all of your muscles simultaneously. Keep your breath shallow while contracting, and pay attention to your body. You may believe that every muscle is fully contracted, but you've likely missed some that are not under proper control. As with the relaxation exercise, scan your body from head to toe to note any muscles you have missed, and contract them. Make sure that no other muscles relax while doing this.

Working on mastering your muscles will allow you to focus less upon lifting heavy weights during resistance training and focus more on feeling the muscles that are doing the work.

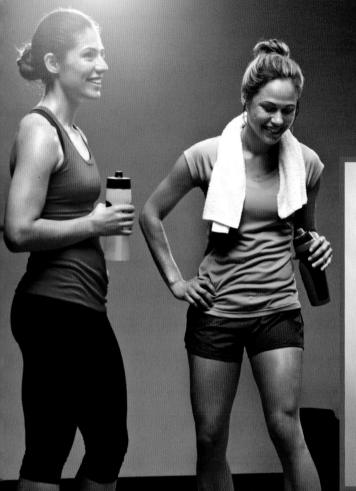

GYM etiquette

064 ASK AN EXPERT

If you notice another gym-goer whose body condition inspires you, or if you have questions on how others reached their goals—goals that you would also like to achieve—simply ask them. Just be sure it's after their workout or while they are resting; it's bad gym etiquette to interrupt anyone during a workout. Most will be flattered that you noticed the result of their hard work and will be happy to offer you assistance and advice when approached in the proper way.

You can also ask for recommendations on specific personal trainers—who works well with those at your level of expertise, for instance, or their opinion of various classes. At the very least you will come away with some useful new knowledge, and (even better) you may have gained a new friend or workout buddy.

TOOLS of the TRADE

065 BRING ON THE BARBELLS

The standard barbell might just be the quintessential piece of resistance-training equipment, so it's smart to familiarize yourself with this tool. Length varies, but a typical bar is about 7 feet (2 m). Even before you add any weight plates, the bar comes in at about 45 pounds (20 kg). Quality varies, but a good steel bar should be able to hold a lot of poundage. Knurling—or grooving—on the bar allows for a better grip. Standard bars are best for squats, overhead presses, and bent-over rows.

Thickness and the amount of whip—the ability to bend a bit and rebound—are two ways to differentiate specialty bars. A thick squat bar has very little whip and also has knurling at its center to help grip the back of your shirt so that it doesn't slide. A narrow deadlift bar has a bit more whip, which gives it greater speed off the floor. Bars for bench presses are slightly thicker with almost no whip, allowing for a more stable exercise.

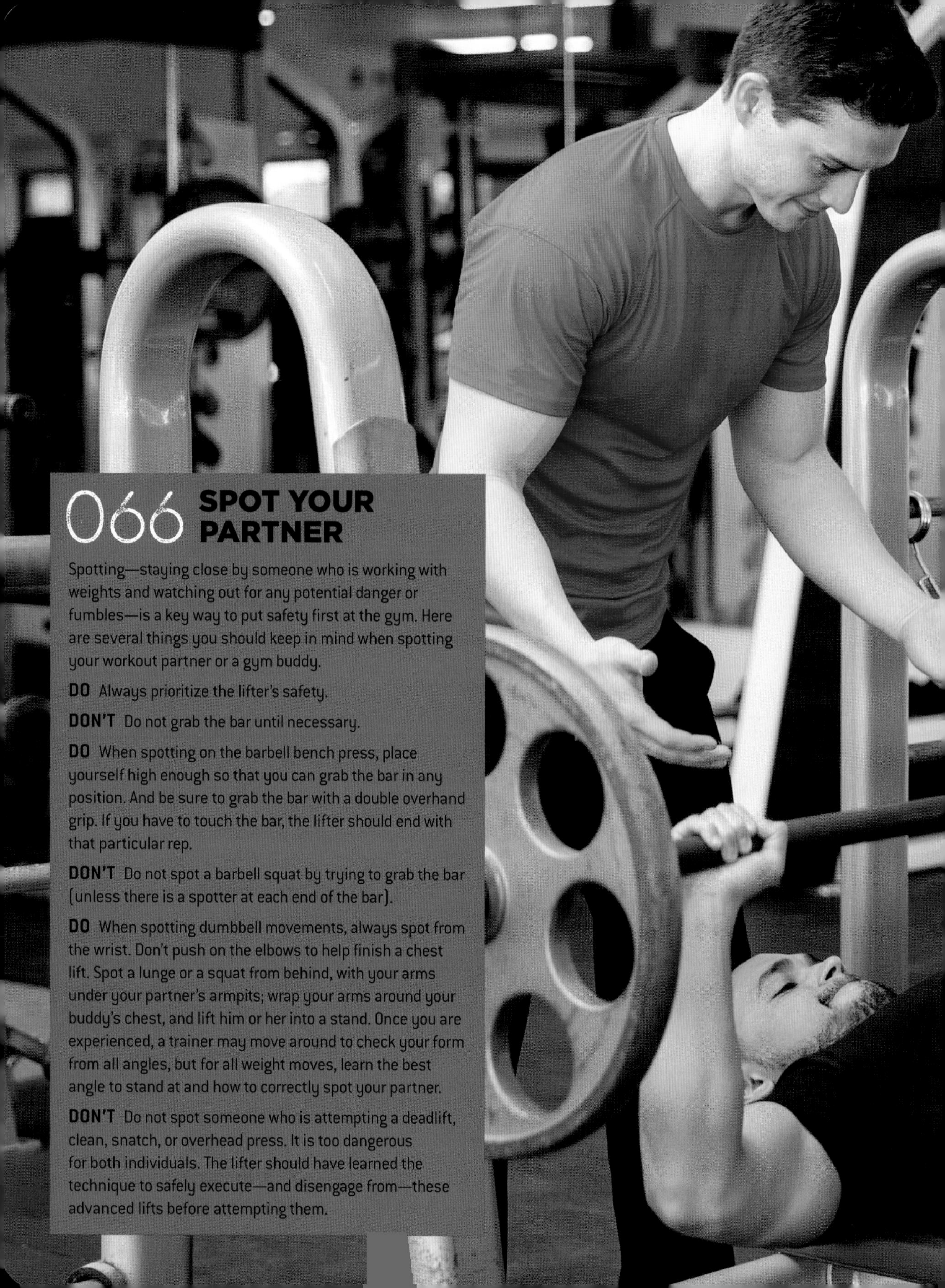

066 SPOT YOUR PARTNER

Spotting—staying close by someone who is working with weights and watching out for any potential danger or fumbles—is a key way to put safety first at the gym. Here are several things you should keep in mind when spotting your workout partner or a gym buddy.

DO Always prioritize the lifter's safety.

DON'T Do not grab the bar until necessary.

DO When spotting on the barbell bench press, place yourself high enough so that you can grab the bar in any position. And be sure to grab the bar with a double overhand grip. If you have to touch the bar, the lifter should end with that particular rep.

DON'T Do not spot a barbell squat by trying to grab the bar (unless there is a spotter at each end of the bar).

DO When spotting dumbbell movements, always spot from the wrist. Don't push on the elbows to help finish a chest lift. Spot a lunge or a squat from behind, with your arms under your partner's armpits; wrap your arms around your buddy's chest, and lift him or her into a stand. Once you are experienced, a trainer may move around to check your form from all angles, but for all weight moves, learn the best angle to stand at and how to correctly spot your partner.

DON'T Do not spot someone who is attempting a deadlift, clean, snatch, or overhead press. It is too dangerous for both individuals. The lifter should have learned the technique to safely execute—and disengage from—these advanced lifts before attempting them.

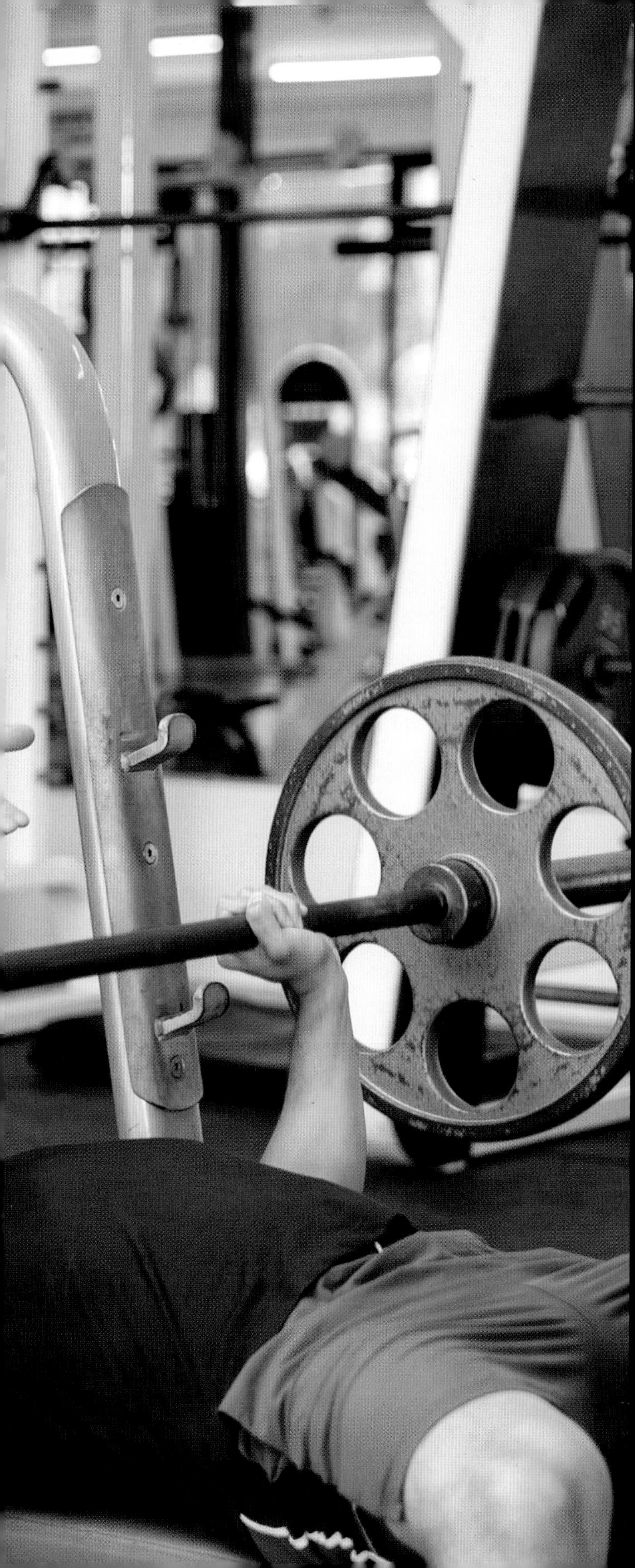

067 COMPLETE THE REP

There are a number of theories on repetition performance ... some experts recommend going slowly, others advocate speed. Perhaps it helps to understand how repetitions work.

THE NEGATIVE During each rep, there is a negative, which means the muscle lengthens (as the biceps brachii does when you lower your arm during the downward motion of a biceps curl, for example).

THE POSITIVE The negative portion of a rep is followed by a positive portion (the upward flexion, or shortening motion, of the biceps during the curl).

THE STATIC Once you have performed the positive portion of the rep, until you move back down into the negative portion, the muscle will then remain static in the contracted position.

Strength-building muscle breakdown happens mostly during the negative phase, so it is critical to complete the full range of motion in order to develop the muscle. You should perform the reps of most exercises with a controlled negative and a more explosive positive for maximum effect, and always work with weights you can handle.

068 BREATHE IN, BREATHE OUT

There are times when breathing becomes more complicated in the course of working out than it needs to be. Ideally, you want to breathe in on the negative movement—the lowering of the weight—and exhale on the positive—or working—portion of the repetition. Breathe in as you lower the barbell in a bench press, for instance, and exhale as you push it back up.

069 WORK TO FAILURE

The gym is perhaps one of the few places where failure is welcome. "Failure"—the inability to do even one more rep—means you've exhausted a muscle to the point where it can temporarily no longer move. Over time, muscle failure coupled with increased lifts and good nutrition will result in larger, firmer, and stronger muscles.

070 WATCH YOUR FORM

Any time you lift weights, you put stress on your back. Paying attention to your form can help you ensure that your workout remains safe and beneficial.

CONTROLLED WEIGHT Make sure to control the weight at all times. Don't swing free weights up and down or allow momentum to drive your movements.

CORRECT TECHNIQUE Ensure that you move the weight through your joint's full range of motion. This not only completely works the muscle, it also reduces the risk of joint injury. If you are unsure of what the proper technique is, consult a qualified trainer or physiotherapist. Incorrect technique can slow your progress or even cause injuries.

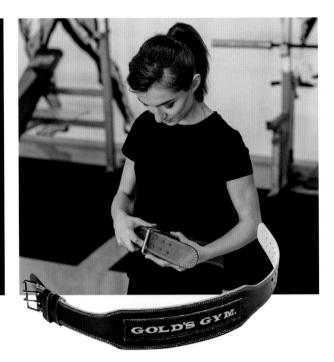

071 WEIGH IN ON WEIGHT BELTS

There are both proponents and detractors of weight-lifting belts. Pro lifters proudly wear specialized belts, yet many folks brag that they never do. The consensus seems to be on the positive side, but you must decide based on your own criteria. Naturally, if you have back or spinal issues, discuss the belt option with a trainer or physiotherapist.

PRO Belts stabilize and reduce stress on the spine. Research confirms that wearing a belt during lifting increases intra-abdominal pressure by as much as 40 percent. This can be compared to inflating a balloon inside your abdominal cavity—the pressure supports your spine from the inside, while the core muscles of the abdominal wall and lower back push on the spine from the outside. It is not so much about the belt providing spinal support, as that the body reacts to wearing the belt in a supportive manner.

PRO Belts aid body biomechanics. Studies also show that wearing a belt while lifting from the ground reduces spinal flexion, spinal extension, and lateral flexion. However, it also increases flexion at the hips and knees. In effect, a belt forces your lower body—legs and hips—to do the lifting, rather than your more vulnerable back. This biomechanic effect is especially important during deadlifts and squats with barbells.

PRO Belts improve performance. Many weight lifters say that wearing a weight belt improves power, strength, and muscle growth, most evidently in lower-body exercises.

CON Belts mean a loss of impact. There are those who believe that weight-lifting belts prevent strengthening of the lower back and possible inhibition of motor learning in the abdominals.

If you do decide to wear a weight-lifting belt, there are three basic types, each with specific pros and cons.

TRADITIONAL BELTS The traditional belts worn by many bodybuilders are made of leather and are wider in the back than in the front. They buckle like powerlifting belts, but are not as strong, providing less internal pressure. They should be considered midway between powerlifting belts and Velcro versions in terms of benefits.

POWERLIFTING BELTS These stiff, heavy-duty belts are the same width all the way around and buckle to adjust tightness. They are specifically designed for the sport of powerlifting—and not so much for safety. Nonetheless, a powerlifting belt's increased contact with the abdomen combined with its tightened, immovable buckle results in a surprising buildup of abdominal pressure. The heightened pressure leads to greater stability, which allows a wearer to lift heavier weights.

VELCRO BELTS These soft, flexible belts are usually made of synthetics. Because they fasten with hook-and-loop closures that can pop open, these are not as force-resistant as buckle belts, and they furnish less intra-abdominal pressure. They are useful for injury protection, but do not offer much of a performance boost.

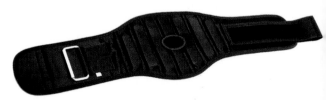

072 ACCELERATE YOUR RESULTS

Every experienced gym-goer understands that there are no true shortcuts, but sometimes certain methods can speed up results—at least enough that you don't become discouraged. The trick, as trainers say, is to work smarter instead of harder. Below are several examples of how to get greater results with less time spent on the floor. (And, as always, get your trainer's permission before attempting any intensive workouts.)

LIFT WITH A 2-4 TEMPO Remember that the speed with which you lift and lower weights is as much of a factor as how much you lift. For best results, follow a 2-4 count during resistance training—raise the weight (the concentric phase of an exercise) for a full two seconds, then take four seconds to return the weight to its starting position (the eccentric phase). According to research, exercisers who lower the weight in this slow, controlled manner gain nearly twice the strength as those who let gravity do the work.

INVESTIGATE INTERVAL TRAINING To get the most out of your gym time, don't just zone out on the same machinery set on the same moderate levels. Look into interval training—mixing periods of short, high-intensity exercise with longer, low-intensity exercise during the same workout. Many studies indicate that interval training boosts your calorie burn and improves overall fitness.

SUPERSIZE WITH SUPERSETS This is another proven way to increase weight-training results. Simply pick a muscle group, say the chest, and perform three or more different exercises for that group without resting in between. This blast of intensity should provide you with maximum results.

Ask the EXPERT

WHY DO SUPERSETS?

Supersets let you get in more work in less time and amp up the cardio benefits, increasing intensity levels, heart rate, and calories burned. This is especially true when supersetting large muscle groups like the chest and back, which places great oxygen demands on the body. You can superset within one body part or you can train two different ones. Effective combos include dumbbell incline chest presses and lat pull-downs, shoulder presses and pull-ups, and chest flies and reverse flies. Start with 5 to 8 reps, and work your way up to 10 or 12. Count three on the way down and two on the way up, and begin with lighter weights than you would normally use.

073 EXPLODE THAT PLATEAU

Explosive movement—those speed-driven exercises that require a strong burst of energy—is the antithesis of the slow, grinding resistance-training workouts many of us perform faithfully at the gym. Explosive training, which includes exercises like Olympic-style lifting, focuses on learning to move from muscle extension to a contraction in a rapid, or "explosive," manner.

Even though slow, controlled, steady weight training is the recommended way to break down muscle fibers, it can lead to plateaus in size and strength. Explosive movements, on the other hand, increase muscle fiber recruitment—how much your muscle is engaged during an activity. By increasing the number of fibers used, lifters can add more weight and affect more fibers—leading to greater changes in growth. Explosive movement can also furnish a welcome change of pace to your possibly stale routine of endless reps. Just remember that these movements should be performed early in your routine, if not right at the beginning.

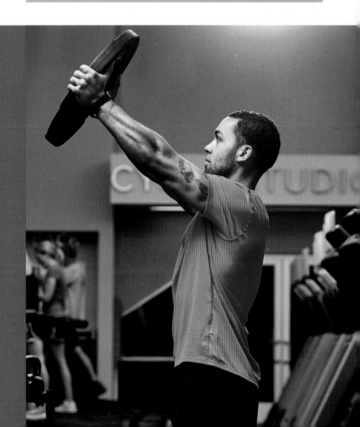

074 LIFT LIKE AN OLYMPIAN

Olympic lifts combine performance and accuracy—the body functioning like a well-oiled machine, the physical components working together in perfect synchronization. Rather than isolating one muscle group, during these lifts, multiple muscles work together to drive the movement.

True Olympic lifts are advanced and require years of dedicated training, but there are a number of modified lifts, called Olympic-style lifts, that are easy to grasp and that can be performed by virtually anyone. The three exercises shown are all Olympic-style powerlifting moves.

Powerlifting is a competitive strength activity that consists of three attempts at maximal weight on three lifts:

the squat, deadlift, and bench press. You don't, however, have to be a competitive weight lifter to benefit from these useful strength exercises. Just make sure you are grounded in resistance training before attempting any complex lifts, and consult with a trainer on how these lifts are properly performed before attempting them.

If you decide to give them a try, keep in mind that your technique and speed are more important that the amount of weight you initially lift. Don't attempt any weights that you can't lift five or six times with perfect form and without slowing down. Beginners may want to keep it light. For sets and reps, follow the chart guidelines for your fitness level.

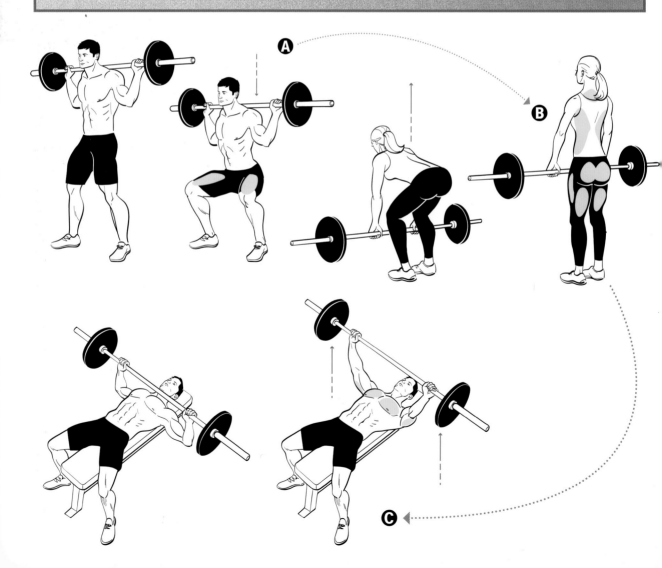

A BARBELL SQUAT The squat is full-body exercise that trains the muscles of the thighs, hips, and glutes, but it has other benefits as well. This multitasking power move also strengthens your bones, ligaments, and insertions of the tendons throughout your lower body. It will also help you develop core strength because your lower back, upper back, abdominals, and arms are all trained isometrically when you perform squats with proper form. To perform, start by resting a barbell across the back of your shoulders, grasping the bar with an overhand grip and standing with your feet shoulder-width apart, your toes slightly pointed out. Push your hips back, and bend at the knees to descend into the squat position. Pause at the bottom of the squat, and then drive your hips upward to return to the starting position.

B BARBELL DEADLIFT The deadlift is a powerful hip movement that helps tone the entire body while simultaneously developing muscle mass in your thighs. Gold's Gym Fitness Institute trainers urge gym-goers to focus on clean technique, meaning a straight spine with perfect posture through the shoulders, rather than maximum weight. Use your lats to really stabilize your spine; the movement should be dominated by your hips. To perform, start with your feet shoulder-width apart and a barbell at your feet. Bend your knees, as if sitting back, while keeping your back straight, and then grasp the bar with a shoulder-width or slightly wider overhand grip. Keeping your lower back straight, take a deep breath, and stand up, thrusting your hips forward as you squeeze your glutes. Exhale, pause, and then lower the bar back to the floor.

C BARBELL BENCH PRESS A resistance-training exercise for the upper body, the bench press works your chest muscles with the support of your arm and shoulder muscles. If your lower body is coming up off the bench during the press, you're probably driving with your legs and hips instead of with your chest and arm muscles. To perform, lie face-up on a flat bench. With an overhand grip, grasp a barbell slightly above the center of your chest with your hands slightly wider than arm's-width and by keeping your elbows pointing out to the side. Aligning your index finger with the first ring on the bar ensures you have a wide enough grip. Bring your elbows back even with your shoulders. Let the bar touch your chest, then drive to full extension in one fluid motion. Keep your body flat and your feet planted on the floor.

EXERCISE	BEGINNER	INTERMEDIATE	ADVANCED
BARBELL SQUAT	Two sets of 10 to 12 reps	Three sets of 12 to 15 reps	Four sets of 12 to 15 reps
BARBELL DEADLIFT	Two sets of 8 to 10 reps	Three sets of 8 to 10 reps	Four sets of 8 to 10 reps
BARBELL BENCH PRESS	Two sets of 8 to 10 reps	Three sets of 8 to 12 reps	Four sets of 8 to 12 reps

BONUS LIFT The high pull, another Olympic-style lift, develops full-body power. A great move for building clean strength, this exercise calls for you to pull the barbell up from a dead stop on the floor. The high pull is an explosive movement—meaning that you mimic the act of jumping without lifting your feet from the floor.

D HIGH PULL Stand with your feet shoulder-width apart in front of a barbell placed about two inches (5 cm) from your shins. Push your hips back, and bend your knees as you grab the barbell with an overhand grip. Explode upward, shrugging your shoulders and trapezius, and bring your elbows back to pull the barbell as high as possible before slowly lowering it back to the starting position.

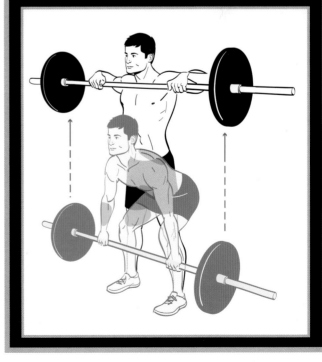

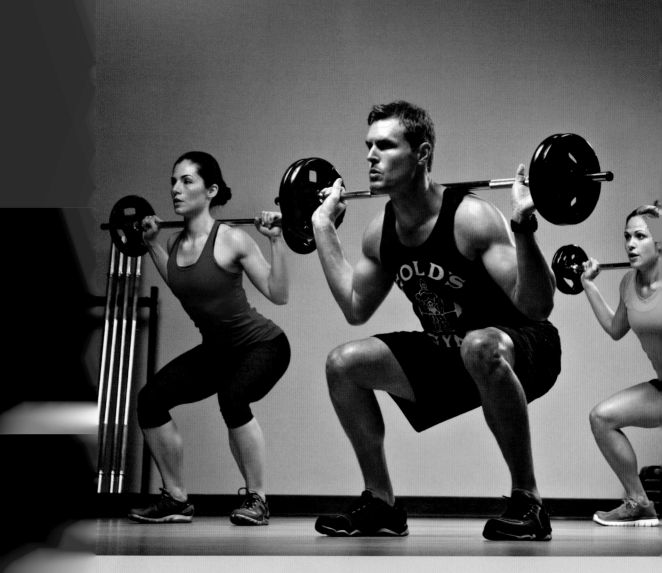

 BURN MORE FAT
Many Challenge participants initially focus on resistance training. Little motivates a gym-goer like seeing those first lines of definition emerge in their arms, legs, and abdominals. And because a pound of muscle can burn up to nine times as many calories as a pound of fat, the more muscle you have, the more calories that your body will burn (even as you sleep). To really get your metabolism going, perform compound exercises that engage the greatest number of body parts in the least amount of time, such as squats, lunges, rows, push-ups, and pull-ups. For an extra boost, instead of resting 45 seconds to a minute between your exercise sets, try doing jumping jacks or lunge jumps in the interim.

 POWER UP WITH FREE WEIGHTS Free weights, like barbells and dumbbells, are popular tools for resistance training. There are several versions of barbells: the Olympic bar is the standard for men's lifting; it is 7.2 feet (2.2 m) long and weighs around 45 pounds (20 kg). Some gyms offer a "women's bar"—33 pounds (15 kg) and 6.9 feet (2.1 m) long. "Beater bars" are inexpensive and often used by fledgling lifters. Fixed weight bars are short—at 4 feet (1.2 m)—and have the weights already attached; they are primarily used for assistance exercises. Other free weights include kettlebells and medicine balls.

 TONE WITHOUT BULK
During the Challenge, you may be striving to improve your conditioning

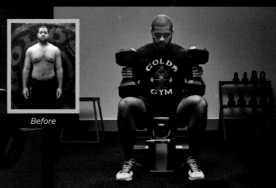

Before

LOST 47.6 pounds (21 kg), 19.9 inches (50.5 cm), and 11% body fat

Since the age of 12, Bradley had struggled with his weight—mostly due to what he calls poor lifestyle choices and terrible eating habits. As he grew older, he cycled through endless diets, gyms, and personal trainers without much success; he never felt he got the results he wanted. Then he joined the Gold's Gym in Kirkland, Washington, and almost at once realized he was leaving the old Bradley—overweight, self-conscious, and insecure—behind.

Bradley competed in the 2014 Challenge and insists it pushed him harder than he'd ever been in his life. "It gave me a purpose for working out and eating healthy and a passion for a healthy lifestyle." He not only dropped more than 45 pounds, but was also finally able to transform his body into lean muscle and gain the results he'd always aspired to. He found that 12 weeks was the perfect amount of time to make these incredible changes in his life.

Bradley's trainer, Andrew, stood by his side through every step of the Challenge, pushing him to succeed, and eventually they became great friends. He feels so grateful to the owners, managers, and trainers at his Gold's Gym, and also to those at all the Gold's Gyms across America.

through strength exercises, and you may also want to increase your muscle mass. This does not necessarily mean "bulking up," with bulging muscles. It simply means that you create micro-tears in your muscle fiber through weight workouts, which then heal to stronger muscle tissue. Even though these repaired muscles will enlarge slightly, they are denser than fat and will make you appear leaner overall. When you start to notice this lean definition, take a progress photo for a visual reminder to keep yourself motivated.

WINNER'S WORDS

"This Challenge is giving people the opportunity to change their lives forever ... I can finally stand proud of who I am!"

~ Bradley Berberich

075 KNOW YOUR...
PECTORALS

Spanning the upper chest from shoulder to breastbone on each side are the large muscles called the "pecs"—short for pectoralis major. This pectoral has two heads: the sternal head creates the bulk of your chest, while the clavicular head is the upper part radiating from your collarbone. Well-developed pecs are most visible on men; on women, they are typically hidden beneath the breasts. Beneath the pectoralis major is the pectoralis minor, which helps pull the shoulder forward and down. Both pecs work to draw your arms forward and in toward the center of the body, and they also work with the shoulders and arms to perform pushing movements, as well as playing a part in breathing, pulling the ribcage to allow the lungs to expand when you inhale.

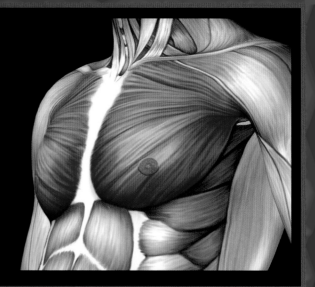

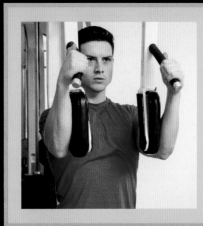

? Ask the EXPERT

HOW EFFECTIVE IS THE PEC DECK?

The pec deck—also known as the butterfly machine—is designed to isolate your chest muscles. Working at a pec deck, you perform a fly exercise sitting upright, with your upper arms spread and parallel to the ground, forearms bent, and your hands grasping the top of two spring-loaded "wings." The arms move forward, bring the wings together, and then guide them back. The machine does, however, have critics. There is some concern that older-style machines yank the arms backward at the end of the range of motion, potentially harming shoulder joints. Make sure your gym is using the newer style of pec deck with handles attached to an axis—or simply stick to free weights and cables.

TOOLS of the TRADE

076 GRASP THE CABLE MACHINE

Just about any gym you wander into will have at least a few cable machines, which are versatile pieces of equipment that are commonly used in weight training and functional training. Its steel frame features cabled weight stacks on each side. The cables that connect the handles to the weight stacks run through adjustable pulleys that can be fixed at any height. The adjustable height and ability to work from all angles means you can perform a wide variety of core and arm exercises, using handles, bars, or ropes.

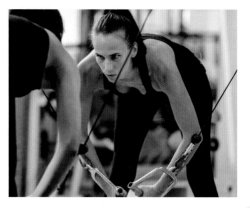

077 PUT YOUR PECTORALS THROUGH THEIR PACES

A smart chest workout, such as this one crafted by the fitness experts at Gold's Gym, will include exercises that target both heads of the pectoralis major, as well as the deep pectoralis minor. This workout will get you started, including moves that target your entire chest. To begin, use weights that you find challenging, but doable. Follow the recommended reps and sets, adjusting the numbers depending on your level of fitness.

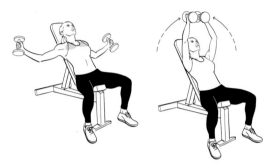

Ⓐ DUMBBELL FLY Most gym-goers default to machines for chest moves like the fly, but don't be afraid of taking up weights. Using free weights is much more effective because you really have to control your body weight, which requires additional energy, so you see results faster. Perform three sets of 10 reps.

HOW Sit on an incline bench holding a dumbbell in each hand, with palms facing in. Extend your arms straight up. Exhale, and lower both arms out to the sides to your shoulder height. Hold briefly, and then slowly raise to return to the starting position.

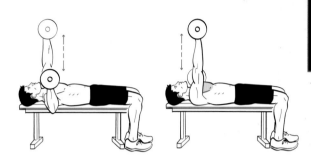

Ⓒ DUMBBELL CHEST PRESS WITH HOLD This version of the classic dumbbell chest press also builds up stamina because you keep your arms and chest engaged at all times. Perform three sets of 12 reps.

HOW Lie on your back on a flat bench. Hold dumbbells with your palms facing forward, and plant your feet on the floor. Lift your arms straight up so the dumbbells are in line with your shoulders. Lower your right arm until your elbow is even with your shoulder while keeping your left arm straight. Lift your right arm back up, then lower your left, alternating sides.

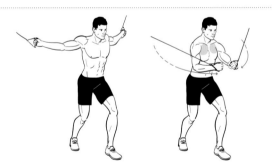

Ⓑ CABLE CROSSOVER Unlike free weights, cables provide you with a continuous and steady level of resistance, which engages the small stabilizing muscles in your chest, as well as the pectorals. Perform three sets with increasing reps of 10, 12, and 15.

HOW Stand with one foot forward and your feet about hip-width apart. Bend your chest slightly forward and grip a cable handle in each hand. Your hands should be slightly above the shoulders and elbows slightly bent. With your arms almost fully extended, slowly bring your hands together in a wide arc. Return to the start position and repeat

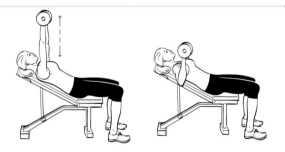

Ⓓ INCLINE BENCH PRESS This dumbbell incline version of the classic flat bench barbell bench press adds angles to your pecs workout, which challenges more muscle groups—the incline position helps you work the top section of the pecs. Perform three sets of 10 reps.

HOW Lie face-up on an incline bench angled between 45 and 60 degrees. Grasp a dumbbell in each hand, and plant your feet firmly on the floor. Hold the dumbbells with your palms facing forward. Press the weights upward to a position over your eyes until your elbows are straight. Lower the dumbbells toward your upper chest, keeping your elbows straight under your wrists. Return to the starting position

MIX UP YOUR PUSH-UPS

From school gyms to military boot camps, the push-up is the go-to exercise. Sure, it builds great pecs, but it also does so much more—it's a powerful core-strengthener that builds power for daily activities and gets you in shape for other fitness pursuits.

This is also an exercise with seemingly endless variations that change up its effects. Balancing on a ball, for instance, forces you to fully engage your core.

Switching leg or arm positions draws the focus from the pectorals to other muscles—bringing your hands together will engage those hard-to-tone triceps, while elevating your legs will get your delts working. And performing it on bent knees, rather than on your toes, is an easier modification perfect for fitness newbies.

Here is just a sampling of some of the many variations of the basic push-up.

Ⓐ PUSH-UP

WHY Works all your major upper-body muscles
HOW Lie prone on the floor with your hands placed as wide or slightly wider than shoulder width, and then rise to a plank position. Lower your body, keeping it in a straight line from head to toe. Keeping your core engaged, exhale as you push back up to the plank position.

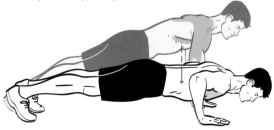

Ⓑ BOSU BALL PUSH-UP

WHY Adds core, arm, and lower-body benefits
HOW Flip a BOSU® ball over onto its dome. Grip the sides or place your hands on top of it, and extend your legs straight behind you. Holding your body in a straight line, lower your chest to the ball, and then return to the starting position.

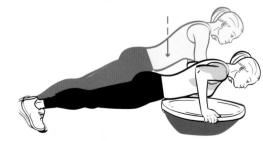

© DIAMOND PUSH-UP

WHY Changes the focus from pecs to triceps
HOW Place your hands on the floor in front of your chest with your fingers and thumbs pressed together to form a diamond shape. Extend your legs straight behind you. Lower your chest to the floor, and then press back into the starting position.

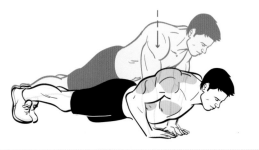

① DECLINE PUSH-UP

WHY Offers a greater challenge and more delts work
HOW Place your feet on a flat bench that is at least a foot off the ground or higher. From there, lower yourself into the regular push-up starting position. Keeping your forearms vertical, lower your chest to the ground, and then return to the starting position.

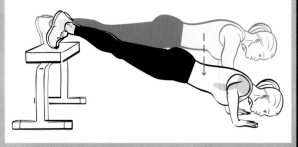

079 KNOW YOUR...
BACK MUSCLES

Strong back muscles are essential—these muscles move the spine, hips, head, arms, and pelvis as you go about your daily life. This group includes the large latissimus dorsi muscles, the fan-shaped muscles located on the back of the torso that function to pull the arms down and back. Well-developed lats give bodybuilders their characteristic V-shaped torsos. The trapezius is the flat, triangular muscle that covers the back of the neck, shoulders, and thorax. The upper part of the trapezius elevates the shoulder and braces the shoulder girdle when you carry a weight. A bundle of muscles lying near the spine is known as the erector spinae. This critical group provides the resistance that allows you to control movements such as bending forward at the waist. Its extensor action then enables you to return your back to the erect position. Other major back muscles and groups are the teres major, rhomboideus, quadratus lumborum, and multifidus spinae.

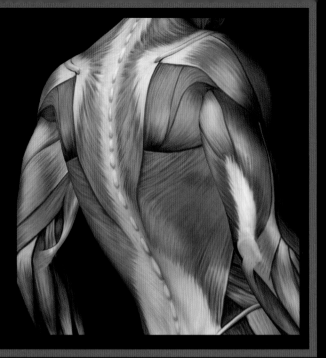

TOOLS of the TRADE

080 LEARN THE LAT PULL-DOWN

The lat pull-down machine is a great tool for beginners and intermediates to strengthen their back muscles in preparation for more taxing movements, like pull-ups and chin-ups. It also allows you to perfect your form for these strength moves while building up your back muscles, especially the latissimus dorsi.

One reason many people have difficulty with pull-ups and chin-ups—to the point where they cannot perform even one—is that they do not know how to engage their back muscles in the movement. The lat pull-down, which is a cable machine that supplies constant tension, acclimates you to using these muscles while focusing on proper posture. The overhand grip, especially, results in a weaker biceps reaction, forcing the body to use the back (lat) muscles.

Train on this machine three times a week, concentrating on proper form. Once reps become easier, start adding weight in small increments.

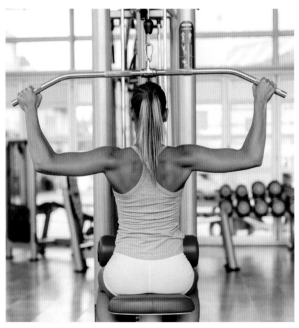

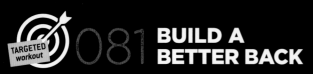

081 BUILD A BETTER BACK

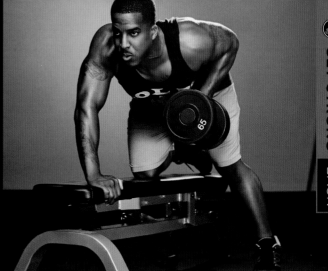

The benefits of a strong back are twofold: a strong back keeps your spine aligned and pain-free; and toned back muscles shape your waist, making it look smaller and more defined. The key to strengthening the back is the appropriate gym equipment, because the back is the hardest body part to work without the right tools. Proper form is also essential, making far more difference than heavy weight.

To prevent back troubles, try performing this multi-target workout from a member of the Gold's Gym Fitness Institute, which allows you to adjust the weight and reps depending on your goal—strength or definition.

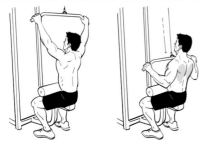

Ⓐ LAT PULL-DOWN MACHINE This machine keeps the focus on your lats. You may sit or stand for this one. For strength, perform four sets of 6 to 10 reps; for definition, four sets of 12 to 15 reps.

HOW Grip the bar with your hands slightly wider than shoulder-width apart, arms straight up and palms facing forward. Pull the bar down to your chest, elbows out. Return slowly to the starting position, arms straight.

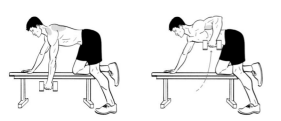

Ⓑ ONE-ARM DUMBBELL ROW This row exercise works your back and arms, including your latissimus dorsi, rhomboids, middle trapezius, rear deltoids, and biceps. For strength, perform four sets of 6 to 10 reps with each arm; for definition, four sets of 12 to 15 reps.

HOW Grab a dumbbell in one hand, and put the opposite knee and hand on a bench so that your torso is parallel to the floor. Start with your arm extended straight down, and pull the dumbbell up to the side of your chest, keeping your arm close to your body. Lower to the starting position.

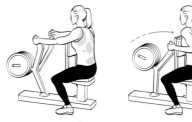

Ⓒ MACHINE ROW The seated row machine is ideal for beginners who want to develop a strong, muscular back. For strength, perform four sets of 6 to 10 reps; for definition, four sets of 12 to 15 reps.

HOW Grab the handles of a seated row machine, and sit with your back straight, shoulder blades back. Pull the weight toward your body until the handles touch your abdomen. Return to the starting position.

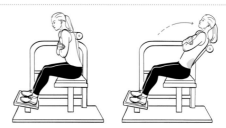

Ⓓ LOWER-BACK EXTENSION Extensions stretch and strengthen your lower back. Perform them as a complement to crunches to develop a strong, balanced midsection. Complete four sets of 6 to 10 reps for strength only.

HOW Adjust the seat of a lower-back extension machine so that the axis is in line with your hips. Seat yourself with your upper back against the roller, and grasp the handles with your feet planted firmly on the footrest. Slowly push back until your spine is naturally erect. Maintain tension as you return to the starting position.

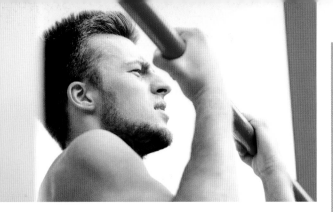

082 PULL YOURSELF UP

To build strength in the back and biceps, the pull-up tops the list of effective exercises. By using your own body weight for resistance, the pull-up works multiple muscle groups, including some of the big guns—rhomboids, biceps, mid and lower traps, obliques, and rectus abdominis—with an emphasis on the latissimus dorsi. Pull-ups not only build up the back, helping you avoid injuries to that vulnerable area, they improve stamina, create lean muscle mass, and strengthen your grip—a necessity for many competitive sports. Most gyms—and many urban playgrounds—feature a pull-up station. You can also purchase door- or wall-mounted bars for home pull-up workouts, if your multipurpose gym machine does not feature one of its own.

Pull-ups may look simple, but they can be a challenge to master; they are even sometimes used by the military in order to determine the fitness level of recruits. Try starting with only a few in the beginning, but hit the bar numerous times a day.

083 GET A GRIP

When performing pull-ups—and certain other exercises—there are three types of grips you will utilize. Each grip emphasizes different muscles: the overhand tends to primarily work the back; the underhand gets the biceps more involved. The placement of your hands on the bar also works different muscles. Positions include shoulder-width apart, slightly narrower than the shoulders, and slightly wider than the shoulders.

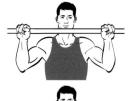

OVERHAND (PRONATED) GRIP Place your hands on the bar with palms facing away from you.

UNDERHAND (SUPINATED) GRIP Place your hands on the bar with palms facing toward you.

NEUTRAL GRIP Place your hands on the bar with palms facing each other. In this position, you perform the pull-up on a special apparatus with both crossbars and perpendicular bars.

084 KNOW THE DIFFERENCE

Closely related to the pull-up is the chin-up. "But aren't they the same thing?" you may ask. No, they are not—small, but crucial, differences in their execution means that they will train your muscles in slightly different ways. Although both exercises train the back and biceps, the chin-up places a bit more emphasis on the biceps. The chart below gives you a quick view of each move's major muscle focus, hand grip, leg position, and movement pattern.

EXERCISE	MAJOR FOCUS	HAND GRIP	LEG POSITION	MOVEMENT PATTERN
PULL-UP	latissimus dorsi	Use an overhand grip with hands just slightly wider than shoulder-width apart.	Bend your knees and cross your ankles.	You rely on shoulder adduction, meaning that your elbows come down and back from the sides.
CHIN-UP	latissimus dorsi/biceps brachii	Use an underhand grip with hands shoulder-width apart.	Let your legs hang straight down.	You rely on shoulder extension, meaning that your elbows come down and back from the front.

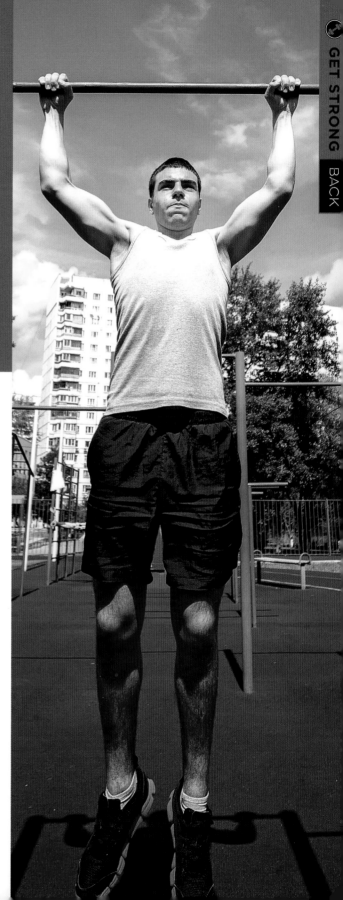

085 FINESSE THAT FIRST PULL-UP

Completing this movement correctly can become the Holy Grail of exercising for many people. For one thing, it requires really good technique—a combination of abdominal muscle control accompanied by powerful back muscles.

HOW Try starting with a dead hang, using an overhand grip with your hands shoulder-width apart. Then lean back so that your chest is pointed toward the bar. Keep your shoulder blades pinched together, and keep your forearms as vertical as you can. Initiate the pull by exhaling forcefully, retracting your shoulders down and back with your lats and using your biceps to flex your elbows. Your aim is to raise your chest, not the tops of your shoulders, to meet the bar. A perfect pull-up tops out with your chin rising just above the bar, and ends with steady inhalations as you slowly lower until your shoulders are at your ears and your elbows are locked straight. Anything less—cheating on either end—will keep you from getting stronger.

086 MIX IT UP

If at first you find you can't perform even one pull-up, there are several ways to increase your upper-body strength before giving it another shot. Try easier, assisted versions—like the band-assisted chin-up—and then move on to simple pull-ups. After mastering those, try the more challenging variations.

BAND-ASSISTED CHIN-UP Loop a resistance band over the bar, and place one foot in the loop. Use an underhand grip with your hands shoulder-width apart. Engage your abs, and then bend your elbows to pull your body up until your chin is above bar. Slowly lower back down.

BASIC CHIN-UP Use an underhand (supinated) grip with your hands placed shoulder-width apart or slightly narrower. The focus shifts to the biceps a bit more than with a pull-up.

CLOSE-GRIP PULL-UP Use an overhand grip with your hands nearly touching. The focus includes your lats, serratus anterior, and humeral muscles.

WIDE-GRIP PULL-UP Use an overhand grip with your hands placed a few inches beyond shoulder-width apart. This keeps the focus on your lats.

MIXED GRIP PULL-UP Place one hand in the overhand position and the other in the underhand position. This changes the way each arm utilizes your elbow flexor muscles.

WEIGHTED PULL-UP Add further resistance by using a dipping belt with a weight plate, grasping a dumbbell or other weight with your feet, or wearing a weighted vest or shorts.

087 KNOW YOUR ROW

An old-school favorite of powerlifters and bodybuilders, the barbell row (a.k.a. bent-over barbell row) is a pull-type compound exercise that is used to strengthen a variety of back muscles, as well as the hips and arms. It is an anti-flexion exercise—meaning that you use your lower-back muscles to keep your torso from folding over—so it builds lower-back strength and stability, which will help you improve your posture. As with any exercise, proper form makes all the difference.

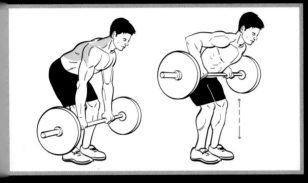

Ⓐ BENT-OVER BARBELL ROW Mastering this basic row will help strengthen your back, especially your lats and traps.

HOW Holding a barbell, stand with your toes pointing slightly outward. Keeping your lower back straight, bend your knees slightly, and hinge forward at the hips. Lead with your elbows, pulling them toward the ceiling until the bar reaches the level of your upper waist. Return the bar to the floor, so that your arms are fully extended and your shoulders are stretched downward.

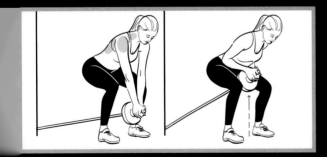

Ⓑ BENT-OVER TWO-ARM LONG BARBELL ROW This row targets the lower and middle back, the lats, and the biceps.

HOW Use an Olympic bar with weight plates on one end only. Put the other end of the bar against a wall or something heavy so it can't slide backwards. Straddle the bar with your knees slightly bent, and bend forward at the waist. Grasp the bar with a neutral grip, your palms facing each other, and pull the bar

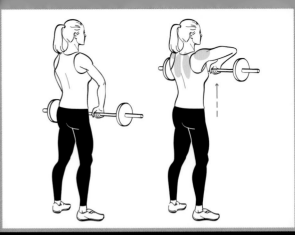

Ⓒ UPRIGHT BARBELL ROW The upright row moves the target upward to the trapezius muscles of your upper back, neck, and shoulders and also works the deltoids and biceps. The narrower the grip, the greater the emphasis on the traps.

HOW Stand upright grasping a barbell with a shoulder-width or slightly narrower overhand grip. With your elbows leading, pull the bar upward to neck height and allow your wrists to flex as you lift the bar. Lower the bar to the starting position.

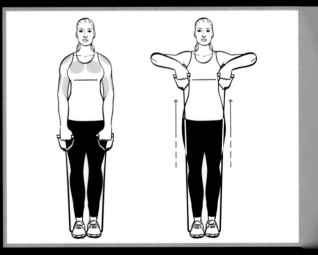

Ⓓ RESISTANCE BAND UPRIGHT ROW Like the barbell version, the resistance-band version emphasizes the trapezius. Because you only need to pack a simple band, it's a great move for those travelers who want to stay in shape on the road without overloading their luggage with heavy weights.

HOW Stand with your feet positioned over the center of a resistance band, and grip each handle with your palms facing the front of your thighs. With your elbows leading, pull the band straight up the front of your body to chest or shoulder height to form a wide V with your elbows. Lower the handles to the

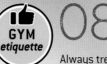

088 SHOW RESPECT

GYM *etiquette*

Always treat the gym's equipment with respect; this is especially important when you are working with barbells and dumbbells. Remember that these are heavy, solid objects, and all it can take is a split second of careless behavior for an injury to occur. So always use respect when handling weights: never swing dumbbells, barbells, or plate weights when there are others nearby, and never toss them onto the floor following a set. When you finish working with weights, re-rack the plates, barbells, and dumbbells for others to use.

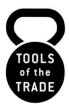

TOOLS *of the* **TRADE**

089 SAY HELLO TO MR. SMITH

The Smith machine, which is used in weight training, consists of a stabilized framework with a movable weight bar that is fixed within two steel tracks. This restricts the weight to vertical or near vertical movement. You can use a Smith machine for a variety of exercises, including bench presses, shoulder presses, and squats. Because the barbell can be secured in any horizontal position with a simple twist of the bar, it is safer for beginners or lifters without spotters. The contained barbell also requires less core stabilization by the lifter, so most individuals can handle more weight on the Smith.

A similar piece of equipment is the power cage (also called a power rack, squat cage, or squat rack), which features four vertical posts with two movable horizontal bar catchers on each side. Many power cages also include pull-up bars. A power cage will allow for a barbell workout without the movement restrictions imposed by the Smith machine.

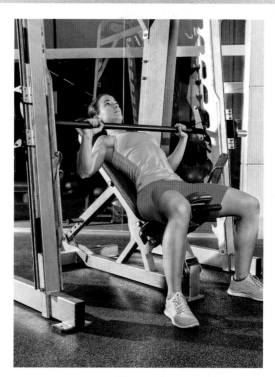

090 SWIM LIKE SUPERMAN ...OR GO TO THE DOGS

Nothing else can sideline you from your workout routine—or even just your daily activities—like lower-back pain. And for good reason: the lumbar region of your spine supports the majority of your body. And an overwhelming majority of us will suffer from a back injury sometime in our lives, most often of the lower back. Inactivity is also a culprit, with those long hours sitting at a desk taking a toll on your spine.

Strengthening the muscles that support your spine is therefore essential. You don't need to be Superman (or Superwoman), but taking a few cues from his midair form is a great way to start a lower-back strengthening routine. Adding in the bird dog exercise will keep your back from going to the dogs.

Ⓐ BIRD DOG

WHY The bird dog primarily targets the erector spinae muscles, which run along your spine and are responsible for extending your torso. This exercise, also called the quadruped arm/leg raise, uses your body weight as resistance to strengthen your lower back.

HOW Start on your hands and knees, with your back straight and abs pulled in. Keep your torso stable and your abs engaged as you contract one of your arms and the opposite leg into your body. Extend that arm outward along with the leg. Hold for up to 15 seconds. Return to the starting position, switch sides, and repeat.

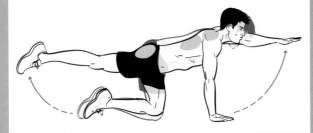

ⓑ SWIMMING SUPERMAN

WHY Also known as land swimming, this exercise combines a stationary Superman exercise with the movements of swimming so that you strengthen your back, core, and leg muscles. Swimming exercises also help improve coordination, thus getting you to move your arms and legs independently from the torso, which should remain solid and stable.

HOW Lie face-down on the floor with your neck parallel to the floor. Lift your right hand and left leg off the floor simultaneously. Repeat with the left hand and right leg, and then continue switching back and forth as if you were swimming on land, making sure to fully engage your back and butt muscles.

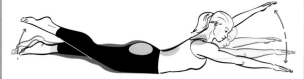

ⓒ STABILITY BALL SUPERMAN

WHY A Superman performed on a stability ball is a smart choice if you are trying to prevent back pain. Any Superman strengthens your back and core, and adding in the ball forces you to use muscles that are often inhibited as you sit at a desk all day, including the glutes, scapular rotators, and posterior deltoids.

HOW Balance on a stability ball with your stomach on top and your toes on the floor. Let your torso fall over the ball, and relax your arms by your sides. Starting with your head and upper back, slowly lift your spine until it's straight. Slowly return to the start.

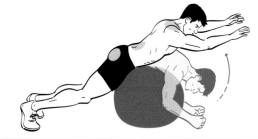

091 KNOW YOUR... DELTOIDS

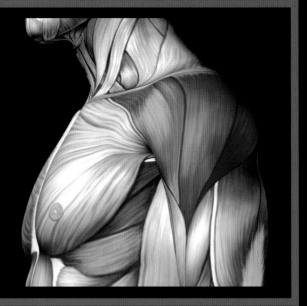

With the greatest range of motion of any joint in the human body, your shoulder needs strong muscles to support it. The deltoids, the largest and strongest of the shoulder muscles, are up to that challenge. Divided into the front, middle, and rear sections called the deltoideus anterior, medialis, and posterior, the delts (as they are known in gym circles) form the outer layer of shoulder muscle. They work to elevate and rotate the arm. The trapezius, located on the back, also works to enable shoulder movement, moving, rotating, and stabilizing the scapula (shoulder blade), while the rhomboid muscle is chiefly responsible for its retraction. Also working the scapula is the serratus anterior, located along your side. This muscle is known as the boxer's muscle because it is largely responsible for the movement that occurs when you throw a punch.

092 PROTECT YOUR SHOULDERS

The rotator cuff is a group of tendons and muscles in the shoulder that connect the upper arm to the shoulder blade. The rotator cuff tendons provide stability to the shoulder, and the muscles allow the shoulder to rotate.

ROTATOR CUFF If you're having trouble reaching during your workout, it may not be the time to work through the pain; it may be a rotator cuff injury. Other signs are tenderness during a military press or when lifting weight away from your body.

WHAT TO DO Avoid lifts that involve raising your hands above your head and shoulders, and work to strengthen the four muscles of the rotator cuff— the supraspinatus, infraspinatus, teres minor, and subscapularis. This is done often through internal and external rotation exercises. For internal rotation, keep your upper arm close to your side with your elbow bent 90 degrees, then bring the hand across your body, as if you were shutting a door. Then, for external rotation, bring your hand in the opposite direction, away from the middle of your body. See Tip #262C for a resistance-band version of this internal and external shoulder rotation exercise.

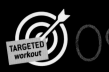

093 SHOULDER THE WEIGHT

This strengthening workout from the experts at the Gold's Gym Fitness Institute targets all three major shoulder muscles, especially the anterior and posterior delts, which will help you to fight off the effects of cubicle crunch. Along with counteracting the consequences of slouching, it tones and defines your upper body and traps. If you're a beginner, start off with a pair of five-pound (2.3 kg) dumbbells.

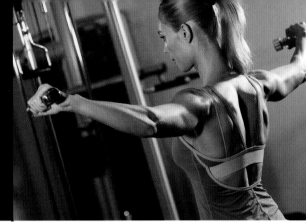

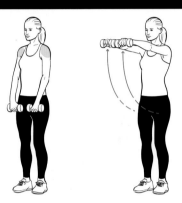

Ⓐ DUMBBELL FRONT RAISE This exercise is an effective move to isolate your anterior deltoid muscles. Perform four sets of 12 reps.

HOW Standing, hold dumbbells in front of you with your palms facing your legs. Keep your elbows and knees slightly bent as you raise your arms straight in front of you to shoulder level. Slowly return to the starting position.

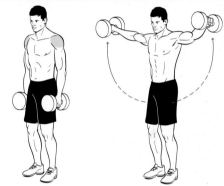

Ⓒ DUMBBELL LATERAL RAISE Lifting laterally activates your posterior deltoids and upper-back muscles. Perform four sets of 12 reps.

HOW Standing, hold dumbbells with your palms facing each other. Keeping your elbows and knees slightly bent, raise your arms out from your sides in wide arcs to about shoulder level. Slowly return to the starting position.

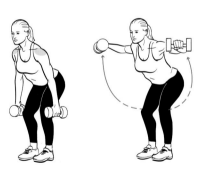

Ⓑ REVERSE FLY This exercise targets your posterior deltoids, along with the rhomboid and middle trapezius muscles of your upper back. Perform four sets of 12 reps.

HOW Standing, hold dumbbells with your palms facing each other. Bend your torso forward, so that it forms a 45-degree angle with the floor. With elbows slightly bent, raise the dumbbells up and out to the sides until they are parallel to the floor. As you lift the weights, focus on squeezing your shoulder blades together.

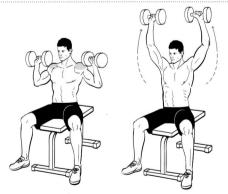

Ⓓ SEATED MILITARY PRESS While building anterior deltoid strength, this exercise also targets the upper back. Perform four sets of 12 reps.

HOW Sit holding a dumbbell in each hand, and raise them to shoulder level with palms facing out and elbows bent. Press the weights up and toward each other as you straighten your arms, keeping a slight bend in your elbows at the top. Slowly bring down the weights, and return to the starting position.

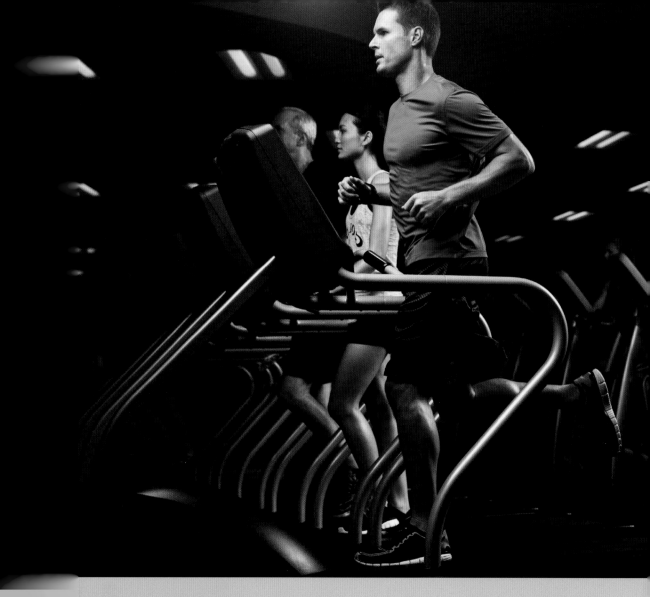

FOCUS ON STAMINA

Cardio workouts—which build up endurance—are the other half of your fitness equation along with resistance training. Three exercise machines offer optimum cardio benefits.

Treadmill The treadmill lets you adjust speed and rate of incline. Keep your gaze forward when running.

Elliptical The elliptical trainer offers a low-impact workout that simulates stair climbing, walking, or running. Don't hunch; stand upright as though there's a glass of water on your head.

Stationary Bike The upright stationary bike works for those without knee or lower-back problems; otherwise opt for the recumbent model. Avoid frantically spinning your legs when pedalling.

BENEFIT FROM CARDIO BURSTS

Try high-energy moves like jumps, hops, or cardio machine sprints in short bursts between strength sets. These intense moves will elevate your heart rate, burn fat and calories, and up the intensity of your workout. And, because you do them between other exercises, your overall gym time isn't extended. Just start slowly, and rest for 60 seconds before resuming.

TRY A UNIVERSAL CARDIO PLAN

This efficient cardio plan allows you to burn roughly 150 calories in less than a half hour on most cardio machines, including the treadmill, elliptical,

FOLLOW A WINNER'S JOURNEY
Darna Magpayo
Female Overall Challenge Winner

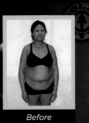
Before

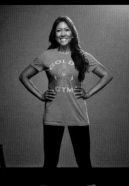

LOST 41 pounds (18.5 kg), 22.75 inches (57.8 cm), and 9.9% body fat

Darna was in a bad place: because of her weight issues, she was on medication for depression, high blood pressure, and palpitations. After another wedding at which she could only fit into a frumpy sundress—and was too heavy to dance with her husband—she signed up at Gold's Gym. Her trainer, Paul, soon had her on the right path. "The times that I slipped up and gained weight or felt like quitting, he would remind me that I was just human. . . . If I had tried to do it alone, I would have quit."

She admits she used to have a drink every night, sometimes two, and saw social occasions as a reason to overindulge, but she soon learned to say no. "I'm no longer on any medications," Darna says. " I lost my uncle recently from diabetes. It makes the gift of health so much more precious to me—more important than any prize."

During a recent vacation, she posed for a photo op. "My son thought it was awesome that I was doing exploding squat jumps. … I never thought in a million years that my body could do the things it does now! Thank you, Gold's Gym, now I have the 'after' picture I have waited for over 20 long years."

and stationary bike. To try it out for yourself, choose your machine, and then start with a slow-paced four-minute warm-up. Follow your warm-up with three minutes at a moderate pace, and then recover at a slow, steady pace for three minutes. Next, blast through an intense sprint for two minutes. Follow the sprint with three moderate minutes, and then three minutes of recovery. Speed up for another two-minute sprint, then two more moderate minutes and, finally, a three-minute cool-down.

WINNER'S WORDS

"I wore a ... fitness band that tracked my calories. My goal was to burn 3,000 calories four days out of the week."

~ Darna Magpayo

094 KNOW YOUR...
BICEPS

Of the diverse and numerous muscles of the arm, the biceps brachii is often the main focus of those who want to get in shape—or show off their great "guns." The biceps, located on the upper arms, consists of two bundles of muscles or "heads." It is a flexor muscle that bends the elbow to bring your lower arm toward the upper arm, and it also acts to turn your palm upward. Because the biceps also crosses your shoulder joint, it helps bring your arm forward and upward or across your body.

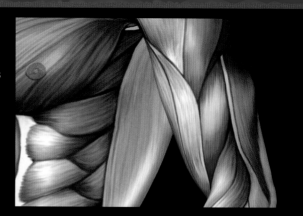

TOOLS of the TRADE

095 DO IT WITH DUMBBELLS

One of the most utilized pieces of weight-training equipment, a dumbbell is a free weight, typically held in the hand, that can be used singly or in pairs. Like smaller versions of barbells, adjustable dumbbells have weight plates that can be changed; other types use fixed weights. They vary in weight from a few pounds or kilos to more than a hundred and can be made from iron, chrome, or other materials, and the weight plates can be round or hexagonal shaped (which prevents them from rolling when you place them on the floor). There are three main categories.

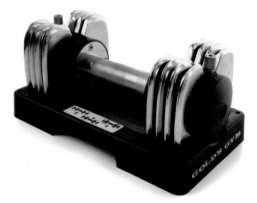

FIXED-WEIGHT Commercial gyms use high-end, fixed-weight dumbbells generally made from bars with securely welded iron plates. The basic fixed-weight dumbbells for home use, however, are weights formed into in a classic dumbbell shape. These kinds of dumbbells are usually the most inexpensive choice, and are often cast iron coated with rubber or neoprene for comfort, or are a rigid plastic shell filled with concrete. Look for sets like the Gold's Gym Dumbbell Set that features color-coded pairs of neoprene weights of 3 pounds (1.36 kg), 5 pounds (2.27 kg), and 8 pounds (3.83 kg).

ADJUSTABLE For space-conscious home exercisers, adjustable dumbbells are a better choice than fixed-weight because they give you a variety of weight levels with a single dumbbell. Adjustable dumbbells consist of a metal bar (which are often knurled, or cross-hatched, to improve grip), upon which you slide disks that are secured with clips or collars. Gold's Gym offers the Transformer Dumbbell set with a Click and Slide System that easily adjusts the weight from 9.9 pounds (4.5 kg) to 44 pounds (20 kg).

SELECTORIZED These dumbbells take adjustable dumbbells a step further, allowing you to easily change the number of plates while the dumbbell is resting in a stand.

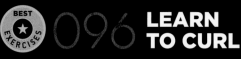

096 LEARN TO CURL

The curl is probably the best-known exercise for the biceps. And the basic curl is one of the easiest resistance-training moves to understand (press up, lower down)—yet getting the form right takes a lot of practice.

Here are four of the many variations of this classic—think about incorporating one or more of them into your workout.

Ⓐ STANDING BICEPS CURL Learning the proper form for the basic biceps curl is essential, helping you to tone your upper-arm muscles and also preparing you for trickier curl variations. As with most curls, you can perform the basic curls

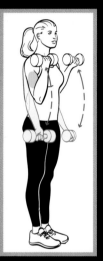

seated or standing. Just be sure to pick the appropriate amount of weight for your fitness level—you'll get more out of well-performed reps at a light weight than you will from sloppily performed reps with more impressive poundage.

HOW Grab a pair of dumbbells, and let them hang at arm's length. Turn your arms so that your palms face forward. Without moving your upper arms, bend your elbows, and curl the dumbbells upward until they are close to your shoulders. Pause, then slowly lower back to the starting position. Each time you return to the starting position, completely straighten your arms.

Ⓑ CONCENTRATION CURL The concentration curl offers a great biceps workout that stimulates the muscle fibers on the peak of the biceps. Taking a seated position limits the degree momentum plays in the execution of the curl, which keeps the focus on where it should be: right on that biceps muscle.

HOW Sit at the edge of a flat bench holding a dumbbell with your left arm. Place the back of your upper arm on top of your inner left thigh, and rotate your palm until it is facing away

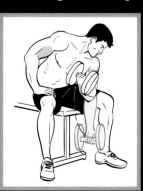

from your thigh. Holding your upper arm stationary, curl the weight upward while contracting your biceps until the dumbbell is at shoulder level. Squeeze your biceps, and hold the contracted position for a second. Slowly begin to bring the dumbbell back to a starting position. Perform the desired reps, and then repeat with the right arm.

097 RACK 'EM UP

Always place your dumbbells in their racks after you're done exercising. It's poor gym etiquette to leave plates loaded on a leg press at the end of your sets or to leave barbells or dumbbells lying on the floor where someone could trip over them. If you're able to lift weights during an exercise, then you're able to re-rack them when you're done. Consideration and courtesy keep things moving smoothly in the gym.

Ⓒ EZ BAR PREACHER CURL The EZ bar is a speciality barbell with a curved bar that allows you to grasp it with your palms in a more natural, less supinated (upward) position. In the EZ bar preacher curl, resting your arms on the sloping pad of a preacher bench will isolate your biceps and force them to work without the help of other upper-body muscles.

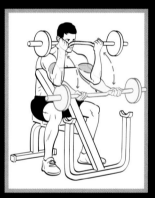

HOW Grab an EZ bar with your hands in the curved sections. Rest your upper arms on the sloping pad of a preacher bench, and hold the bar in front of you with your elbows slightly bent. Without moving your upper arms, bend your elbows, and curl the bar toward your shoulders. Pause, then slowly lower the weight back to the starting position.

Ⓓ HAMMER CURL The hammer curl is all about the angles—flipping your basic curl grip to its side. This small change in

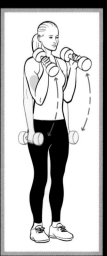

your grip transfers more of the work from your biceps brachii to your brachialis—a muscle that can make your arms look thicker.

HOW Grab a pair of dumbbells, and let them hang at arm's length next to your sides with your palms facing your thighs. Keeping your upper arms still, bend your elbows, and curl the dumbbells as close to your shoulders as you can. Maintain the contracted position for a second, and then slowly lower the weight back to the starting position. Make sure to completely straighten your arms each time you return to the starting position.

098 KNOW YOUR…
TRICEPS

The triceps brachii is a three-headed extensor muscle located on the back of the upper arm. It is the extensor muscle of your elbow joint, and it also fixates your elbow when you use your forearm and hand for fine movements, such as writing. Its long head comes into play when you need to generate sustained force; the medial head enables more precise, low-force movements; and the lateral head allows for movements requiring occasional high-intensity force. The triceps is the antagonist of the biceps. With antagonistic pairs, one muscle contracts as the other relaxes—in this case, the triceps relaxes while the biceps contracts to lift the arm.

099 TIGHTEN UP
THOSE TRICEPS

As most gym-goers know, certain parts of the body stubbornly resist toning and conditioning. Perhaps the most notorious of these are the triceps, the muscles located at the back of your arms. They are not only a tricky spot to create definition, they can become saggy, especially after a period of weight loss.

Unfortunately, we often ignore our triceps. One possible reason is that we tend to "only work the muscles we see"—that is, we can't view our triceps with the same clarity that we see our abs, biceps, and chest and so don't give them priority. Furthermore, these muscles require deliberate movement to exercise them, making them difficult to work effectively. Weight training is the answer to taming those triceps, using either free weights or weight machines. Conditioning them is also important because any time there is a deficiency in one muscle group—in this case the triceps—other muscles—like the biceps—have to work harder, tiring you out more quickly. So include a triceps exercise in your weekly routine, and before long you'll notice sleek, lean underarms taking shape.

THINK *about it*

There was a time when many gym-goers focused only on building "show" muscles, but the current approach is to aim for long, lean, functionally strong muscles. That's the new sexy.

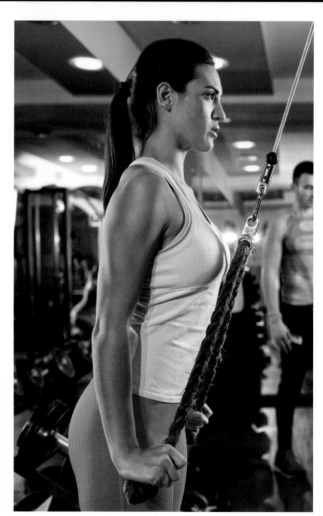

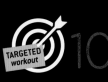

100 TONE AND DEFINE YOUR TRICEPS

The key to sleek-looking arms is a targeted triceps routine. These four exercises utilize weights—dumbbells, barbells, and cable machine—to work all three heads of the triceps, preparing them for the next level of training. To allow for adequate recovery, perform this workout once a week only. Start with one set of each, and work your way up to four.

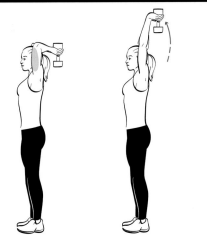

Ⓐ OVERHEAD TRICEPS EXTENSION To keep the focus on your triceps, keep your shoulders down and your elbows as close to your ears as possible, and avoid arching your back. Perform one to four sets of 12 reps.

HOW Stand with your knees soft and your arms straight up with your elbows next to ears, holding a dumbbell with both hands. Bend your elbows to a 90-degree angle. Squeeze your triceps to straighten your arms, pressing the dumbbell up. Slowly lower back to the starting position.

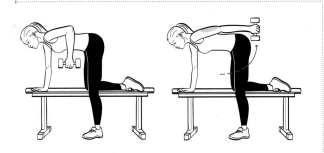

Ⓑ ONE-ARM KICKBACK To perfect your form, be sure not to lock your elbow at the top of the movement. Straighten your arm, but keep your elbow slightly bent. Perform one to four sets of 12 reps with each arm.

HOW Holding a dumbbell in your left hand, place your right knee on a flat bench, and bend forward, bracing yourself with your palm. Bend your right elbow to a 90-degree angle, and then slowly straighten your arm. Hold for a moment, and then return to the starting position.

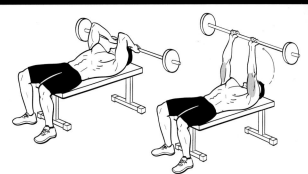

Ⓒ BARBELL SKULL CRUSHER Be sure to recruit a spotter for this exercise—its name is a reminder of what can happen if you do the exercise improperly and drop the barbell. Perform one to four sets of 10 reps.

HOW Lie face-up on a bench, and extend both arms overhead, grasping barbell with an overhand grip. Bend your elbows so that your forearms are parallel to the floor. Slowly straighten your arms, and then lower to the starting position.

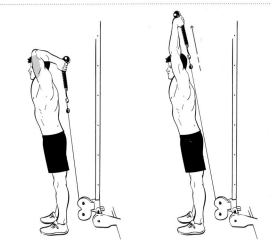

Ⓓ CABLE ROPE OVERHEAD EXTENSION If you are performing this exercise properly, you'll feel a distinct stretch in your triceps. Perform one to four sets of 12 reps.

HOW Stand with your feet shoulder-width apart, and keep your back straight and abs tightly drawn in. Grab the ends of a cable rope with both hands with your palms facing up, and then raise the rope over your head. Once your arms are fully extended, slowly lower the rope in an arc behind your head. Hold for a count, then slowly raise the rope back to the start.

101 CHOOSE THE BEST BENCH

Visit any gym, and you're sure to see the three basic varieties of benches: the flat, incline, and decline. Each has its uses and can change how the same exercise works your muscles.

Any bench must be sturdy enough to hold you and a range of training weights. You can do flat-bench exercises and lifts on any flat, raised surface, even a park bench or sturdy picnic table bench, but the ideal weight-training bench is adjustable. It will allow you to switch positions to optimal incline or decline in order to increase strength demands during your workouts. Gold's Gym has a variety of benches, including multi-position benches that include racks to hold barbells, curl yokes, and four-roll leg developers.

FLAT BENCH The basic bench of resistance-training, you can use it for exercises like barbell and dumbbell presses. When you perform a bench press on a flat bench, you evenly work both the upper and lower heads of the pecs.

INCLINE BENCH This is the position if you really want to develop chest definition. Performing a bench press on an incline puts more stress on your upper pecs and anterior deltoids.

DECLINE BENCH A bench press on a decline works much the same as a flat press, but you can lift a little more weight, but also lose some range of motion.

102 DO A BENCH DIP

One of the most effective exercises for the triceps is the bench dip. This medium-intensity exercise allows you to use your body's own weight to strengthen this hard-to-work muscle. You can use any bench, from your gym's flat bench to a convenient park bench.

Plan on doing two to three sets of 10 reps three days a week for six to eight weeks. A more advanced version of the bench dip involves propping your heels on another bench or a sturdy box across from where you are seated before lowering yourself down.

HOW Position your hands shoulder-width apart behind you on the edge of a secured bench. Walk your feet out in front of you until you are resting on your heels. Bend your elbows to lower your upper body toward the ground until your upper arms are parallel to the ground. Slowly press off with your hands to push yourself back up to the starting position.

103 SCULPT YOUR ARMS

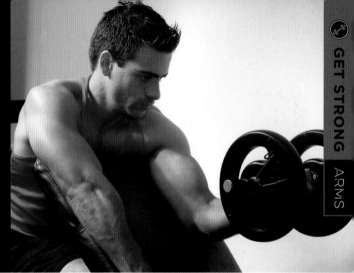

You don't have to work each muscle in isolation to sculpt your arms. These three exercises challenge every major arm muscle, working the biceps, triceps, and forearms in tandem.

Gold's Gym has designed this workout so that you can also work this group for different purposes—defined bulk or toned sleekness. Just follow the recommendations for the goal of your choice. For bulk, perform four sets of 8 to 12 reps, resting for one to two minutes between sets; for toning, do four sets of 16 to 25 reps taking no more than 30 seconds to rest between sets.

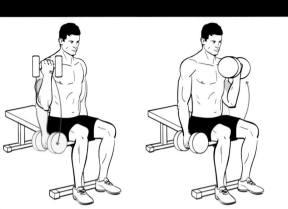

ⓐ SEATED ALTERNATING DUMBBELL CURLS Curls will work your elbow flexors, which comprise the biceps brachii, brachialis, and brachioradialis.

HOW Sit with a dumbbell in each hand, your arms at your sides and palms facing in. Starting with the right arm, curl the dumbbell up, rotating your wrist 90 degrees so that you finish with your palms up. Squeeze your biceps for one second before lowering. Repeat on the left side. That's one rep.

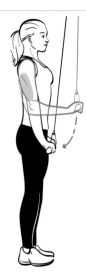

ⓑ STANDING TRICEPS PUSH-DOWN This exercise uses a weighted cable machine to efficiently work out your triceps.

HOW Stand with your feet shoulder-width apart in front of a triceps push-down or cable machine with the straight bar, rope, or cable hanging at about chest level. Grab on with both hands, keeping your elbows pinned to your sides. Push your hands toward floor, fully extending your arms in front of your body to touch the tops of your legs. Hold for a second, reverse the movement, and then return to start.

ⓒ TWENTY-ONES This is a highly effective biceps and forearm exercise. The number in its name refers to the total number of reps you perform in a set, which is divided into three, seven-rep segments. With so many reps using three different ranges of motion, twenty-ones are a compound exercise that truly challenges your stamina. With those extra demands that this exercise places on your arms, it's best if you choose a weight that is about 40 percent of what you can comfortably curled 10 times, and perform it as the last exercise of your upper-body workout.

HOW You can use a barbell or dumbbells for this exercise that combines three kinds of curls. Do 7 repetitions of each kind, for a total of 21 reps.

Set 1 Standing, hold weights at your thighs, palms facing up, and lift to waist height.

Set 2 This time, start at waist height, and lift to your chest.

Set 3 Finally, do a full curl, starting with the weights at your thighs and finishing with them at your chest.

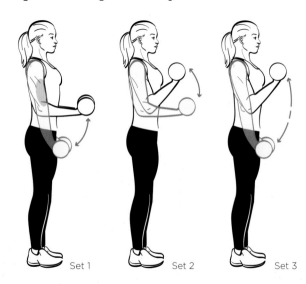

Set 1   Set 2   Set 3

104 KNOW YOUR... ABDOMINALS

The main abdominal muscle, the rectus abdominis, is a paired muscle running vertically along your abdomen, beginning at the pubic bone and ending at the sternum. The abs work to contract your body forward and are important postural and core muscles. A targeted abdominal workout, paired with a proper diet, results in the highly defined look known as "six-pack" or "washboard" abs.

Along with the rectus abdominis is the transversus abdominis, a deep muscle in the abdominal wall lying beneath the internal oblique muscle. Nicknamed the corset muscle, a well-toned transversus abdominis works to pull in your abdomen, preventing it from protruding. The external obliques, the side abdominals, are located on each side of the rectus abdominis, and lying beneath the external obliques are the internal obliques. This muscle group flexes the rib cage and the pelvic bones together, bends the torso sideways, and rotates the torso.

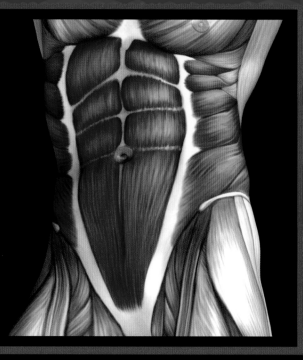

105 RIP YOUR ABS

In recent years, a spate of ultra-fit Hollywood hunks—and hunkettes—popularized the look of extremely defined abdominal muscles, the infamous "six pack." This sculpted appearance is not achieved without concentrated effort, but it can be worth all the hard work, especially if you spend a lot of time at the beach or poolside.

To trim your midsection, you must watch your nutrition. Try to eat the proper amounts of protein and healthy fats, and remember your post-workout complex carbs. At the gym, forget doing thousands of crunches and add in core-centric exercises, such as the captain's chair knee raise (see #106) that employs more than twice the abdominal activity of basic crunches. Be sure to include exercises that work your obliques—those side abs that are too often hidden behind fat deposits (those pesky love handles).

High-intensity, whole-body resistance training will also promote post-exercise fat burning. Try to maintain proper sleep habits, and keep stress levels low to avoid hormonal changes that affect waist size. This is one reason many women have trouble getting ripped—their hormonal makeup contains less testosterone, making it more difficult to build muscle mass and burn calories during and after exercise.

Result may vary, but most individuals will start to see results in 12 weeks. Finally, don't think that all you need is a fat-burning supplement. There are no shortcuts to ripped abs.

106 SALUTE THE CAPTAIN

If you are serious about strengthening your abs, try the captain's chair knee raise. In recent studies, this exercise stimulated 210 percent more ab activity in the study's participants than the traditional crunch. It also engages the hard-to-work lower abs.

HOW Stand on the captain's chair machine or power tower. Grip the handles, and press your back against the pad. Keeping your feet close together, remove them from the support steps so that your legs dangle freely. Engage your abs, and bring your knees up toward your chest, keeping your upper back and shoulders strong. Then, with slow, controlled movements, lower your legs back to the starting position.

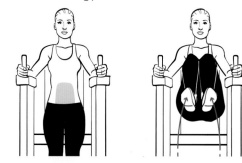

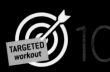

107 WHITTLE YOUR WAIST

Choosing a workout to tone your midsection means including exercises that target the obliques, the muscles that define and shape your waist.

Just about any move that calls for you to reach to the side will work these muscles, but ones that also incorporate your rectus and transversus abdominis will more effectively sculpt and slim your waistline. Exercises that target the obliques and the intercostals—several additional groups of muscles that run between the ribs—also help to get you in top shape for rotational sports like tennis and golf.

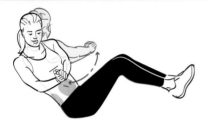

Ⓐ SEATED RUSSIAN TWIST This ab exercise really works your obliques, while also engaging your back muscles. Perform three sets of 10 reps.

HOW Sit on the floor with your knees bent, pull your abs to your spine, and lean back a few inches while lifting your feet off the floor. Keep your back straight, reach your arms out in front of you, and twist your torso to the right, then to the left.

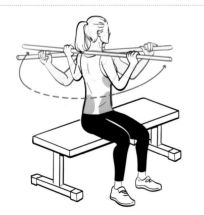

Ⓑ BROOM TWIST This twist is a great abdominal exercise for increasing flexibility and working out your obliques. Perform three sets of 10 reps.

HOW Place a broomstick across the back of your shoulders, holding it with an overhand grip with your hands, and sit with your back straight, abs tight, and chin up. Twist your upper body to one side, and then slowly twist to the other side. Continue without stopping for the full number of reps.

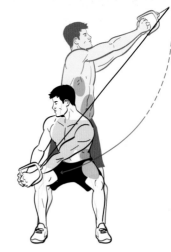

Ⓒ CABLE WOOD CHOP The wood-chop motion engages your obliques, back, shoulders, and legs. Repeat on the opposite side for a total of two sets of 10 reps on each side.

HOW Stand sideways to a cable stack with a D-handle set low. Squat, and hold it with both hands, arms extended toward the anchor point. Extend your legs, and twist through your waist to bring the handle above your opposite shoulder. Return to the start, following the same path of motion.

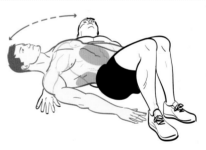

Ⓓ PENGUIN CRUNCH This reaching exercise uses extension and lateral movement to target your abs and obliques. Complete three sets of 10 reps.

HOW Lie on your back with your knees bent and feet flat, hip-width apart, and arms at your sides. Crunch, and slightly lift your upper body, and then rotate your torso to one side, trying to touch your fingertips to your heel by sliding your hand across the floor. Then rotate to the other side with your other hand. Continue alternating fingertip-to-heel touches.

THINK *about it* To make the penguin crunch a little more challenging, just move your heels farther away from your body, so you extend more in order to touch them. To make it easier, scoot them in closer.

108 CUSTOMIZE YOUR CRUNCH

When you think of exercises for the abs, what's the first one that comes to mind? Yeah … it's the crunch. A basic crunch is simple in theory, but not always easy to execute properly in reality. Form is everything, especially if you have lower-back or neck problems.

PULL IN YOUR ABS Keep your abs pulled in. This places greater tension on them, so that you don't overarch your lower back.

DON'T PULL ON YOUR NECK Don't pull on your neck with your hands or draw your elbows in, as it may strain your neck muscles and vertebrae.

CURL AND LIFT Curl forward as if doubling over, as well as lift your torso and shoulders. Don't just yank your head, neck, and shoulder blades off the floor.

KEEP IT SMALL The crunch is a small movement. No need to touch your head to your knees—lifting just a few inches off the floor is high enough to effectively engage your abdominal muscles.

Once you've mastered the basic moves, try the variations below that amp up the basic crunch to really maximize your abs workout.

Ⓐ BASIC CRUNCH

WHY Strengthens the abdominals.

HOW Lie down on your back with your knees bent and feet flat on the floor, hip-width apart. Cross your hands over your chest or bring them together behind your head. Keeping your neck relaxed, roll your upper back off the floor so that your head, neck, and shoulder blades lift off the floor. Hold for a moment at the top, and then lower slowly.

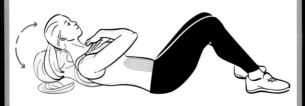

Ⓑ REVERSE CRUNCH

WHY This exercise has been shown to stimulate more than twice as much abdominal activity than the traditional basic crunch.

HOW Lie on your back, and extend your arms at your sides. Raise your knees and feet so that they create a 90-degree angle. Contract your abs, and exhale as you lift your hips off the floor; your knees will move toward your head. Inhale, and slowly lower.

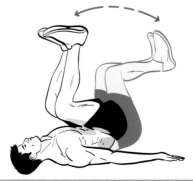

C BICYCLE CRUNCH

WHY One rep reaps the benefits of many crunches.

HOW Lie on your back. Put your hands behind your head. Lift your legs off the floor, and then extend your right leg while bringing your left knee up toward your chest. Lift your head, neck and shoulders up and reach with your right elbow across your body toward your left knee. Lower back down. Keep alternating sides in a pedaling motion.

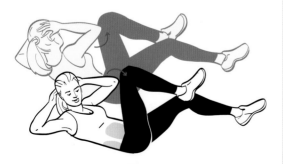

D DOUBLE CRUNCH

WHY Combines the moves of a basic crunch with the power of a reverse crunch that will target your lower abdominals.

HOW Lie on your back with your legs bent, hands behind your head and feet flat on the floor. While exhaling, contract your abs and simultaneously raise your head and torso with your hips and knees, bringing them toward each other to touch.

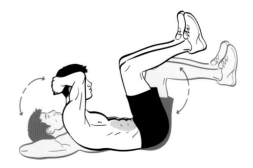

109 CULTIVATE YOUR CORE

Strengthening your core is an age-defying activity that should be a consistent part of your weekly workout routine. Having strong core muscles makes even everyday activities like holding your kids, climbing stairs, and carrying your groceries much easier. A great way to strengthen this important group is the Gold's Gym Ultimate Core Workout of Six Essential Exercises shown below.

You may ask, what is the core? Don't confuse the term *core* with *abdominals*. The core is a complex series of muscle groups that includes far more than your abs, and you rely on it for almost every move you make. Along with the abs and obliques, major core muscles include the pelvic floor muscles, multifidus spinae, erector spinae, and the diaphragm. Minor core muscles include the latissimus dorsi, gluteus maximus, and trapezius. These muscles act as stabilizers for movement, transfer force from one limb to another, or initiate movement itself.

To complete this workout, start with 10 minutes of cardio, then follow the chart's recommended reps and sets for your fitness level, and end with 5 minutes of stretching. Don't forget to hydrate throughout. Do this routine three times a week, and you should see results within a month.

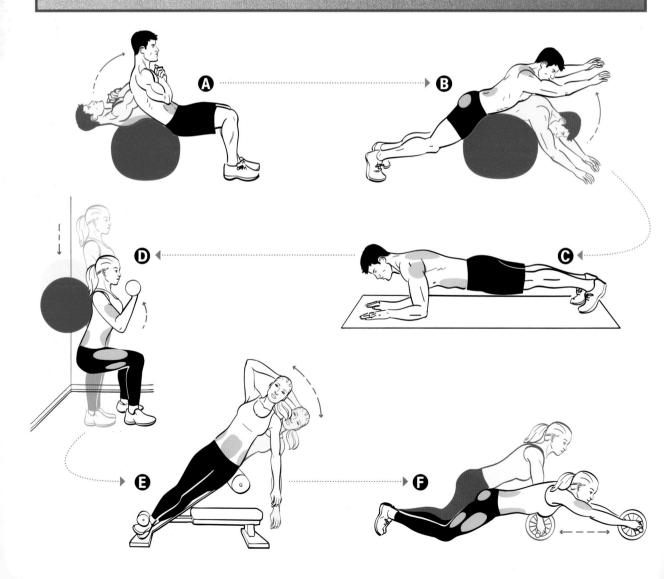

A STABILITY BALL CRUNCHES Lie back on a stability ball, with feet flat on the floor and your torso forming a 45-degree angle with the ball. Cross your hands, and place them on your upper chest. Contract your abs to lift your torso, keeping your feet and neck stable, and then slowly lower back down.

B STABILITY BALL EXTENSION Lie facedown on a stability ball, with your feet supporting you about hip-distance apart. Hold your arms out Superman-style, and slowly lift yourself up. Drop your chin to the ball, and elevate your upper torso so that your back and rear are in a straight line; be sure not to overextend into a curve.

C ELBOW PLANK Lie facedown on a mat as if you were about to perform a push-up. Keep your arms bent so that your palms and forearms rest flat on the mat. Your legs should be extended straight out with your feet resting on your toes. Contract your abdominal muscles, and slowly lift your torso off the floor, keeping your palms, elbows, forearms, and toes grounded on the floor.

D STABILITY BALL WALL SQUAT WITH CURL Place a stability ball between your mid-back and a wall. Stand with feet hip-distance apart. With your arms relaxed at your sides, grasp a dumbbell in each hand. Maintaining contact with wall, squat down until your thighs are at parallel with the floor. At the same time, perform a biceps curl. Push through your heels to stand back up, while lowering the weights to the starting position.

E SIDE TRUNK RAISE Position yourself sideways on a hyperextension bench so that one hip rests on the large pad, and hook your feet under the foot pads. Let one arm hang straight down relaxed, with the other resting behind your head. Exhale, contract your oblique muscles, and then lower your free arm toward the floor. Keep your neck straight, and don't twist your upper body. Inhale, and then return to the starting position. Alternate sides between each set.

F THE AB WHEEL An ab wheel is a small wheel with a handle on either side. With your knees bent and resting on the floor, contract your core, and slightly tilt your pelvis back to prevent arching your lower back. Grab the handles on the wheel with both hands, and hold it directly below your shoulders, keeping your arms straight. Roll the wheel straight out in front of you, moving it far enough to work all your ab muscles. Squeeze your abs, use your lower-back muscles, and pull the wheel back toward you.

EXERCISE	BEGINNER	INTERMEDIATE	ADVANCED
STABILITY BALL CRUNCH	One sets of 10 reps	Two sets of 10 reps	Three sets of 10 reps
STABILITY BALL EXTENSION	One sets of 10 reps	Two sets of 10 reps	Three sets of 10 reps
ELBOW PLANK	Hold for 15 to 30 seconds	Hold for 30 to 45 seconds	Hold for 45 to 60 seconds
STABILITY BALL WALL SQUAT WITH CURL	Two sets of 10 reps	Two sets of 12 reps	Three sets of 12 reps
SIDE TRUNK RAISE	Two sets of 10 on both sides	Two sets of 12 on both sides	Three sets of 12 on both sides
THE AB WHEEL	One set of 10 reps	Two sets of 10 reps	Three sets of 10 reps

MORE THAN SKIN DEEP Many of your core muscles are deep muscles well hidden beneath the layers of the exterior muscles that your workouts so often target—like the rectus abdominis. But your core most often acts as a stabilizer and force transfer center, rather than as a prime mover, so it is essential to mix up exercises like crunches, which target the external rectus abdominis, with other functional exercises like planks, which hit the deeper muscles, such as the transversus abdominis.

MORE THAN JUST STRENGTH Research is showing that strengthening your core does more than just tighten your midsection. It can also improve cognitive functioning and help prevent bone and muscle weakening. And not to mention that a well-conditioned core will give you a confidence-boosting midsection that looks good in (and out of) your clothes.

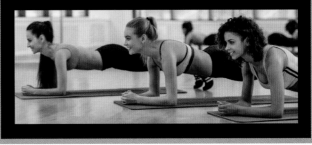

KNOW YOUR…
QUADRICEPS

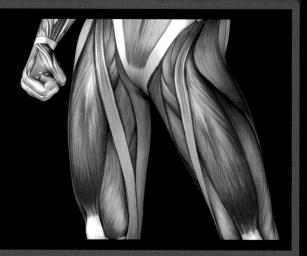

Among the strongest muscles in your body, the four-headed quadriceps femoris covers just about all of your femur—the long bone of your thigh. The quadriceps femoris actually includes four front thigh muscles—the rectus femoris vastus lateralis, vastus medialis, and vastus intermedius. This group functions to extend your leg. The rectus femoris attaches to the ilium bone of the pelvis, so it also flexes the hip—an action essential to walking or running as it swings the leg forward into the next step you take. The vastus medialis, the innermost muscle of the quads, stabilizes your kneecap and joint during walking or running.

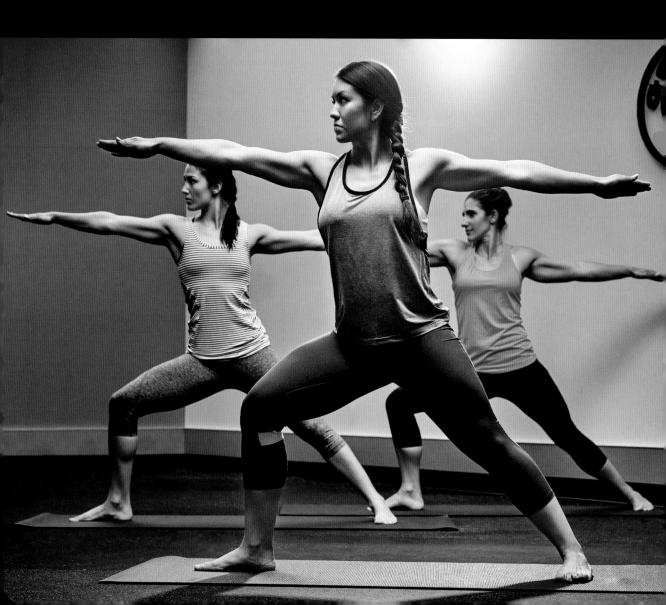

111 TONE YOUR QUADS

Having strong quads yields multiple benefits: your quads help to stabilize and protect your knee and hip joints, strengthen your bones, and increase muscle mass (which will help your body to burn calories more efficiently). And any endurance activity (in fact, just about any physical activity), such as walking, climbing, or running, relies on strong leg muscles. Here are three effective exercises to target your quads that require no extra equipment.

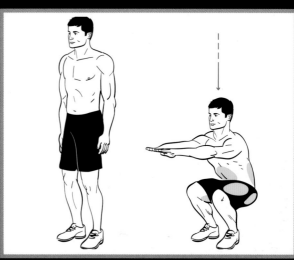

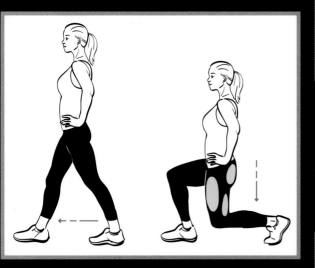

A STATIONARY LUNGE The lunge is one of the best leg exercises around, working nearly every part of your lower body. This version places an extra emphasis on your quads.

HOW Stand with your feet hip-width apart. Take a large step forward with your right foot. Keep your back straight and your right foot flat on the floor, and lower straight down until your right thigh is parallel to the floor. Hold for a count of two, and then slowly rise. Repeat for the desired reps, then switch legs.

112 TRY IT WEIGHT FREE

You don't actually need barbells, dumbbells, or weight machines to perform effective quadriceps exercises—you can instead use your own body weight to supply resistance. These body-weight quads moves also work several muscle groups at once, which can make your leg workout more efficient when you're short on time. Because they require no equipment, you can perform a complete lower-body workout just about anywhere, and they are ideal for those days when you can't make it to the gym, but want to maintain your workout schedule.

B NARROW-STANCE SQUAT Like any squat, the close-stance squat will strengthen your entire lower body, with an added emphasis on the quads and outer-thigh muscles.

HOW Stand with your feet slightly closer than hip-distance apart. Keeping both feet completely flat on the ground, squat as low as you can. Hold the bottom position for a few seconds before returning to the top to begin the next rep.

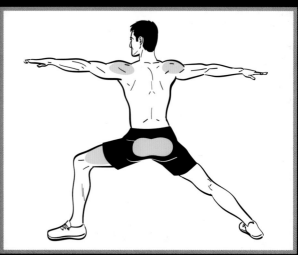

C WARRIOR II POSE The series of yoga stances known as the Warrior poses calls for you to hold a lunge position. Warrior II stretches and strengthens the legs, while also building stamina.

HOW Stand with your feet facing forward and your legs wide apart. Turn your right foot 90 degrees so that it points straight out to the side. Raise your arms out to your sides so they are parallel to the floor, and then lower until your thigh is also close to parallel with the floor. Hold for 30 seconds to a minute, and then release the pose. Turn to the left, reversing the position of your feet, and repeat on the opposite side.

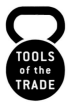

TOOLS
of the
TRADE

113 IMPRESS WITH THE LEG PRESS

Despite how much we use our legs every day, it can be difficult to strengthen or sculpt them to the level we desire, even at the gym. The leg press machine, which is found in most gyms, health clubs, and fitness centers, enables you to both build strength in your lower body and tone your muscles from ankle to hip—give it a try, and you'll soon see results in your quadriceps, hamstrings, calves, and glutes. The leg press is also a useful tool for evaluating an athlete's overall body strength from knee to hip. There are two types of leg press machines.

DIAGONAL OR VERTICAL SLED LEG PRESS In this version of the leg press, you recline seated below a sled that has weight disks attached and is mounted on two rails, and you push the weight upward with your legs.

CABLE OR SEATED LEG PRESS In this version of the leg press, you sit with feet hip-width apart and flat against a footplate. You bend your knees to 90 degrees. and then extend your legs until they are straight but not locked.

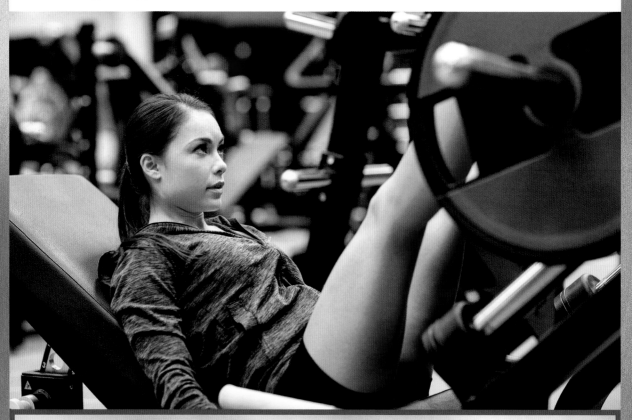

GYM
etiquette

114 FOCUS ON YOURSELF

No matter what level you might have reached in any given endeavor, there will always be someone more advanced. That, in part, is why the gym is a good place to better yourself—there are so many success stories all around you. But no matter how admirable any other person's physique or definition may be, remember not to stare openly at anyone working out or resting between sets. Conversely, if you see someone noticeably unfit or fumbling with the equipment, unless they're doing something unsafe, simply leave them to find their footing in the gym. Whether you're a fitness pro or a rank beginner, always be polite—and give others their space.

115 WEIGHT FOR IT

Want to work on your quads at the gym? You'll find plenty of options. Along with the leg press machine, most gyms offer leg extension and hack squat units. Free-weight exercises using barbells and medicine balls also give your quads a real workout. As with any resistance exercise, start with lighter weights, and work your way higher as your strength increases.

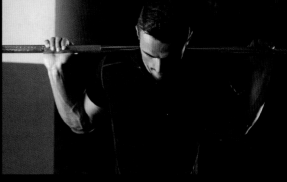

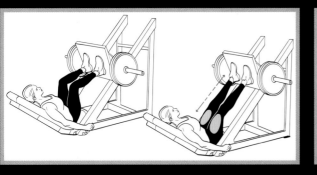

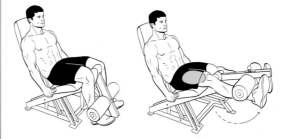

Ⓐ LEG PRESS Leg presses are effective, but don't work with too-heavy weights, which may put you at risk for back problems.

HOW Sit on a leg-press machine with your back against the pad and your feet placed hip-width apart. Set the weight on a challenging, yet doable, resistance. Bend your knees to a 90-degree angle, keeping your feet flat against the footplate. Extend your legs until they are straight but not locked. Slowly return to the starting position.

Ⓒ LEG EXTENSIONS Another gym staple, the leg extension machine allows you to target the your quadriceps.

HOW Sit down on the seat of a leg extension machine, and hook your legs behind the padded bar. Adjust the bar so that it rests on your lower leg. Select a weight, and slowly lift the bar until your legs are almost straight, then lower your legs back down. Make sure to keep your back straight, and grip the handles on each side of the seat.

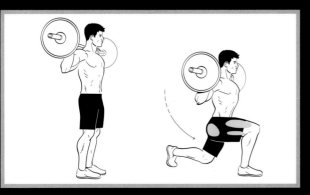

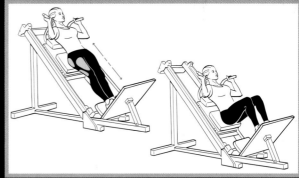

Ⓑ BARBELL WALKING LUNGE The exercise not only engages your quads, but also your glutes and hamstrings.

HOW Squeeze your shoulder blades, and place the barbell on top, making sure that the bar is resting on your muscles, not your spine. Grasp the bar with an overhand grip, step forward, and land first on your heel and then the forefoot. Keep your chest up, then lower your body by flexing the knee and hip of your front leg until the knee of your rear leg is almost in contact with the floor. With assistance from your rear leg, stand up on your front leg, and then lunge forward with the opposite leg.

Ⓓ HACK SQUAT Like the leg press, the hack squat machine allows you to effectively target your quadriceps.

HOW Lie back with your shoulders under the pads. Position your feet shoulder-width apart on the platform. Place your arms on the side handles, and disengage the safety bars. To get into the starting position, straighten your legs without locking your knees. Inhale, and bend your knees to slowly lower the unit until your upper legs are below parallel to the floor. Exhale, and push the sled with your heels to straighten your legs, and raise the unit back to the starting position.

116 FLEX YOUR MUSCLES

Your muscles do more than flex, functioning in a variety of ways to let your body to move through your daily life, as well as allowing you to pursue a fitness regimen and other athletic pursuits. There are a few terms that you should know in order to understand just how your muscles work.

FLEXION The bending of a joint: the contraction of a flexor muscle decreases the angle between two bones. For example, the elbow flexor muscles (the brachialis, biceps brachii, and brachioradialis) bend your arm by decreasing the angle between the forearm and upper arm. You perform this action when you lift a dumbbell during the upward phase of a biceps curl.

EXTENSION The act of straightening; the contraction of an extensor muscle extends or straightens a limb or other part of the body. For example, the forearm extensors (the triceps brachii and anconeus) straighten the arm. You perform this action when you lower a dumbbell during the downward phase of a biceps curl.

ABDUCTION Movement away from the body, the contraction of an abductor muscle moves a limb away from your body's midline or from another part. For example, the hip abductors (the gluteus maximus, gluteus medius, gluteus minimus, and tensor fasciae latae) spread the legs away from the midline and away from each other. Developing strong hip abductors lets you to quickly move from side to side—an ability that can give you an edge in sports like basketball.

ADDUCTION Movement toward the body, the contraction of an adductor muscle moves a limb in the direction of the midline of the body or toward another part. For example, the adductor muscles of the hips (the adductor longus, adductor brevis, adductor magnus, pectineus, and gracilis) pull the legs toward the midline of the body so that the legs are closer together. The hip adductors also allow you to cross your legs across the midline of the body—well-trained adductors are useful for kicking a soccer ball.

ROTATION The rotation of a joint, a rotator muscle assists the rotation of a joint, such as the hip or the shoulder. For example, the medial, or internal, hip rotators (mainly the tensor fasciae latae and gluteus medius) turn your leg in toward your hip, while the external rotators (piriformis, gemellus superior, obturator internus, gemellus inferior, obturator externus, and quadratus femoris) allow you to move your leg backward and out and to rotate your leg outward. Both kinds of rotators are important for maintaining balance and stability when running.

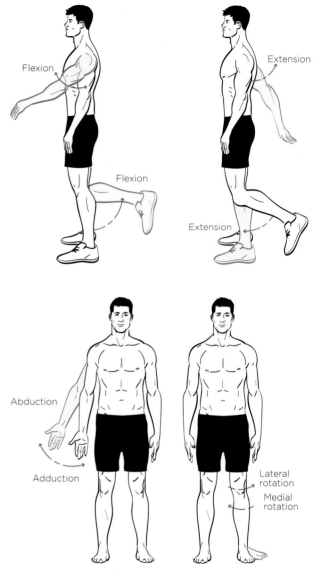

AGONISM AND ANTAGONISM Muscles close in proximity often work in concert to create functional movement. An agonist muscle is the primary mover, initiating the major movement by contracting, or shortening. Its antagonist is the secondary mover. For example, during a biceps curl, your biceps brachii and triceps brachii work in opposition to flex and extend your elbow joint. During the lifting (flexion) phase, your biceps works as the agonist, engaging in a shortening contraction as it brings the dumbbell closer to your upper arm, while at the same time, the antagonist triceps is lengthening. In the lowering phase, the triceps kicks in as the agonist, lowering the dumbbell while the biceps functions as the lengthening antagonist.

117 WORK YOUR HIPS AND THIGHS

To work your inner and outer thighs, look for exercises that target your hip abductors and adductors. There are good reasons to train these muscle groups—it will improve muscular imbalances, strengthen your core, and help prevent injury.

Leg-openers such as the clamshell or the fire hydrant strengthen the abductors. A move like lateral bounding will work just about all of your lower body, while adding a plyometric boost to strengthening your adductors.

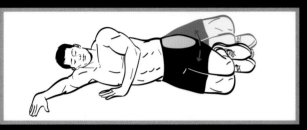

Ⓐ CLAMSHELL The clam shell is an effective exercise if you suffer from knee or lower back pain.

HOW Lie on your side with your knees and feet together and knees bent. Keeping your feet together, slowly raise your knee. Return to the start position, repeat for the desired reps.

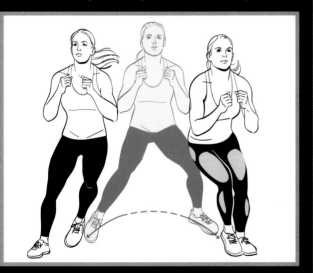

Ⓑ LATERAL BOUNDING Here's an example of a power-producing plyometric exercise, a quick, powerful move that starts with an eccentric (muscle lengthening) action immediately followed by a concentric (muscle shortening) one.

HOW Start in a shallow squat with your weight on your right foot. Leap sideways as far as you can go to the left, landing on your left foot, then bringing the right foot over to the left as well. Immediately reverse directions, and jump to the right. Continue jumping side to side.

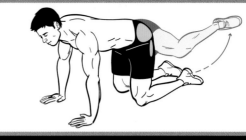

Ⓒ FIRE HYDRANT This exercise works as both an abductor strengthener and a core stabilizer.

HOW Get on all fours. Keeping your knee bent, left your leg away from the midline of the body. Pause at the top of the motion, and then slowly return to the starting position.

 Ask the EXPERT

SHOULD I USE THIG MACHINES?

The inner thigh machine, also known as the thigh adductor, helps you focus on the hip adductor muscles, as well as the glutes and the hamstrings. Your inner-thigh muscles work to stabilize your pelvis and promote good balance, and the adductor magnus, one of the largest muscles in the body, helps promote stability at the knee. Keeping these muscles fit and healthy is important. Controversy surrounds these machines, though, with detractors convinced that they don't work. Most authorities agree, however, that although an adductor machine won't spot reduce fat, it will help to strengthen inner-thigh muscles and also to develop greater bone density and stronger connective tissue. It is one of the easiest machines to use during your lower-body circuit, but many pros prefer the standing multi-hip machine for strengthening both the inner and outer thighs because it engages the actual muscles you use while walking, running, and twisting.

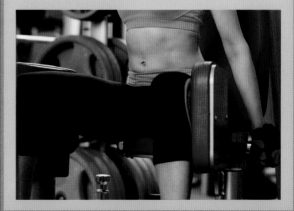

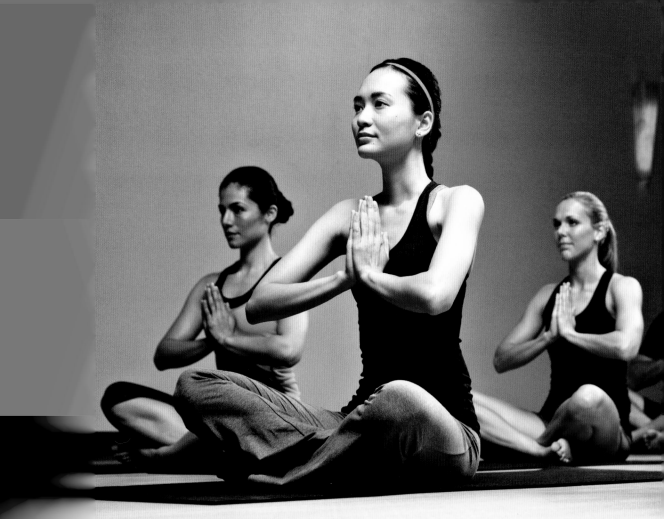

 BEND AND STRETCH
Building strength
and improving cardio
health are difficult tasks if your
body is stiff and unyielding
when you work out, so it is
vital to develop supple joints
and muscles as you tone and
oxygenate. Stretching yields
results: better flexibility can
improve your performance in
sports, training, and in everyday
life. And because it helps your
joints move through their full
range of motion, it can also
decrease your risk of injury.
Stretching increases blood flow
to your muscles, as well.

The loss of the ability to
comfortably flex and stretch

is a side effect of aging—but
it is one that can be kept at
bay with the right exercises.
Optimum flexibility can be
achieved (and maintained)
at any age with a proper
regular regimen. For example,
perform 10 to 15 minutes of
body stretches, work out
with stability balls and foam
rollers, and perform exercises
that concentrate on flexibility
and mobility (try taking a
yoga or Pilates class).

Maintaining a balanced
diet that includes adequate
amounts of both protein and
calcium is essential. Also, be
sure to drink plenty of water
to stay hydrated.

 MIRROR THE MOVES
Include both negative
and positive motions
when you're stretching: for
example, follow up a stretch to
the left with one to the right; if
you bend forward, be sure to
bend backward.

To get the full benefit of your
exercises, stretch until you feel
a little strain in your muscles—a
bit of strain is normal. Never rush
stretches or overextend them.
You should gradually increase
the difficulty of your stretching
regimen—duration of hold or
length of reach, or both. Try
warming up beforehand with 8
or 10 jumping jacks.

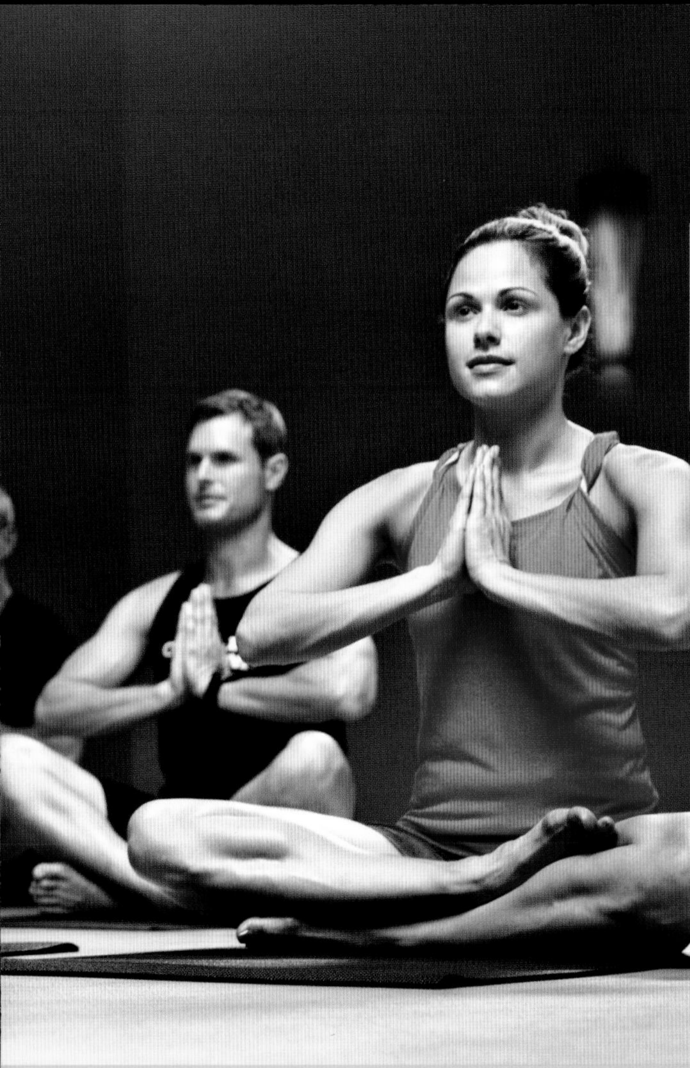

FOLLOW A WINNER'S JOURNEY
Steve Bingham
Male Winner, Ages 60+

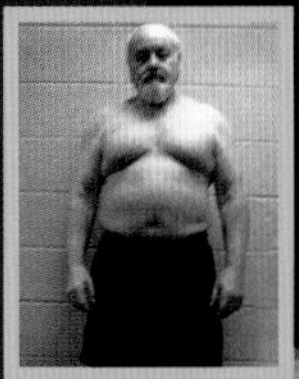

Before

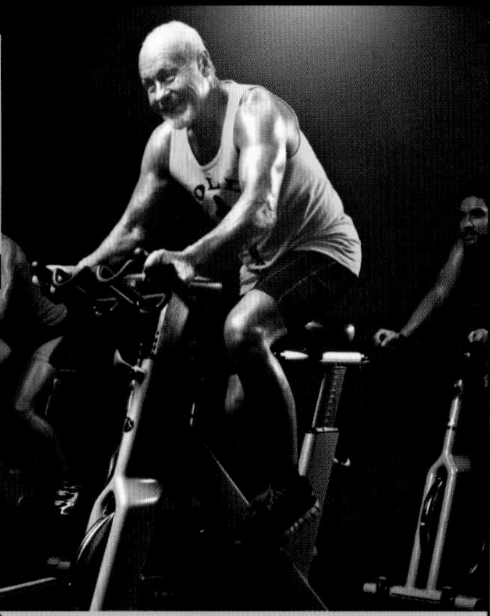

LOST 60 pounds (27.2 kg), 18 inches (45.7 cm), and 12.6% body fat

When he was in his mid-60s, Steve took the Challenge because he wanted to be less than 200 pounds when he turned 70. He felt the Challenge would motivate him; otherwise, he says, "it would have taken me three years instead of three months."

His regimen was intense. He completed five or six hours of classes a day—including body pumping and spinning—which, he says, helped him to strengthen and stretch. Three times a week he did body training. He also used a fitness website to track his exercises and calculate how many calories he could eat and still achieve his goal.

Steve believes that making this choice must be a very personal thing, that you have to desire deep down. For himself, he wanted to enjoy his 24 grandkids and also be healthy enough to go skiing, swimming, boating, and biking, and take part in other physical activities. "I want to enjoy the rest of my life," he proclaims, then adds, "and I really want to climb Mount Everest."

RELAX AND SAY "OMMM" To keep muscles limber and joints fluid, try yoga. Yoga has grown from a niche pursuit into a worldwide health practice approved by doctors—and gurus—alike. Forget your fears of looking silly—everyone who's ever stepped on a mat has probably felt this way. You don't need to be a contortionist to practice yoga; you'll gradually work up to the more complicated poses. Start with a beginner's class, which often includes aids, such as blocks or stretching straps, to help you to achieve the proper alignment during poses.

WINNER'S WORDS

"The best thing that happened to me was yoga, because it got me standing on one foot and stretching my lower back."

~ Steve Bingham

118 | KNOW YOUR…
HAMSTRINGS

The group of muscles on the back of the thigh is known as the hamstrings. This group is made up of the semitendinosus, semimembranosus, and biceps femoris. When your trunk is fixed, the semitendinosus and semimembranosus extend the hip, and they flex the knee and rotate your lower leg inward when you bend your knee. When you take a step, the biceps femoris extends your hip and also flexes your knee and rotates your lower leg outward when your knee is bent. Along with the quadriceps, the hamstrings enable you to walk, run, jump, and squat.

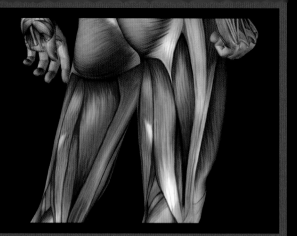

119 | GUARD YOUR HAMSTRINGS

Many of us have jobs that require long hours seated at a desk; others spend a lot of time working or relaxing at their home computers. If this is the case, your hamstrings are likely to be tight—the result of muscles held in a static, shortened position. This tightness puts you at risk for hamstring injuries, knee injuries, and back pain. Hamstring injuries can also occur during athletic pursuits, such as jogging, soccer, baseball, volleyball, and basketball—as a result of over-training, falls, dehydration, and inflexibility. Support your hamstring strength work with a plan to keep these muscles supple. By creating a stretching routine involving both static and dynamic stretches, incorporating yoga or Pilates classes into your weekly routine, and focusing on training for balance, you will keep your hamstrings flexible and supportive.

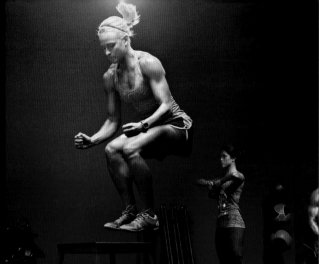

120 HONE YOUR HAMSTRINGS

Whatever your athletic pursuit, to stay at the best performance level, you have to pay attention to your hamstrings. A regimen of exercises that target this group will help keep your legs strong and flexible. A typical plan is to start with two days of leg workouts per week, concentrating on the hamstrings work before you move on to more quad-dominant exercises. Start slow, and work up to the recommended sets and reps. With dedication, not only will you eventually be able to run faster, jump higher, and squat and deadlift a heavier weight, you also reduce your chances of sustaining a knee injury.

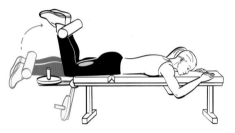

Ⓐ HAMSTRING CURL MACHINE Lying leg curls work the hamstrings with particular emphasis on the biceps femoris. Perform three sets of 15 reps.

HOW Set a hamstring curl machine to a challenging, but doable, weight. Lie down on your stomach on the bench, and hook your ankles in place behind the padded leg rests. Draw your ankles toward your buttocks until your legs form a 90-degree angle. Slowly return to the starting position.

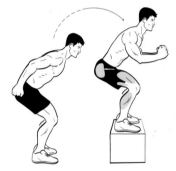

Ⓒ BOX JUMP AND SQUAT Depending on your skill, choose a box between 15 to 30 inches (38–76 cm) high. Perform one set of 10 reps.

HOW Start in the squat position about a foot from the edge of the box. Power off both legs, landing in the middle of the box in a half-squat position. Return to the starting position.

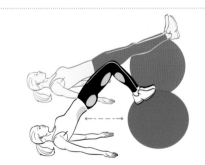

Ⓑ STABILITY BALL HAMSTRING CURL This hamstring curl utilizes a ball to help raise your legs and hips off the floor. It precisely targets your hamstrings and also engages your hip and back muscles. Perform one set of 20 reps.

HOW Lie with your calves on the ball, arms by your sides, palms up. Raise your hips until your body forms a straight line from shoulders to heels. Bend your knees to roll the ball toward you until your feet are flat. Straighten your legs to roll the ball back, and then lower your body to the floor.

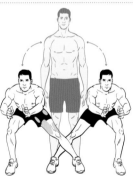

Ⓓ LATERAL SQUAT Adding lateral movement to a squat improves rotational strength and flexibility in your hips and knees, while also refining your balance and coordination. Perform one set of 20 reps on each side.

HOW Start by taking a wide stance. Squat down to the right, keeping your weight on your right heel. Your left leg should remain straight. Sit as low as comfortable for one second, and then power up and alternate legs.

121 GET KEEN ON KETTLEBELLS

The kettlebell, a cast iron ball with a handle, is a versatile training tool for men and women of all fitness levels. Its range of movements includes the carry, the rack, the swing, and the press, performed with one or two bells. This simple weight is known for the efficiency of its workouts, which offer both strength and cardio benefits. It also improves balance, coordination, flexibility, burns fat, builds core strength, and increases muscle tone. Slow presses yield fast gains, and swings generate greater endurance. It's no wonder some trainers consider it a miracle fitness aid, akin to a complete portable gym. The kettlebell's recent surge in popularity does not make it a gimmick or fad at all. These weights, which originated in Russia as the crop-weighing *girya*, have been around since the early 1700s. The design has not changed much over time—picture a cannon ball with a thick, rounded handle. Because its weight is

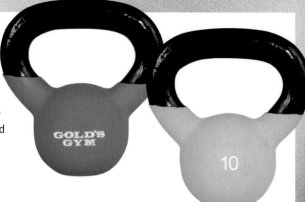

not evenly distributed like a dumbbell, a kettlebell requires users to stabilize their body and maintain balance during exercises, giving the core a good workout. Its small size means that it can travel with you to hotel rooms or to the park or beach. Bells range in weight from 9 pounds (4 kg) to more than 100 (45 kg); most women beginners start out with a bell of 18 pounds (8 kg) and men 35 pounds (15.8 kg). Gold's Gym offers a wide array of kettlebells.

122 DETONATE THE DEADLIFT

What is a deadlift? Well, if you've ever lifted a heavy box from the floor or picked up a small child, you've already performed this standard resistance-training move.

It may seem like a simple "I pick things up, and I put things down" bodybuilder exercise, but the deadlift works in far from simple ways. There are also many different versions of this move to add plenty of variety to your workout routine and amp up its already impressive list of benefits, like those below.

WORKS MULTIPLE MUSCLES Deadlifts work your lower body—your hamstrings, quads, glutes, and calves—and your upper body—your arms, core, back, trapezius, and shoulders.

BURNS CALORIES You burn a lot of calories doing deadlifts because they work so many muscles.

IMPROVES YOUR POSTURE By strengthening your core and back muscles, deadlifts can improve your posture and can help you prevent lower-back pain and injury.

RAISES YOUR HEART RATE Performing deadlifts adds a cardio component to a strength workout, raising your heart rate and improving your ability to transport and efficiently use oxygen during exercise.

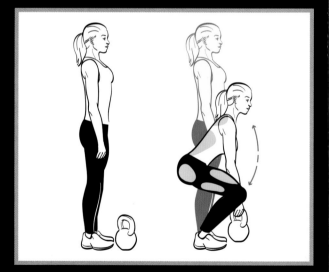

A KETTLEBELL DEADLIFT The kettlebell deadlift is a great beginner's exercise for strengthening the hamstrings, lower back, and glutes.

HOW Stand with a kettlebell at your feet. Squat, and grab the kettlebell with both hands. Rise, and then return to the squat, lightly touching the kettlebell to the floor. After one set, hold the squat position for 30 seconds, keeping the kettlebell just slightly above the floor.

WHY USE KETTLEBELLS?

Most advanced gym trainees use free weights for much of their workout routine. Many beginners can be put off by the various movements possible, and the proper technique required, so they make very little use of these valuable tools. Kettlebells' unorthodox design may seem intimidating, but you can add muscle, burn fat, increase mobility, improve endurance, and boost metabolism, all in the same workout. So, why not give them a try? Be sure to follow the tips in this book or ask a personal trainer to teach you how to get the most from kettlebells and free weight training.

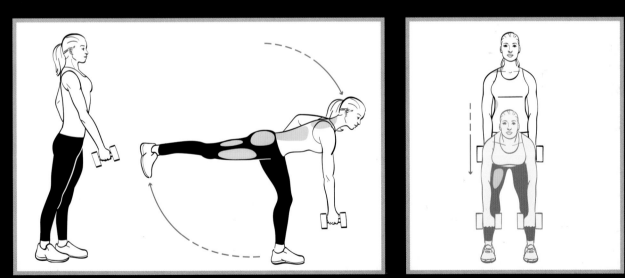

Ⓑ SINGLE-LEG ROMANIAN DEADLIFT Single-leg versions of the deadlift are especially great for dancers—or anyone who wants to increase their hip and core strength.

HOW Stand holding a dumbbell in your right hand. Slightly bend your left knee as you lean forward, and raise your right leg behind you in a straight line. Return to the starting position, and then switch, holding the dumbbell in your left hand and bending your right leg.

Ⓒ STRAIGHT-LEG DEADLIFT This deadlift helps you to learn how to stabilize the spine and pelvis under load while properly hinging at the hips—a skill needed for many exercises.

HOW Stand tall with your feet shoulder-width apart. With an overhand grip, grasp a dumbbell in each hand letting them hang in front of your thighs. Hinge forward at the hips to lower them down, keeping your back straight and your chest out. Slowly return to the starting position.

123 KNOW YOUR...
GLUTES

Your glutes are a group of three muscles: the gluteus maximus, medius, and minimus. Located at the back side of each hip or buttock, these hard-working muscles have many functions, including the extension, abduction, external rotation, and internal rotation of the hip joint. Connected to the coccyx, or tailbone, as well as other surrounding bones, the gluteus maximus is the largest muscle in the human body, contributing most of the mass of your buttocks. As well as being the largest, it is also one of the most powerful muscles, keeping your trunk in an erect posture and acting as a sort of antigravity muscle that aids you in walking up stairs. It is also responsible for movement of the hip and thigh, and it supports your extended knee through the iliotibial band (see #224). Situated on the outer surface of the pelvis and partially covered by the gluteus maximus is the smaller gluteus medius muscle. It works to provide rotation of the thigh outward from the center of the body, which enables you to walk with a steady gait. The gluteus minimus is a deep muscle located anterior to the gluteus medius. This broad, triangle-shaped muscle plays a secondary role in extending the hip.

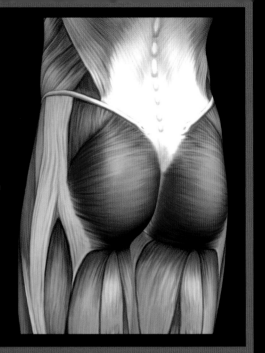

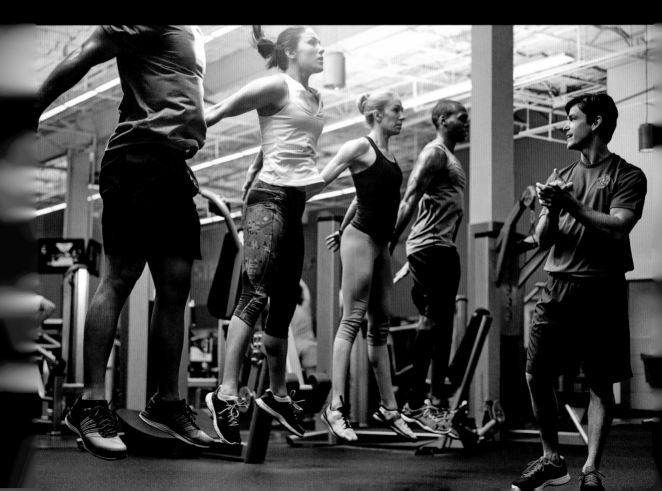

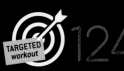

124 WORK YOUR BUTT OFF

The hours-long pressure put on your buttocks each day—whether sitting at the office, in the car, or in front of the TV—can cause the glutes to atrophy and sag. Yet your glutes are the biggest muscle in your body for a reason—they provide the stabilization and power required to perform any upright motion, acting as the powerhouse of your lower body.

To get your glutes in top shape, follow this targeted workout, which combines machine-weight, free-weight, and body-weight exercises with plyometrics—or jump training—for added power. For the weight exercises, find a weight that you are comfortable with, and then go one step further. For the best results, do this routine three times per week. Start with 10 minutes of slow cardio, followed by 5 minutes of moderate stretching. First perform three sets of 15 reps on the hamstring curl machine (see #120A), and then continue with the exercises below.

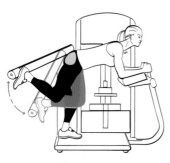

Ⓐ MACHINE GLUTE ISOLATOR This machine will help you isolate your glutes for strengthening and toning. Perform three sets of 15 reps on each leg.

HOW Stand at a glute isolator, and rest your chest on the pad in front of you. Place one foot against the pedal behind you. Push back with your leg, and then slowly return to the starting position. After completing one set, switch sides.

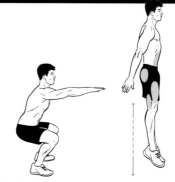

Ⓒ JUMP SQUATS This high-energy plyometric exercise strengthens your glutes and revs your metabolism. Perform three sets of 10 reps.

HOW Start in a squat position with your feet shoulder-width apart and your arms extended parallel to the floor. Swinging your arms down and back, jump as high as you can, and come down with your knees bent. Jump again with no rest.

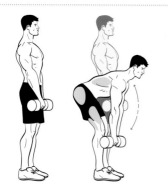

Ⓑ STANDING DEADLIFT Deadlifts will target your entire lower body. Perform three sets of 10 reps.

HOW Stand with a dumbbell at your feet. Squat, and grab it with both hands. Rise, and then return to the squat, and touch the dumbbell to the floor. Complete one set, and hold the squat for 30 seconds.

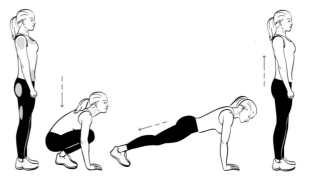

Ⓓ SQUAT THRUST As it strengthens your glutes, this classic gym exercise incorporates aerobic training and resistance training into one sequence to really give your cardiovascular system, legs, and upper body a thorough workout. It also helps you to improve your coordination. Perform three sets of 15 reps.

HOW Begin in a standing position with feet apart. Squat, and place your palms on the floor in front of you. Kick your feet back as if you were going to do a push-up. Quickly return to the squat position, and then stand up.

125 LEARN TO SQUAT

To really target your lower body muscles, including your quads, hamstrings, glutes, and core, the squat is a can't-miss compound exercise. It not only improves muscular strength and power, it also works almost every joint in your body while efficiently burning calories.

The basic squat is a great move no matter what your level of fitness, and there are many variations that increase its difficulty or add emphasis on particular muscles. You can also perform them anywhere with no special equipment. The following squats use your own body weight for resistance, but you can add other weights, like barbells, kettlebells, or dumbbells, to lower your center of gravity and help you maintain balance.

Executing this exercise with proper form is essential, so keep in mind the following tips, which will help you get the maximum benefits from your squat reps.

HEAD UP Face forward with your head in a "neutral" position, meaning it should balance directly over your spine and not lean forward or be cocked to one side.

SHOULDERS BACK Keep your chest up and shoulders back.

ARMS BALANCED Extend your arms in front, parallel to the floor or hands entwined. You can also place your hands on your hips or bring them behind your head. The key is to keep balanced.

ABS TIGHT Engage your abs throughout the exercise.

KNEES IN LINE Make sure your knees are in line with your feet, and they should not come past your toes.

HEELS DOWN Keep your weight firmly on your heels—you should be able to lift your toes and wiggle them.

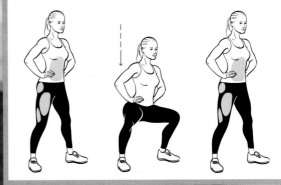

Ⓐ BASIC SQUAT

WHY The squat is a great lower-body exercise that give you fast gains in size and strength.

HOW Stand with your feet hip-width apart. Slowly lower your bottom as you would to sit in a chair. While keeping your back straight and chin up. Lower as far as you can while keeping your knees parallel with your ankles, then slowly stand back up.

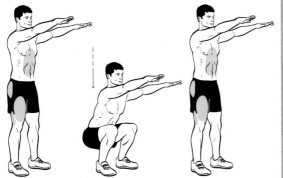

Ⓑ SUMO SQUAT

WHY The sumo squat adds emphasis on the inner-thigh adductors.

HOW Stand with your feet wide, toes facing outward. Bend your knees and hips to slowly squat. Once you feel the stretch in the glutes and hamstrings, push up through your heels, and squeeze your glutes at the top.

© WALL SQUAT

WHY Wall squats have the same benefits as basic ones; practicing these will help perfect your form.

HOW Stand with your back against a wall, placing your feet about two feet in front of you and hip-width apart. Bend your knees, and slide your back down against the wall until your knees are at 90-degree angles. Hold for 30 to 60 seconds.

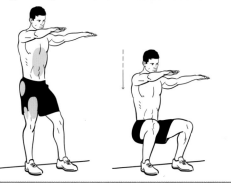

© BULGARIAN SPLIT SQUAT

WHY Split squats will help you develop balance and hip flexibility as they strengthen your lower body.

HOW Stand tall, and place one foot on a bench or similar sturdy platform. Keep your weight centered on your front foot and bend your legs to lunge. Bring your rear knee close to the floor, then drive up through your front heel to return to starting position.

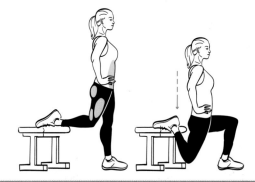

126 KNOW YOUR...
CALF MUSCLES

Located on your lower legs are several muscles that move your ankles, feet, and toes. Giving your calves their characteristic shape is the gastrocnemius, the larger calf muscle. The gastrocnemius has two heads, which together create a diamond shape. Lying beneath the gastrocnemius is the soleus, a smaller, flat muscle. These muscles join to form the strong calcaneal tendon—also known as the Achilles tendon—and attach to the calcaneus bone in your heel. The gastrocnemius and soleus contract to flex the toes and also move your foot or toes to flex downward toward the sole, such as when you stand on tiptoes. On the front of your calves, the shin muscles, such as the tibialis anterior and extensor digitorum longus, are what bend the foot upward and extend the toes. All of your calf muscles also work to stabilize your ankle joint and feet and help you to maintain your balance.

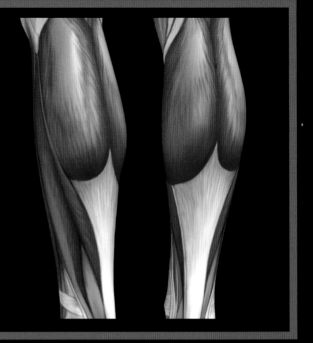

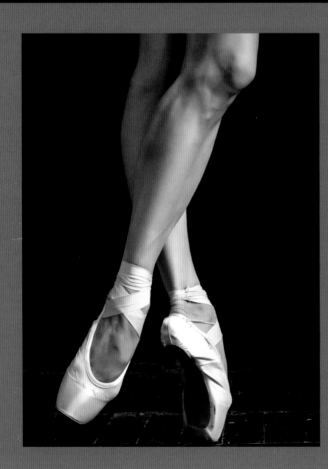

127 STAND ON TIPPY-TOES

Genetics ultimately determines just how much you can build the size of your calves, whether you are trying for the bulging appearance of a bodybuilder or the long, sleek look of a dancer. Whatever your goal, training your calf muscles will enhance your performance in many athletic pursuits.

HIKING, WALKING, AND RUNNING These pursuits are all excellent calf-strengthening exercises. Uphill walking or running is particularly beneficial—your calf muscles will really get a workout the steeper you climb.

RUNNING SPORTS Just look at the calves of a soccer player, and you'll be convinced that this kind of sport demands lower-leg strength. When you participate in running sports like soccer, tennis, lacrosse, field hockey, and basketball, you run, jump, and push off your calf muscles to accelerate or change direction quickly—and these kinds of moves will tone your calves.

DANCING Whether at a step or salsa class or pursuing ballet, dancing works calf muscles in ways few activities do, demanding that you step up and down or bend your knees and push off as you move from high to low positions.

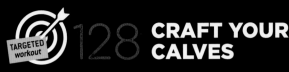

128 CRAFT YOUR CALVES

To get a complete leg workout, incorporate calf resistance-training exercises into your fitness routine. Be warned, though: your calf muscles can be hard to work, mostly because the Achilles tendon comes into play when you lower or lift your heel. It acts similar to rubber band, transferring energy during the heel-lowering and heel-lifting phases of calf exercises, which means your muscles do less work. To counteract this effect, pause for about five seconds at the bottom of each rep and three seconds at the top.

Perform this routine about once a week. Gym newbies should perform just one set of each exercise. As your strength increases, work up to two and then three sets, resting for about two minutes between sets.

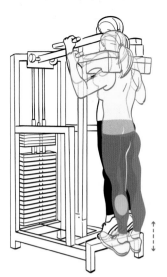

ⓑ STANDING CALF RAISE MACHINE A standing calf raise, which you do with straight legs, will target the gastrocs more than the soleus muscles. Perform one to three sets of 12 reps on each leg.

HOW Stand on the footplate of a calf raise machine with your shoulders squared. Slowly rise up onto your toes, pause, and then lower your heels until fully extended. To work your calves one at a time, simply cross one leg over the other.

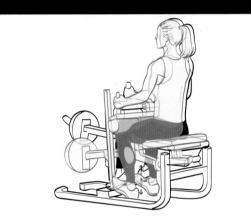

ⓐ SEATED CALF RAISE MACHINE A seated calf raise, by bending the knee, will relax your gastrocnemius muscles, placing more emphasis on your soleus muscles. Perform one to three sets of 12 reps.

HOW Sit at calf raise machine with your thighs under the leg pad and the balls of your feet on the foot rest, allowing your heels to hang off the edge. Slowly raise your heels up as high as you can go, pause, and then lower them.

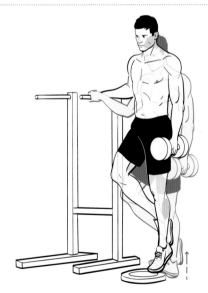

ⓒ ONE-LEG DUMBBELL CALF RAISE Standing calf raises place tension on both the lateral and medial heads of the gastroc muscle—resulting in thickness and definition. Perform one to three sets of 12 reps.

HOW Stand on one leg with your foot on a block, holding a dumbbell in the same-side hand, the other gripping a support for balance. Raise yourself up on to the ball of your foot, pause, and then lower your heel. Repeat on other leg.

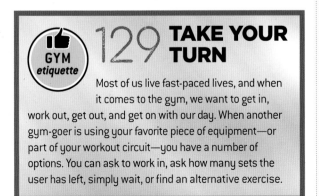

GYM etiquette

129 TAKE YOUR TURN

Most of us live fast-paced lives, and when it comes to the gym, we want to get in, work out, get out, and get on with our day. When another gym-goer is using your favorite piece of equipment—or part of your workout circuit—you have a number of options. You can ask to work in, ask how many sets the user has left, simply wait, or find an alternative exercise.

130 SNAP BACK INTO SHAPE

You don't have to rely on iron to add resistance to a workout. Pick up a set of elastic resistance bands to provide muscle-building tension for just about any resistance-training exercise, whether a press, row, extension, curl, fly, or squat.

Bands offer you safe, effective workouts—physical therapists often recommend them for rehabilitation. And they are portable, so you can take them anywhere.

Try these moves to add a new twist to a full-body workout.

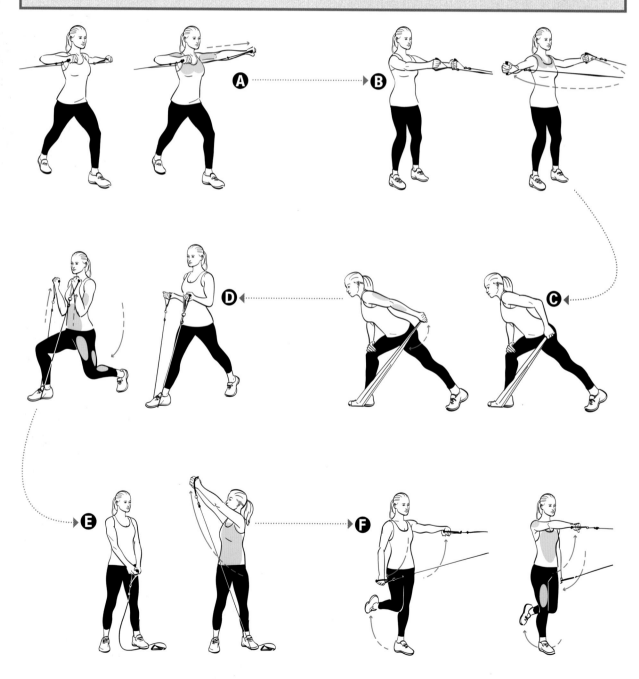

Ⓐ RESISTANCE BAND CHEST PRESS Run the band around a stable object. Stand facing away from the object, holding both ends of the resistance band in front of your chest. Extend one arm straight in front of you to full lockout position, keeping the other arm steady. With control, bring your arm back to the starting position.

Ⓑ RESISTANCE BAND REVERSE FLY Run the band around a stable object. Stand upright, with your feet planted shoulder-width apart and your knees soft. Grasp both of the handles of the band, and extend your arms in front of you to near shoulder height, holding the band taut. With control, bring both arms out to the sides. Return to the starting position.

Ⓒ RESISTANCE BAND TRICEPS KICKBACK Stand in a lunge position, with your front leg bent and your back heel off the floor. Place one end of the band beneath your front foot, and grasp the other end in your opposite hand. Lean forward, keeping your back flat so that your torso and back leg form a line. Bend your elbow to position the band next to your hips. While keeping your upper arm in place, straighten your arm behind you to full lockout. Lower, and repeat.

Ⓓ RESISTANCE BAND SPLIT SQUAT WITH CURL Position the band beneath one foot. Grasp both handles. Step back so that one leg is several feet behind the other, your front foot anchoring the band and your back heel off the floor. Bend your elbows, and hold the band taut just in front of your torso. Drop your back knee, bending both legs until your front thigh is parallel to the floor. At the same time, curl the band upward with palms facing your shoulders. With control, straighten your legs as you rise, and return your arms to the starting position.

Ⓔ RESISTANCE BAND WOOD CHOP Stand with your feet a little wider than hip-distance apart, the band anchored beneath one foot. Hold one handle with both hands, positioning it in front of your body slightly closer to the anchoring foot. Smoothly rotate your core, and raise your arms away from the anchoring foot. In a controlled "chopping" motion, return to the starting position.

Ⓕ RESISTANCE BAND ONE-LEGGED DOWNWARD PRESS Run the band around a stable object and face the anchoring object. Grasp the handles, and extend your arms straight at shoulder height, with your hands a few inches apart. Bend one knee at a right angle lifting the foot behind you. Keeping one arm stable, lower the other arm to your side. Return your arm to the starting position.

EXERCISE	TARGETS	REPS/SETS
RESISTANCE BAND CHEST PRESS	Strengthens and tones pectorals, chest, shoulders, and triceps; stabilizes core	Three sets of 15 reps per arm
RESISTANCE BAND STANDING FLY	Strengthens and tones shoulders and upper back	Three sets of 15 reps
RESISTANCE BAND TRICEPS KICKBACK	Strengthens and tones triceps	Three sets of 15 reps per arm
RESISTANCE BAND SPLIT SQUAT WITH CURL	Strengthens and tones glutes, thighs, and biceps	Three sets of 10 reps
RESISTANCE BAND WOOD CHOP	Tones abs and obliques; improves core strength and support	Three sets of 20 reps per side
RESISTANCE BAND ONE-LEGGED DOWNWARD PRESS	Strengthens and tones abs, deltoids, and triceps	Three sets of 15 reps per arm

HOW RESISTANCE BANDS WORK Elastic resistance bands act in a similar way to free weights, but unlike weights, which rely on gravity to determine the resistance, bands rely on the consistent tension supplied by your muscles. They are made from elastic rubber and usually come in two forms: wide and flat or tubular with handles. You can use either type to achieve the same results, and both come in several levels of tension, from very stretchy to very taut, allowing you to adjust the intensity of your workouts. You can further adjust the intensity by giving the band more or less slack.

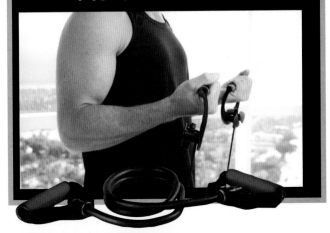

131 PLAN YOUR RESISTANCE PROGRAM

Now that you're familiar with the parts, cogs, and goings-on inside the gym, it's time to put your resistance-training program together and get results. Before constructing a resistance training program, there is one basic question you need to ask yourself: What are my goals?

CONDITIONING AND TONING If you're looking for general conditioning and overall body toning, the full-body program might be for you. This will include working each of the major muscles of the body to some capacity and in some instances working them together within the same workout. An example is a push-up performed on dumbbells combined with an alternate row at the top of the movement, which will work all the major muscles of the torso. Those workouts are based more on conditioning and stamina.

MUSCLE DEVELOPMENT If you're looking for more muscular development, quality of muscle separation, and greater control over working muscles, perhaps a workout split based on traditional bodybuilding is ideal for you. In workout splits, during a session you work one or two muscles to temporary muscle failure, while primarily recruiting major muscles with little ancillary help from nearby muscles. These workouts are based more on prioritization and individuality.

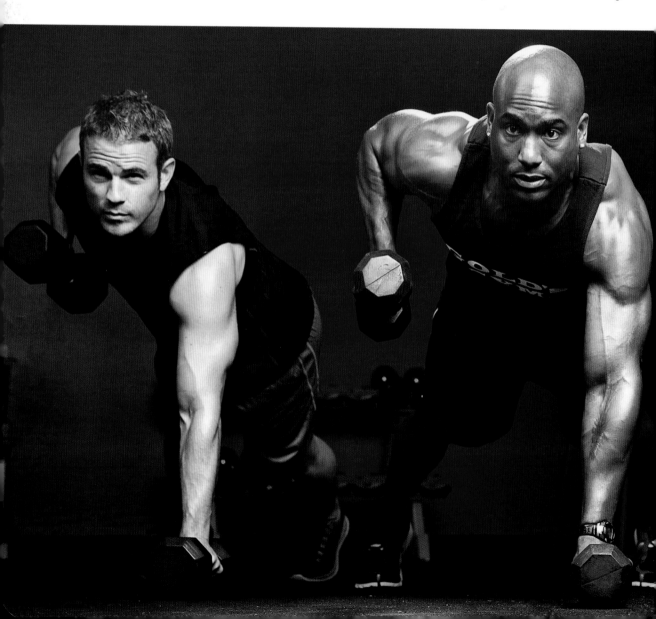

132 STRATEGIZE FOR SUCCESS

Whatever your goal, there are a few strategies to keep in mind that will help you to make the most of your workout plan.

PUT YOUR WEAKER SELF FIRST Work your weaker muscle groups earlier in the week when your strength and reserves are high. If your upper body is weaker than your lower body, for example, work your pecs or shoulders on Mondays, and save the legs and glutes for Friday.

STAY FOCUSED WHILE YOU WORK For each and every set and rep, pay attention to how your muscles are working. Five haphazard sets will always be inferior to two driven and focused sets. Give your all to your working sets, keeping tension on the proper muscles. Up your weights when you are able, and you will improve over time.

TRACK YOUR TRAINING PROGRESS Write in a journal or use an app, but keep track of your numbers. Increased lifts will let you know how well you are developing your muscles. Record workouts, reps, and even changes to your diet in order to keep the path to progression smooth.

KEEP YOUR FITNESS PLAN FUN Keep it progressing, keep it safe, but also keep it fun. Don't hesitate to change up a stale workout. Maybe substitute hack squats for basic squats or dumbbell rows for barbell rows. Keep it interesting.

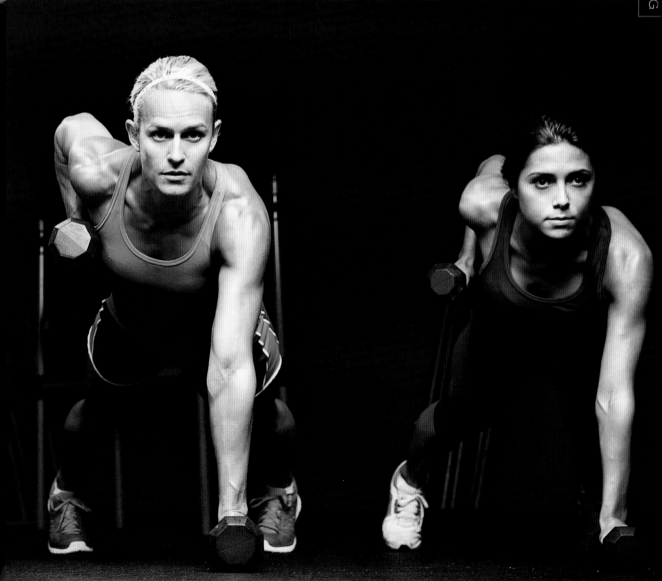

133 CUSTOMIZE YOUR WORKOUTS

It's easy to create a program tailored to your personal goals and schedule. The examples below show a full-body three-day-a-week workout for overall conditioning and a four-day-a-week split plan that has you working different muscles groups each workout day. You can use the sample exercises listed or use the charts at right, which also show recommended sets and reps, along with where to find the specific exercises in this book (the "TIP #" column at right will guide you to which of the numbered exercises from earlier in the chapter you should be studying).

FULL BODY WORKOUT

Perform the full workout three times a week, on alternating days.

- Push-up
- One-arm dumbbell row
- Stability ball wall squat with biceps curl
- Stability ball Superman
- Basic crunch
- Resistance band upright row
- Pull-up
- Reverse fly
- Hack squat
- Straight-legged deadlift
- Hamstring curl machine
- Barbell walking lunge
- EZ bar preacher curl
- Standing triceps push-downs
- Stability ball extension

BODY SPLIT WORKOUT

Work out each muscle group once a week.

MONDAY: LEGS/ABS

- Basic squat
- Leg press
- Stationary lunge
- Leg extensions
- Hamstring curl machine
- Straight-legged deadlift
- Standing calf raise machine
- Plank
- Stability ball crunch

TUESDAY: CHEST/ SHOULDERS

- Incline bench press
- Barbell bench press
- Dumbbell fly
- Pec deck
- Push-up
- Seated military press
- Dumbbell lateral raise
- Reverse fly
- Upright barbell row

THURSDAY: BACK/ABS

- Pull-up
- Lat pull-down machine
- Bent-over barbell row
- Machine row
- Stability ball extension
- Reverse crunch
- Penguin crunch

FRIDAY: BICEPS/TRICEPS

- Biceps curl
- Hammer curl
- Skull crusher
- Overhead triceps extension

UPPER BODY			
TARGET	EXERCISE	SETS/REPS	TIP #
CHEST	Barbell bench press	3/8-10	074C
	Bosu ball push-up	2/12-15	078B
	Cable crossover	2/12-15	077B
	Decline push-up	2/12-15	078D
	Diamond push-up	2/12-15	078C
	Dumbbell chest press with hold	2/8-10	077C
	Dumbbell fly	2/12-15	077A
	Incline bench press	3/8-10	077D
	Push-up	2/12-15	078A
	Resistance band chest press	3/10-15	130A
BACK	Bent-over barbell row	3/8-10	087A
	Bent-over two-arm long barbell row	3/8-10	087B
	Bird dog	2/12-15	090A
	Lat pull-down machine	3/8-10	081A
	Lower-back extension	2/12-15	081D
	Machine row	3/8-10	081C
	One-arm dumbbell row	3/8-10	081B
	Pull-up	3/8-10	085
	Resistance band upright row	2/12-15	087D
	Stability ball Superman	2/12-15	090C
	Swimming Superman	2/12-15	090B
	Upright barbell row	2/12-15	087C
SHOULDERS	Dumbbell front raise	2/8-12	093A
	Dumbbell lateral raise	2/8-12	093C
	Reverse fly	2/8-12	093B
	Seated military press	3/8-10	093D
BICEPS	Biceps curl	3/8-10	096A
	Concentration curl	2/12-15	096B
	EZ bar preacher curl	2/8-10	096C
	Hammer curl	2/8-10	096D
	Seated alternating dumbbell curls	2/8-10	103A
	Twenty-ones	2 sets	103C
TRICEPS	Barbell skull crusher	3/8-10	100C
	Bench dip	3/12-15	102
	Cable rope overhead extension	3/12-15	100D
	One-arm kickback	3/10-15	100B
	Overhead triceps extension	2/12-15	100A
	Resistance band triceps kickback	3/10-15	130C
	Standing triceps push-down	4/12-25	103B

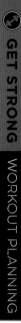

LOWER BODY			
TARGET	**EXERCISE**	**SETS/ REPS**	**TIP #**
ABDOMINALS	The ab wheel	2/12–15	109F
	Cable wood chop	3/20	107C
	Basic crunch	3/25	108A
	Bicycle crunch	3/20	108C
	Broom twist	3/20	107B
	Captain's chair knee raise	3/20	106
	Double crunch	3/15	108D
	Side trunk raise	2/12–15	109E
	Penguin crunch	3/15	107D
	Resistance band wood chop	3/20	130E
	Reverse crunch	3/20	108B
	Seated Russian twist	3/20	107A
	Stability ball crunch	2/20	109A
QUADRICEPS	Barbell walking lunge	3/12–15	115B
	Hack squat	3/12–15	115D
	Leg extensions	2/12–15	115C
	Leg press	3/12–15	115A
	Narrow–stance squat	3/12–15	111B
	Stationary lunge	2/12–15	111A
	Warrior II pose	3/15– 30 sec.	111C
INNER/OUTER THIGHS	Clamshell	2/12–15	117A
	Fire hydrant	2/12–15	117B
	Lateral bounding	2/12–15	117C
HAMSTRINGS	Box jump and squat	2/12–15	120C
	Hamstring curl machine	3/12–15	120A
	Lateral squat	2/12–15	120D
	Stability ball hamstring curl	2/12–15	120B
GLUTES/LEGS	Barbell squat	3/12–15	074A
	Basic squat	3/12–15	125A
	Bulgarian split squat	3/12–15	125D
	Machine glute isolator	2/12–15	124A
	Sumo squat	3/12–15	125B
	Wall squat	3/12–15	125C
CALVES	One–leg dumbbell calf raise	3/12–15	128C
	Seated calf raise machine	2/12–15	128A
	Standing calf raise machine	3/12–15	128B

COMBINATIONS			
TARGET	**EXERCISE**	**SETS/ REPS**	**TIP #**
ABDOMINALS/ SHOULDERS/ ARMS	Resistance band one-legged downward press	3/10–15	130F
BACK/ SHOULDERS	Resistance band standing fly	2/8–12	130C
CORE/BACK	Stability ball extension	2/12–15	109B
CORE/ARMS/ LOWER BODY	Stability ball wall squat with curl	2/12–15	109D
CORE/CHEST/ SHOULDERS/ BACK	Elbow plank	1–3/30– 60 sec.	109C
LOWER BODY/ABS	Jump squats	2/12–15	124C
LOWER BODY/ UPPER BODY	Barbell deadlift	3/8–10	074B
	High pull	2/12–15	074D
	Kettlebell deadlift	3/8–10	122A
	Resistance band split squat with curl	3/10–15	130D
	Single-leg Romanian deadlift	2/8–10	122B
	Squat thrust	2/12–15	124D
	Standing deadlift	3/8–10	124B
	Straight-leg deadlift	2/12–15	122C

134 GET A THIRTY-MINUTE WORKOUT

By deciding to get in shape and joining a gym, you've taken the most important step toward leading a healthy lifestyle. Now you need the ultimate roadmap to get you started. Robert Reames, Gold's Gym Fitness Institute member and author of the book *Make Over Your Metabolism,* offers a guide for beginning your new fitness routine, putting together simple, easy options that you can mix and match to get you going and get you results.

Your goal is to make the best use of your time, obtaining the maximum bang for your buck whenever you go to the gym. This program offers you a three-phase 30-minute total-body workout that will also familiarize you with your gym's facilities and the possibilities available.

As you build momentum, schedule a session or two with a personal trainer to further consult with you on a specific program(s) that meets your individual abilities and goals so that you can continue to open up opportunities for yourself. Keep in mind that this is just the start—your fitness program is a process that will continue to develop and evolve in the coming weeks, months, and years of your life.

Here's the main breakdown of the three phases. Follow the chart opposite for specific recommendations. When you have completed the workout from warm-up to cardio, take a minute or two to walk around the gym, and give yourself kudos for a job well done!

PHASE 1: WARM-UP (4 TO 5 MINUTES) The purpose of the warm-up is simply to elevate your body temperature, increase circulation, and to get your body ready to move.

PHASE 2: STRENGTH (12 TO 15 MINUTES) This part consists of resistance training to develop lean muscle—the fat-burning machinery that works for you 24/7. Pick out three machines: one pushing unit, one pulling unit, and one leg press unit. Strength train on alternate days, allowing 36 to 48 hours of rest and recovery for the major muscle group worked.

PHASE 3: CARDIO (8 TO 10 MINUTES) Your third part is where you begin to increase stamina, endurance, and overall cardiovascular capacity.

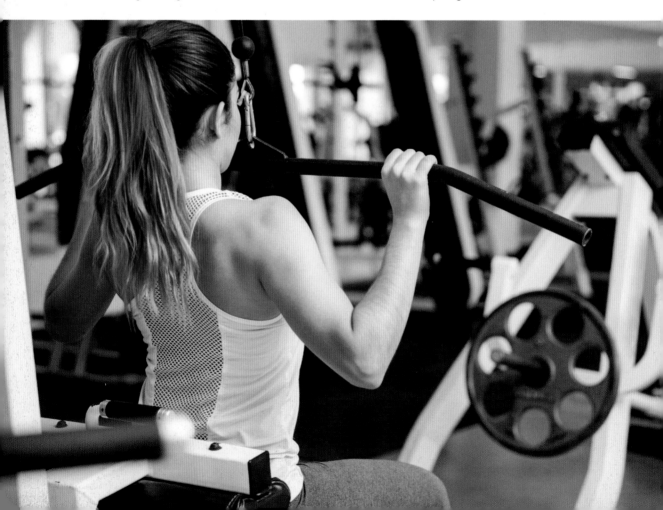

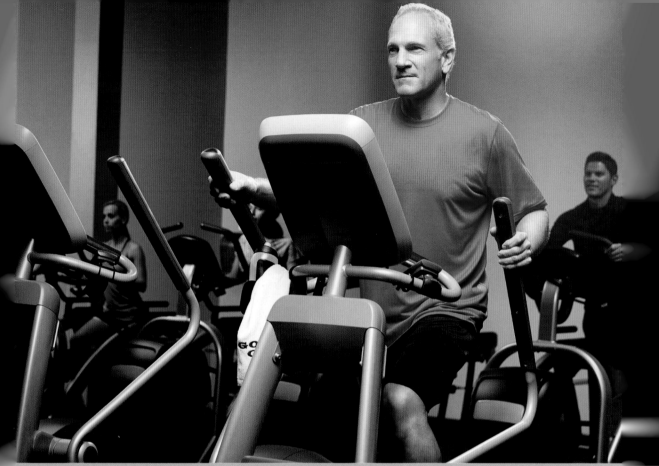

PHASE	EXERCISE	TIME/SETS/REPS	NOTES
WARM-UP	Treadmill, elliptical, bike, rowing machine, or other cardio option	4 to 5 minutes	Start at a moderate intensity, gradually increasing as you go.
STRENGTH: UPPER BODY (PUSH)	Chest press	1 to 2 sets 10 reps each 45–60 second rest between sets	Pushing exercises will work your chest, shoulders, and triceps. See exercises #074C, #077C, #77D, and #130A for options and for full descriptions of how to do them safely and effectively.
STRENGTH: UPPER BODY (PULL)	Lat pull-downs or rows	1 to 2 sets 10 reps each 45–60 second rest between sets	These exercises will work the muscles of your back, biceps, and all elbow flexors. See exercises #081A–C and $087A–D for options and for full descriptions of how to do them safely and effectively.
STRENGTH: LOWER BODY	Leg press	1 to 3 sets 10 reps each 45–60 second rest between sets	This exercise will give you a comprehensive lower-body workout See exercise #115A for full description of how to do it safely and effectively.
CARDIO	Treadmill, elliptical, bike, rowing machine, or other cardio option	8 to 10 minutes	Take one or two minutes to escalate your intensity. Use the next six to seven minutes to work at your peak level, then take one to three minutes to cool back down to where your heart rate is back to a normal resting level.

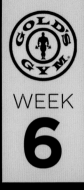

WEEK

6

Evaluate Your Progress

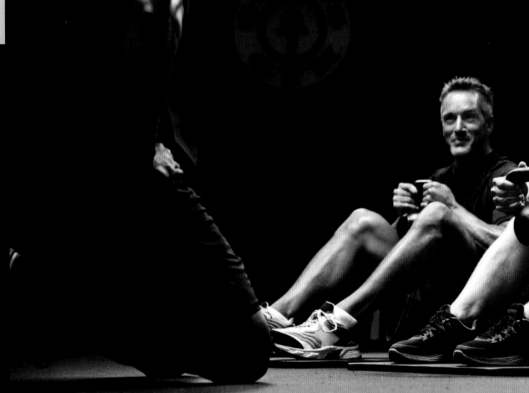

DO A MID-CHALLENGE CHECK-IN You've now been participating in the Challenge for six weeks, and it's time to assess just how far you've come. It's time to step back on the scale and take out the tape measure to compare these numbers with those of week one, or take out a camera for a pictorial progress report. It is also time to consult your trainer about any concerns you might have. Is there lingering soreness in a joint or is some portion of your anatomy stubbornly resisting improvement? Is there

unfamiliar equipment you want to explore, but need a hands-on demonstration first? Your trainer is the go-to person to handle these issues, as well as rev you up for the next six weeks. Rest assured that, in spite of any minor setbacks, you are well on the way to accomplishing your 12-week goal.

TACKLE WEAK SPOTS Whether it's skinny calves, weak biceps, or unflattering triceps, everyone has some part of their body that resists conditioning. Trust

a trainer to come up with effective answers; he or she has experience dealing with stubborn areas and can guide you toward weight-loss plans, muscle-specific exercises, and conditioning equipment or machines that will help you win that particular battle.

AVOID ACHES; ADJUST ATTITUDE The temptation, especially during the Challenge, is always to do more, to try to "hurry up" the results. But be patient—impatience can leave you vulnerable to exercise-related

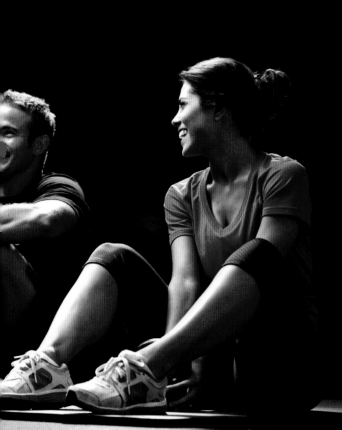

FOLLOW A WINNER'S JOURNEY
Adam Lucas
Male Winner, Ages 18-29

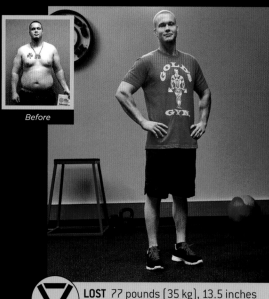

Before

LOST 77 pounds (35 kg), 13.5 inches (34.3 cm), and 32% body fat

Adam felt that the pressures of his everyday life meant that getting in shape was just not in the cards for him. As a full-time student and the father of 8-year old twins who'd been diagnosed with nonverbal autism he told himself that he didn't have time for fitness. "The day-in and day out life I was leading was plagued with unhealthy eating and a lack of self-worth," he says. "What I came to realize throughout this journey is that healthy eating habits coupled with exercise can improve my life in every aspect."

He found the first week of the Challenge grueling but he promised himself that he would stick with it so that he could be a better, more energetic father.

He and his wife began spending more time on outdoor activities with their sons, which was fun for the whole family. And after 12 weeks he was able to say with confidence that the Challenge had made him a better father, husband, and student.

injuries—sprains, strains, and even tears that will only slow your progress by keeping you out of the gym. Always consult a trainer if you are increasing your number of reps or weight load, or if you have muscle pain that lingers. Another stumbling block you might face is boredom—from performing the same safe circuits over and over. It's time to be bold and adventurous. If your training is becoming stale, ask your trainer to recommend some new equipment or unfamiliar classes to help give you a fresh new perspective.

WINNER'S WORDS

"I came to realize that healthy eating habits coupled with exercise can improve your life in every aspect."

~ Adam Lucas

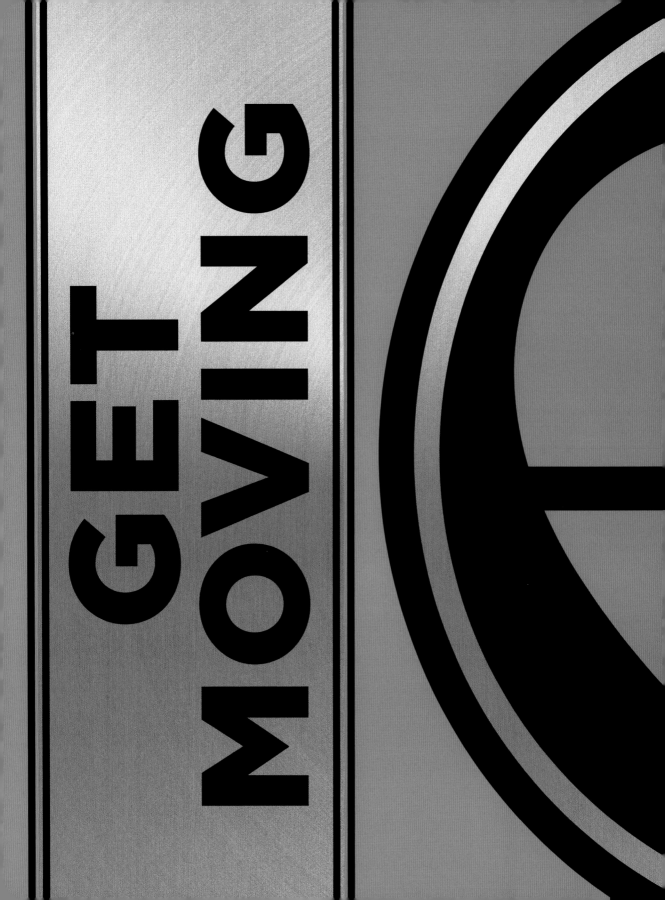

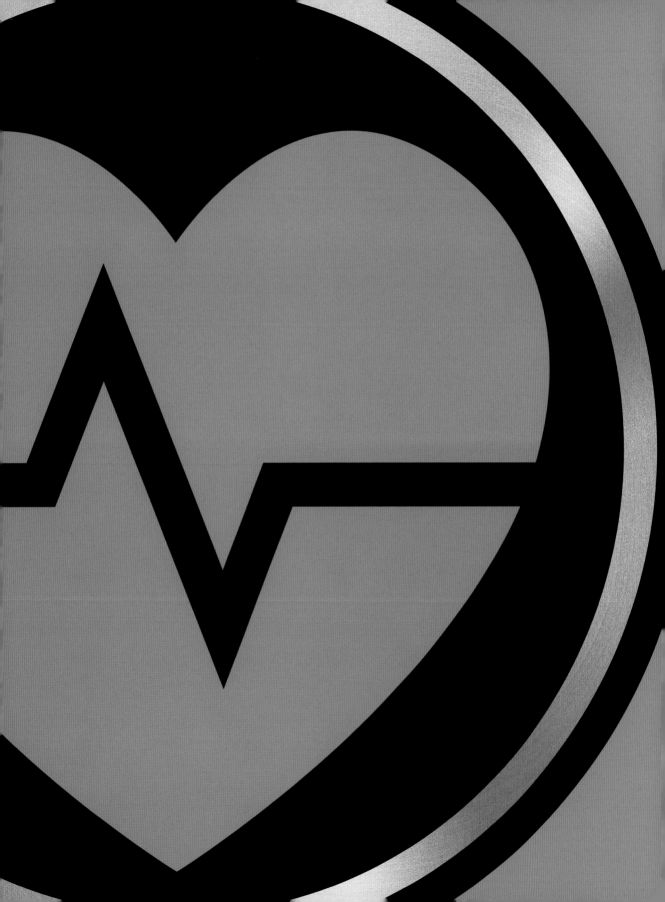

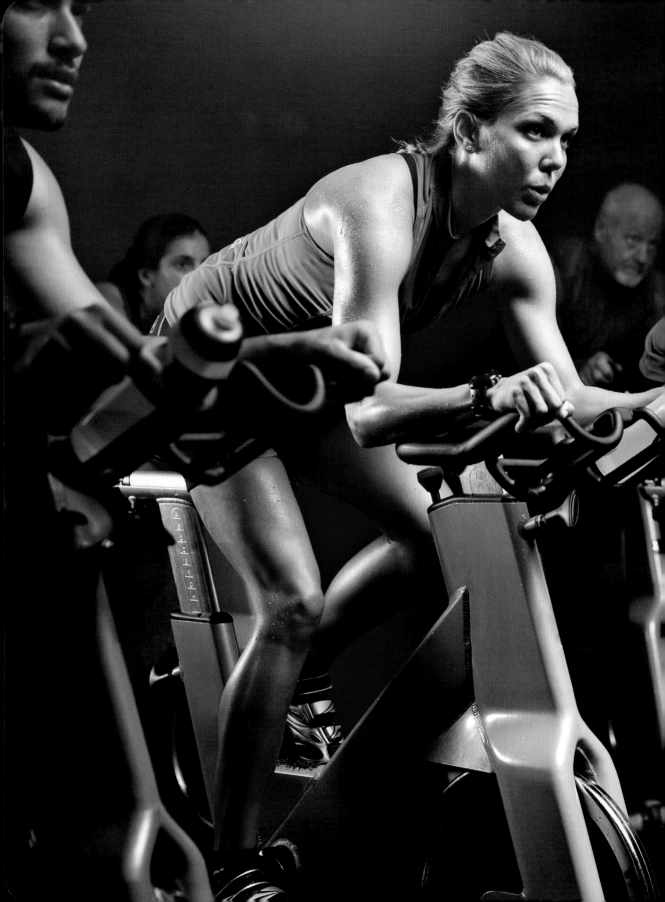

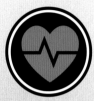 Cardiovascular training—any activity that raises your heart rate and increases the circulation of blood—can speed up metabolism, improve stamina, and strengthen both the heart and lungs. As such, cardio should be considered a necessary component of a balanced fitness regimen.

KNOW YOUR CARDIO

There are various forms of cardiovascular exercise—biking, walking, running, rowing, aerobics, dancing, swimming, martial arts, and boxing, among many others—and different methods for performing them that offer specific benefits. When creating a cardio routine, consult with a trainer to make sure your plan is providing the benefits you seek.

UNDERSTAND THE BENEFITS

Although some forms of cardio are slightly more effective for weight loss, all will efficiently burn calories. More moderate methods of cardio can also decrease workout recovery time—after an intense session with weights, a relaxed stint on the treadmill will help eliminate the by-products created by your body. Eventually you might want to investigate advanced forms of cardio, such as interval training, tempo training, and HIIT sprints.

The benefits of cardio workouts are manifold. In addition to weight loss and a stronger heart and lungs, you will increase your bone density, gain more energy, develop better sleep habits, lower your stress levels, find temporary relief of depression and anxiety, reduce risk of heart disease and some types of cancer, manage your diabetes by utilizing more glucose, and increase your confidence. You will also be setting a good example for others in your family and circle of friends by staying active.

BUILD YOUR PROGRAM

You'll hear a lot of opinions about how much cardio to include in your regimen; a commonly accepted guideline suggests 30 minutes of moderate cardio five days a week or 20 minutes of more intense exercise three days a week. To achieve weight loss, you might find that you need as much as 60 to 90 minutes per session.

135 GET YOUR HEART PUMPING

Your heart is a muscle, and it benefits from exercises that give it a workout and make it strong, just like any other muscle in your body. By asking the heart to pump at a faster rate on a regular basis, you can get it into shape and keep it healthy. If you find you are winded just from performing simple tasks like walking up the stairs or lifting a basket of laundry, you're probably neglecting to work your heart muscle—and that's something to remedy. Cardiovascular disease can affect anyone, and heart health is not to be taken lightly. The good news is that finding solutions is easy—anything aerobic that gets you moving and elevates your heart rate—like walking briskly, jumping rope, or riding a bike—will work. You might have to start slow, but before long you can tackle exhilarating cycling workouts or compete in charity runs.

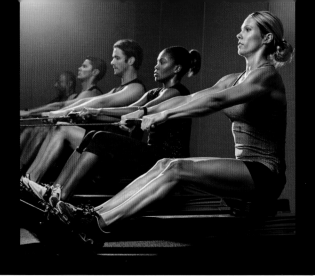

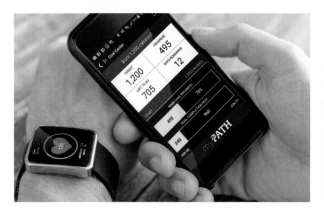

136 MONITOR YOUR HEART

During any taxing exercise, it's important to watch your heart rate and record your progress. A heart rate monitor (HRM) will track your pulse, and it will also help you figure out when you're at maximum exertion levels, will track calories burned, and will let you know if you hit fat-burning zones. It's a great tool regardless of your fitness level, and dependable models can be purchased for as little as $35.

CHEST STRAP HRMs These include a wireless sensor on a chest strap that detects your pulse electronically and then sends that data to a wrist receiver that displays your heart rate. Basic chest-strap HRMs will also time your workout and give you continuous, average, high, and low heart-rate data.

STRAPLESS HRMs A sensor in the wrist unit's band detects your pulse. You may find strapless HRMs more comfortable, but they tend to be less accurate than chest-strap HRMs, and they don't typically sync with speed and distance sensors.

137 GET IN THE ZONE

Determining the optimal heart-rate target zone for your specific goal is essential. The target zone is the percentage range you will aim for and is based on your maximum heart rate (MHR). The simplest calculation is: MHR = 220 minus your age. A more precise figure is 216 minus 93% of your age for men and 200 minus 67% of your age for women. There are four zones. The highest, or VO$_2$ Max, enhances speed, but for short bursts only because the muscle groups subject to this much effort will soon become deprived of oxygen.

ENDURANCE (60 TO 70 PERCENT) This range works for endurance and weight loss and develops cardio and muscular efficiency. In this zone, your body burns stored fat as fuel.

AEROBIC (70 TO 80 PERCENT) This range is ideal for overall cardio fitness, weight management, and muscle strength. In this zone, your body burns mostly fat and carbs.

ANAEROBIC (80 TO 90 PERCENT) This is the range for interval workouts or consistent speed. You will breathe heavily and feel your muscles tire out in this zone, but you'll increase lung capacity and get other long-term benefits.

THINK *about it* To take your own pulse, place two fingers between the bone and the tendon over the radial artery, on the thumb side of your wrist. Count the number of beats for 15 seconds, and multiply by four.

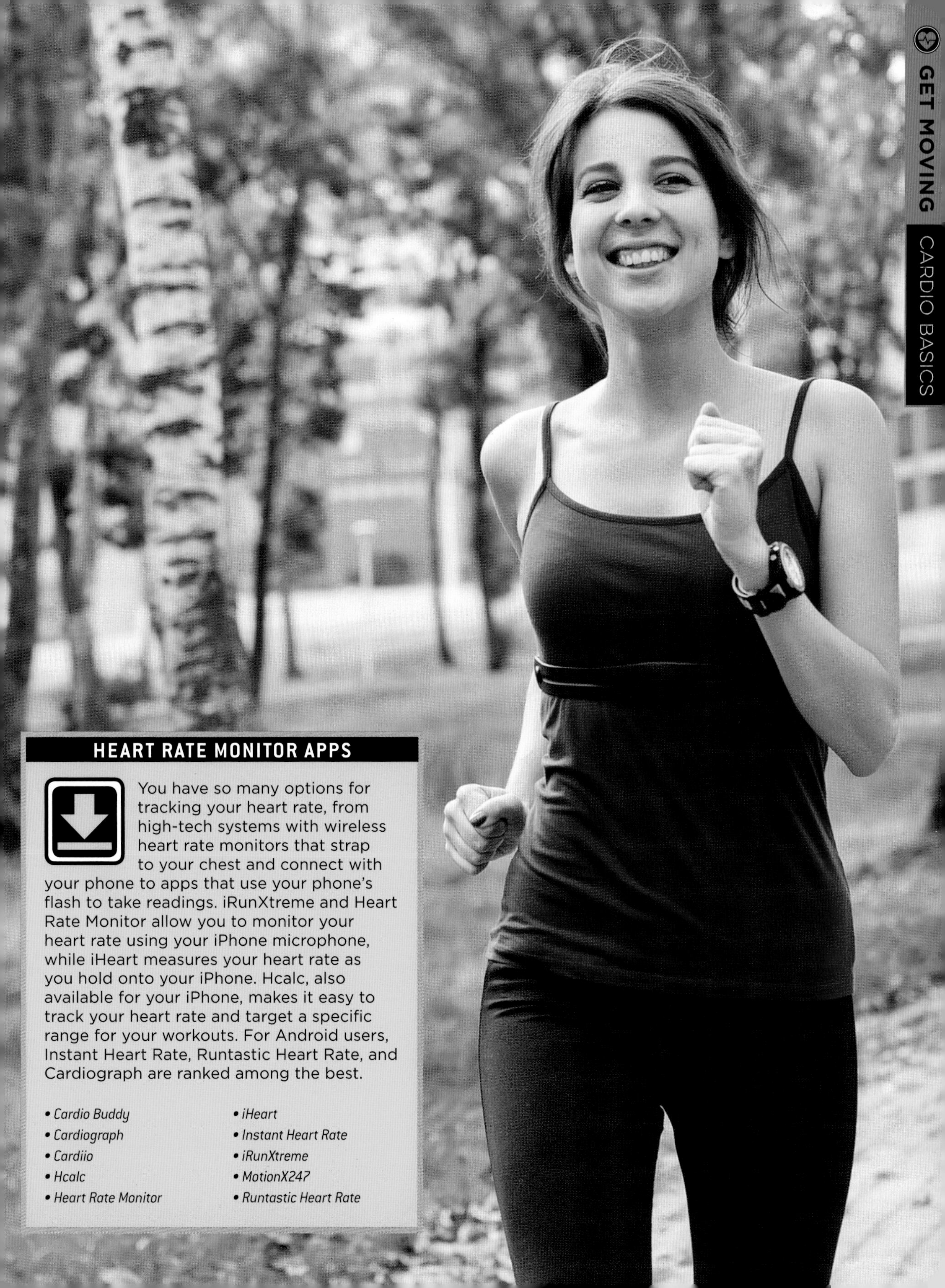

HEART RATE MONITOR APPS

You have so many options for tracking your heart rate, from high-tech systems with wireless heart rate monitors that strap to your chest and connect with your phone to apps that use your phone's flash to take readings. iRunXtreme and Heart Rate Monitor allow you to monitor your heart rate using your iPhone microphone, while iHeart measures your heart rate as you hold onto your iPhone. Hcalc, also available for your iPhone, makes it easy to track your heart rate and target a specific range for your workouts. For Android users, Instant Heart Rate, Runtastic Heart Rate, and Cardiograph are ranked among the best.

- Cardio Buddy
- Cardiograph
- Cardiio
- Hcalc
- Heart Rate Monitor
- iHeart
- Instant Heart Rate
- iRunXtreme
- MotionX247
- Runtastic Heart Rate

138 TRACK YOUR ACTION

Wearable devices that allow you to track your mileage, intensity levels, heart rate, and more, while you run, walk, bike, swim, or perform other forms of cardio exercise are a firm part of the fitness scene. These trackers can also act as motivators, encouraging you to keep moving and meet your daily goals.

The simplest device is a basic pedometer, a portable electronic or electromechanical device that you can clip on or attach to a lanyard so that it counts the steps you take each day by detecting the motion of your hands or hips. Pedometer functionality can also be introduced to smartphones, iPods, and MP3 players that have integrated accelerometers.

The current stars of the fitness world are the various wearable activity monitors ("wearables") that count steps and may display distance traveled, goals met, calories burned, and the intensity of the workout. When worn in an armband at night, certain versions measure the length and quality of your sleep; some can even wake you with a vibrating alarm. Most wearables connect to your computer via USB, where your data is automatically uploaded and displayed on a profile web page. Depending on the manufacturer, some versions can access a wide range of fitness apps. Microsoft and Apple both have their own devices; popular platform-agnostic brands include Fitbit, Garmin, and Polar. Certain devices are tailored to specific activities such as swimming or cycling, so do some online research to see which device will best suit your needs.

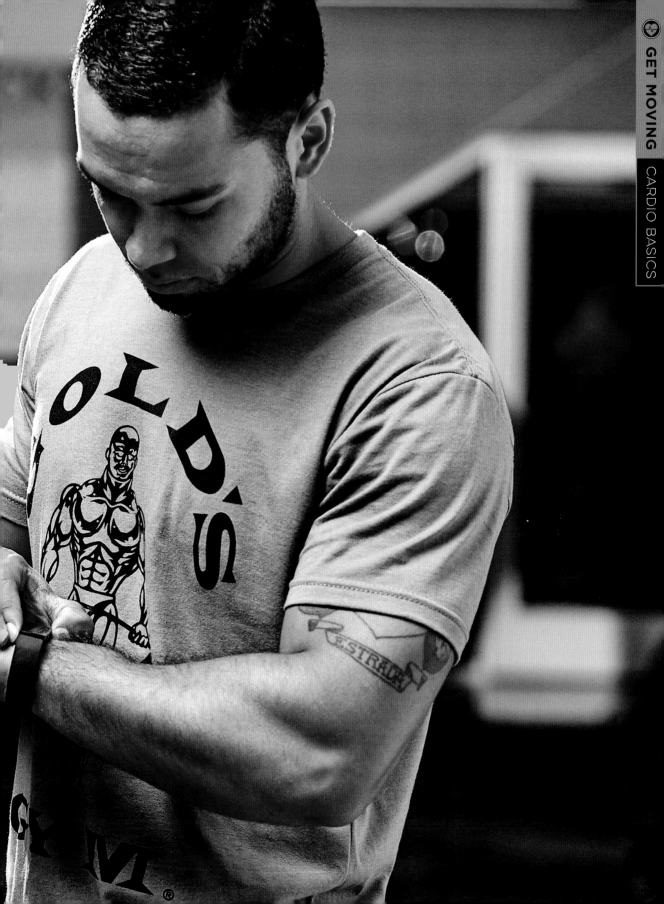

139 AMP UP YOUR ENDURANCE

Many people who work out regularly complain that they eventually become fatigued while exercising or even while doing chores at home. The trick to improving endurance and staying power is to add strength moves to your cardio workout—cardio will make you aerobically fit, while strength training will propel you through demanding workouts. If you are a runner, adding muscle will also help absorb the impact of your feet hitting the ground that would otherwise stress your joints. Here are some strength-boosting suggestions.

COMBINE STRENGTH DAYS WITH CARDIO DAYS Do bench presses and pull-ups followed by a speedy circuit of the track, or jump rope for a minute, and then do a series of squats, overhead presses, and crunches.

REDUCE YOUR REST Give yourself only a minimal break or no break at all between sets. Perform three sets of 10 back-to-back exercises such as pull-ups, squats, push-ups, and crunches. By the end, you should be sweating and your muscles should be burning.

OPT FOR COMPOUND MOVEMENTS Get more bang for your buck with exercises that use more than one joint—such as squats, step-ups, pull-ups—instead of isolated movements.

ADD EXPLOSIVES Incorporating explosive plyometric movements, like box jumps and jumping knee tucks, into your session will soon have you moving faster—and longer.

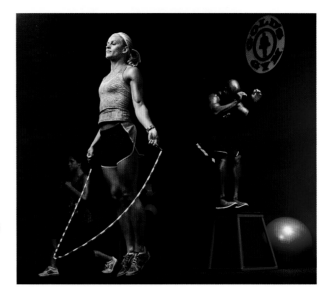

CHANGE YOUR ROUTINE Your body will adapt to a particular workout after only two weeks, so it's important to move your muscles in a different way by incorporating new activities into old routines—in other words, keeping your body guessing. Runners could try martial arts disciplines; cyclists might move onto the stair climber machine.

CHECK OUT HYBRIDS These exercises take two separate movements and combine them—a squat with an overhead press, a jumping pull-up, or a lunge with bicep curls are some examples. The more muscles you engage, the more your heart is stimulated, increasing your stamina.

140 SPIKE YOUR METABOLISM

In addition to working your heart, cardio exercise can also increase the rate of various other processes in the body, known as your metabolism. The more intense your cardio session, the more you'll notice an uptick in your metabolic rate. The experts at Gold's Gym offer several ways you can amp up your metabolism, which means you'll have an easier time maintaining your weight—or shedding excess pounds.

JETTISON THE STRESS Stress is a well-known cause of midriff and belly weight. Relaxation therapy, like yoga, can lower stress levels and bring back your metabolic oomph.

GET QUALITY SLEEP People who sleep at odd hours or who don't get enough sleep can stress their bodies and disrupt their metabolism. Try to maintain a consistent sleep

FOCUS ON NUTRITION If you eat a protein along with a fiber, some carbohydrates, and a good fat, you're keeping your insulin levels steady, so you're burning fat instead of storing fat. Eating protein at every meal is also key—it builds muscle, and more muscle leads to higher metabolic rates.

SPICE IT UP Hot, spicy seasonings, such as cayenne pepper or turmeric, will jump-start your metabolism. Add them to meat and fish rubs, egg dishes, soups, stews, and salad dressings.

DRINK EIGHT GLASSES Water, which is the foundation of so many chemical reactions in the body, is necessary for proper metabolic functions. Drinking green tea and

141 LEARN YOUR CARDIO OPTIONS

Determining the best cardio exercises to include in your routine depends on many factors. Do you like doing cardio in the gym, or would you prefer to take it outside? Other than the cardio benefits, are you also looking to lose weight or tone muscle?

The chart below can serve as a basic guide, indicating how many calories some typical exercises and cardio machines burn and listing their main health benefits. The calories burned are based on a person of average weight.

MODALITY	CALORIES BURNED	BENEFITS
WALKING	200/hour moderate pace	Heart, lungs, weight control, blood pressure, bones and muscles, balance and coordination
RUNNING	270/half hour at 10 MPH	Heart, lungs, muscle mass, weight control, blood pressure, and reduces stress
CYCLING	650/hour moderate pace	Heart, lungs, muscle strength and tone, balance and coordination, mental health, and low impact
ROWING	200/half hour moderate pace	Heart, lungs, muscle tone, reduced strain on back and joints, weight loss, and reduces stress
SWIMMING	250/half-hour slow freestyle	Heart, lungs, muscle strength, weight maintenance, and low impact
AEROBICS	195/half hour moderate pace	Heart, respiration efficiency, improves blood volume and delivery to muscles
STAIR CLIMBER	180/half hour moderate pace	Heart, lungs, muscles, slows bone loss, and low impact
TREADMILL	350/half hour moderate-pace jog	Heart, lungs, muscle tone, weight loss, insulin control, and reduces stress
ELLIPTICAL	330/half hour moderate pace	Heart, lungs, weight control, blood pressure, bones and muscles, balance and coordination, and low impact

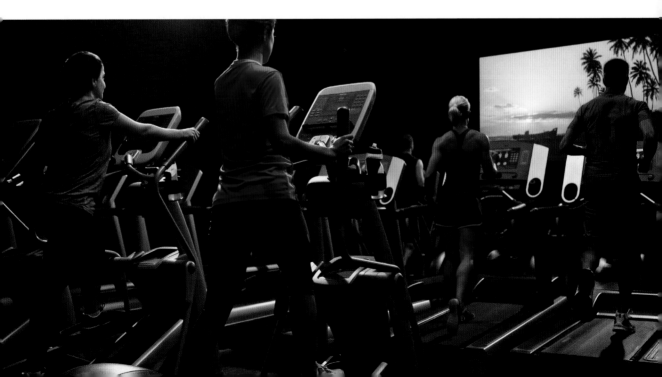

142 HIIT IT HARD

Just 20 minutes of explosive high-intensity interval training exercise can help turn your body into a powerful calorie-burning machine. This is the power of plyometrics—exercises designed to boost athletic performance.

"Explosive movements target the fast-twitch muscle fibers that don't get accessed during traditional training at the gym," says Adam Friedman, a trainer for Gold's Gym. Fast-twitch fibers are found in muscle groups throughout the body and are used for short bursts of intense activity such as in weight lifting or sprinting. Targeting these fibers will

help to add more lean tissue to your muscles, which is where fat is burned.

Adding a quick 20- to 30-minute workout like this one can also help maximize strength gains. These moves engage muscle groups in your core and lower and upper body—at times simultaneously. Plus, they'll develop your eccentric strength (when a muscle contracts and lengthens under tension), an important component of injury prevention. Anyone at any fitness level can tackle this highly adaptable routine, and it is great to perform with a partner.

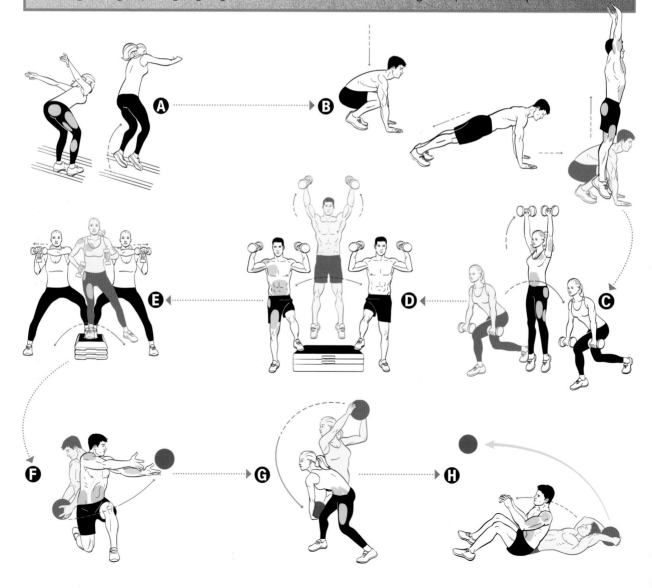

A STAIR HOPS Keep both feet together, bend your knees slightly, and swing your arms backward. Jump upward to land on the next higher step, and swing your arms forward. When you reach the top, walk down.

B BURPEES Start in a squat position with your hands on the floor in front of you. Kick your feet back to a push-up position, and perform one full push-up. Immediately bring your feet back to the squat position, and jump up on tiptoes with your arms overhead. That's one rep.

C ALTERNATING SPLIT SQUAT JUMPS WITH DUMBBELLS Stand with your feet staggered, holding a pair of light dumbbells by your sides, palms facing behind you. Lower into a lunge, bending your knees until your back knee is almost touching the floor, and then jump in the air, switching the front leg. During the upward motion of the jump, perform one clean swing with the dumbbells above your head.

D ALTERNATING BOX PUSH-OFF WITH SHOULDER PRESS Place your left foot on a plyometrics box, with your heel close to the edge, and hold a pair of lightweight dumbbells at shoulder level. Push off with your left foot to explode vertically, pressing the dumbbells overhead as you jump, and land with your feet reversed.

E SIDE-TO-SIDE BOX SHUFFLE With Dumbbell Punch Stand with one foot on a low box, holding a pair of dumbbells. Jump sideways so that the opposite foot is on the box. Repeat this side-to-side shuffle. As you jump, alternately punch forward with a dumbbell, using the same-side arm and leg.

F MEDICINE BALL KNEELING SIDE THROW Start in a kneeling position holding a medicine ball with both hands. Twist your torso, and throw the ball sideways to a wall or a partner, using your abdominals to move the ball, and not your arms.

G MEDICINE BALL WOOD CHOPS Start with your feet more than hip-width apart. With both hands, hold a medicine ball by your left hip. Turn your torso to the right, and lift the ball overhead on the right. Move it from high to low across your body, ending on the left side, as if you were chopping wood.

H SIT-UP MEDICINE BALL THROW WITH PARTNER Sit facing a partner, holding a medicine ball in both hands. Lie back with the ball overhead, and tap the floor behind you with the ball. As you sit up, immediately throw the ball to your partner from overhead. Your partner should catch the ball in front of their head.

EXERCISE	SETS/REPS	TARGET
STAIR HOPS	One set of 10 reps	Quads, calves. hamstrings, hips, and glutes
BURPEES	One set of 10 reps	Core and upper and lower body
ALTERNATING SPLIT SQUAT JUMPS WITH DUMBBELLS	One set of 20 reps	Core and upper and lower body
ALTERNATING BOX PUSH-OFF WITH SHOULDER PRESS	One set of 20 reps	Shoulders, chest, triceps, abs, hips, and quads
SIDE-TO-SIDE BOX SHUFFLE WITH DUMBBELL PUNCH	One set of 20 reps	Shoulders, chest, hips, and quads
MEDICINE BALL KNEELING SIDE THROW	One set of 10 reps on each side	Core, shoulders, and forearms
MEDICINE BALL WOOD CHOPS	One set of 10 reps on each side	Abs, obliques, and quads
SIT-UP MEDICINE BALL THROW WITH PARTNER	One set of 10 reps	Core

CATCH AND RELEASE Why not add a medicine ball to your fitness toolbox? This sphere, which measures about 7 to 14 inches (18–35 cm) in diameter, weighs from 2 to 25 pounds (1–12 kg), and adds resistance to an exercise like other free weights. Yet, unlike metal weights, you can safely throw and catch them, allowing you to develop explosive power. When you use a dumbbell or kettlebell, your muscles must work to accelerate and decelerate the load, but with a medicine ball, the power comes from releasing it, so you can add a plyometric boost to a strength move that will up its metabolism-boosting benefits.

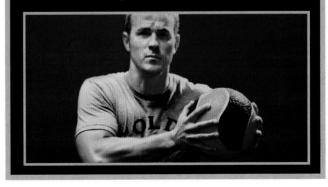

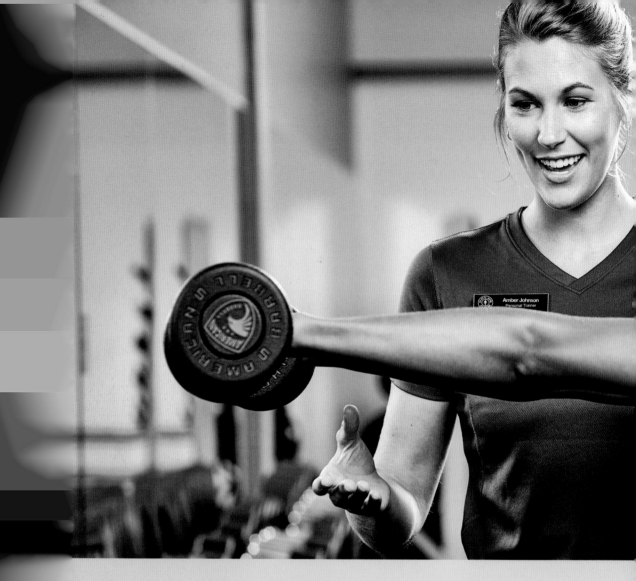

DON'T GO IT ALONE

Even if you began the Gold's Gym Challenge on your own, there will be times when you need to seek expert advice, especially once you start to increase intensity and add new modalities to your workout. It is critical to perform even the simplest exercises with proper form, and as you advance to more complex movements and compound lifts, it's wise to enlist a pro. Along with your personal training session, if you want to mix it up, take a yoga or Pilates class—ask your current trainer to recommend an instructor who has an appropriate background in flexibility training.

UNDERSTAND THE STAGES

Another reason to consider enlisting a trainer is that they often have fitness "shortcuts"— methods of training that can boost metabolism and create sleek contours relatively quickly. Trainers who have worked with Challengers before also understand the various stages of the competition. For instance, when you hit a plateau or feel you are losing motivation, your trainer can help you overcome these obstacles and forge ahead. And during the final weeks, when you might be starting to burn out, your trainer can keep you motivated, focused, and revved up for the finish line.

STAY ACCOUNTABLE

One way to stay accountable is by sharing with friends, family, and your personal trainer, the person who has invested in

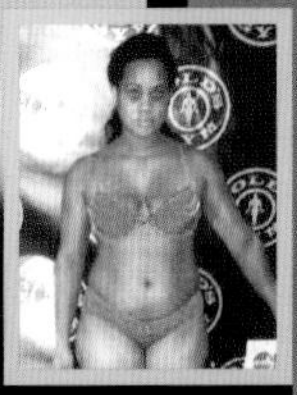

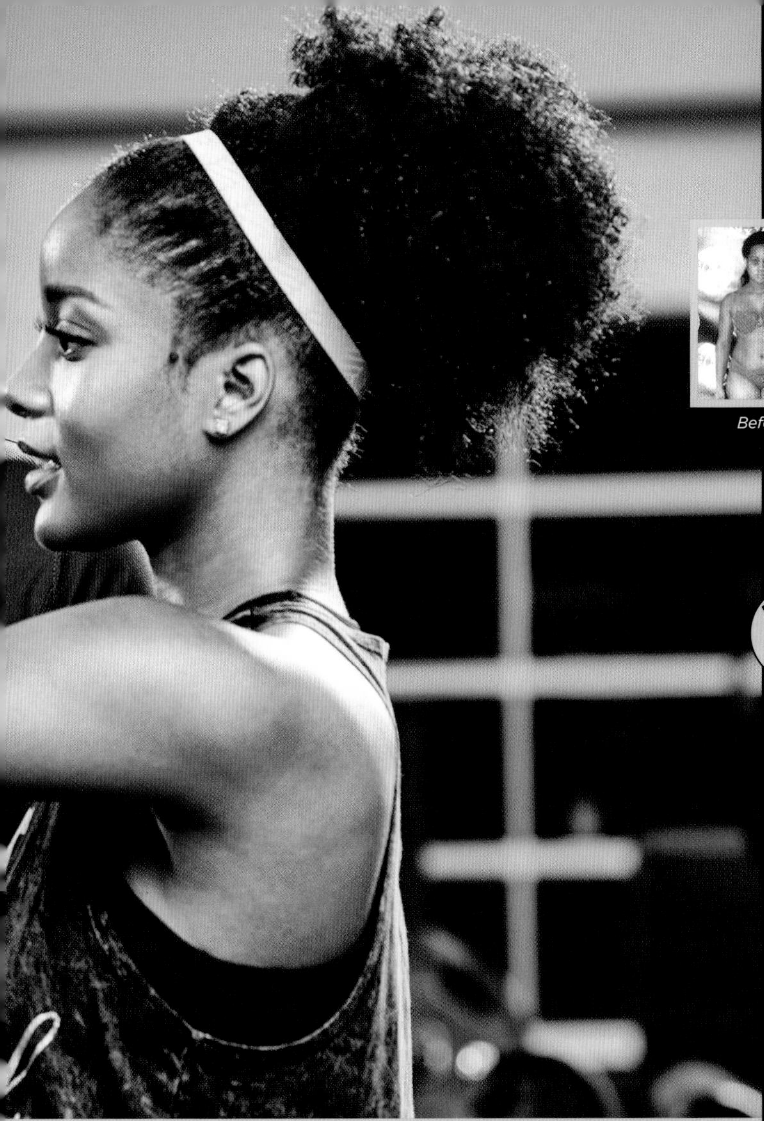

Before

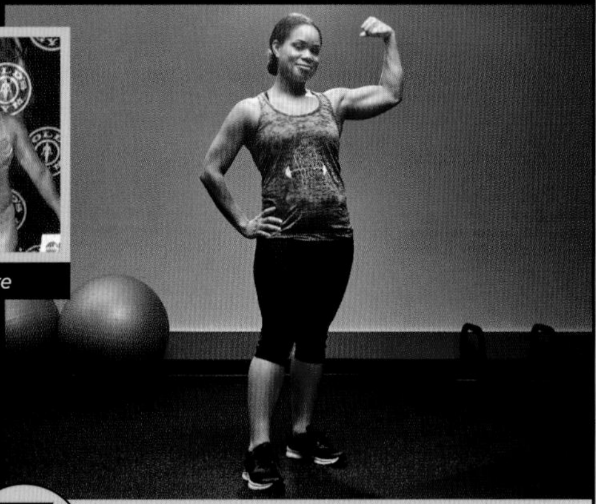

LOST 17.6 pounds (7.98 kg), 15.1 inches (38.5 cm), and 10.9% body fat

Texan Denae Quintera is one of 11 siblings, all of them athletes except for her. Even while serving in the military, her weight was an issue: she barely passed her body-fat percentage tape test. When she and her husband found out she was pregnant, they were ecstatic—until her doctor warned them that her extra weight might cause her to miscarry. Devastated, she made the necessary life changes and delivered a healthy baby girl. But her old bad habits soon returned—and so did the weight.

Then, at a high school reunion, she realized that her classmates were thinking, "She let herself go." Denae determined to make a lasting change. She was a member of Gold's Gym, yet rarely went. Now, armed with new resolve, she began to work with her trainer, Carla, on the Challenge. "I wanted to be skinny," Denae explains. But Carla told her the correct goal was to become fit and healthy. After weeks of intense workouts, sweat, and tears, her weight decreased and muscles started to form. When Carla moved, Ana volunteered to train Denae and introduced her to weights. "She has really helped me in pushing myself when I think I can't," Denae says.

you and becomes someone that you don't want to disappoint. When Gold's Gym expert trainer Eddy Campbell looked at who finished the Challenge and those who didn't, he discovered that "very few of the people who never met with a personal trainer finished. I think it's because those Challengers weren't accountable to anyone." Campbell suggests two personal trainer sessions a week or enlisting some gym buddies to take the Challenge so you can encourage one another to go the distance.

WINNER'S WORDS

"Both my trainers … taught me the importance of being fit, healthy, having confidence, and never giving up. "

~ Denae Quintera

143 TACKLE THE TREADMILL

TOOLS of the TRADE

The treadmill is a piece of equipment used for walking or running in place. It consists of a wide, conveyor-belt footbed, and a sturdy frame with a front stability brace topped by a console. The tread, which offers different levels of resistance, can be self-propelled or, in more expensive models, motorized. The console of electronic models typically features a lit display with different speed and terrain settings, a timer, and a mileage counter. Some even have programs that monitor calories burned and heart rate, as well as touch-screen access to TV, the internet, popular fitness apps, and interactive courses.

Over time, this mainstay of the commercial gym has become one of the most valued additions to the home gym. Advantages of the treadmill include the ability to complete your cardio session no matter the weather; a cushioned tread that is easier on the feet and legs than running on a hard roadbed, incline settings that allow you to run "uphill" for additional toning benefits, and rate settings that allow you to maintain a steady pace or choose variable speeds. Look for models like the Gold's Gym Trainer 430i, which is iFit Bluetooth Smart Enabled, iPod compatible, and combines quick speed with incline control. Many users also watch TV or DVDs while on the treadmill, turning a once-sedentary activity into a healthy workout.

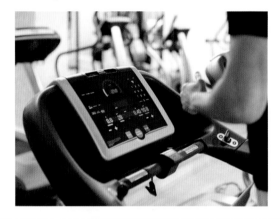

144 MAKE THE MOST OF YOUR TREADMILL WORKOUT

The treadmill can offer a comprehensive cardio workout to gym-goers of all levels, especially if you follow these suggestions.

WARM UP PROPERLY Never just climb onto the machine and kick it into high gear. A typical session would be warming up first with three minutes of walking. Follow with three minutes of jogging and then three sets of 20-second speed sprints with 40 seconds of recovery in between.

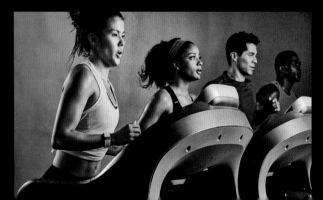

PLACE GEAR NEARBY The point of the treadmill—or any cardio machine—is to exert yourself until you sweat, so keep a hand towel on the console, and pat yourself dry as needed. A water bottle that opens with one hand is a great way to stay hydrated without stopping to fiddle with a screw cap.

PAY ATTENTION TO CADENCE There are two ways to run faster—lengthening your stride or upping the number of smaller strides, thus increasing cadence. The treadmill is perfect for the latter: you have a timer in front of you, and you can hear your foot strike the tread in order to find the sweet spot, which should be fairly quiet. Count the strikes of one foot in 15 seconds, and multiply times 4. You should be aiming for 90 beats per foot per minute.

UP THE INCLINE Because, by many accounts, running on a treadmill actually feels similar to running slightly downhill, keep the incline on your machine set to 1 percent to compensate.

RECOVER SLOWLY The general rule of thumb for ending your session is to cool down one minute for every mile run, so a five-mile (8 km) workout requires an easy-paced five-minute walk

145 SET YOUR TREADMILL ON AN INCLINE GRADE

Uphill workouts are among the best exercises you can do because they provide a high-intensity cardio session while also having a low impact on your joints. Recent studies have shown that incline work—even walking up steep angles—has a wide variety of benefits. Your sessions, whether walking or running, have the potential to build strength and power, burn fat, tone muscle, and increase the stroke volume of your heart, while at the same time strengthening the lower back, glutes, quads, hamstrings, and calves. This machine even speeds up the pace at which your brain sends messages to your muscles.

Gold's Gym Fitness Institute member Robert Reames configured these three workouts that combine walking and running. A treadmill is the best place for hill workouts because it removes the most troublesome aspect: the downhill. Most hill-related injuries actually occur on the downslope—the reverse incline adds a gravity-induced load. So the treadmill has all the great uphill benefit with none of the, well, downside of the downhill.

As a general guide, you should set the treadmill incline between a 4- and 10-percent grade, and set your sprint speed from 7.5 to 10 miles per hour (12–16 kph). Focus on pushing yourself, but be sure to maintain good posture, keeping your hips, shoulders, and neck relaxed. Add one of these workouts to your current routine or pair them up for even more intensity.

THE 10-MINUTE WORKOUT
- 3 minutes warm-up
- 1.5 minutes high-incline power walk
- 1 minute rest interval
- 1.5 minutes sprint
- 3 minutes cool-down

THE 15-MINUTE WORKOUT
- 2 minutes slow warm-up
- 1 minute moderate warm-up
- 1.5 minutes high-incline power walk
- 1.5 minutes high-incline sprint
- 3 minutes rest interval
- 1.5 minutes high-incline power walk
- 1.5 minute high-incline sprint
- 2 minutes moderate cool-down
- 1 minute slow cool-down

THE 20-MINUTE WORKOUT
- 2 minutes slow warm-up
- 2 minutes moderate warm-up
- 2 minutes high-incline power walk
- 2 minutes rest interval
- 2 minutes high-incline sprint
- 2 minutes rest interval
- 2 minutes high-incline power walk
- 2 minutes rest interval
- 2 minutes cool-down on flat grade
- 2 minutes cool-down interval on flat grade

146 OVERCOME OBSTACLES

Many competitive runners and recreational joggers who run outdoors are resistant to the treadmill at first. Here are some challenges they've noted, and how to overcome them.

SIZE The treadmill is not a portable piece of equipment that can be folded up and stored under a bed. So, if you have a small apartment, maybe keep your treadmill sessions to the gym.

VARIETY If you're used to running outdoors in all kinds of weather, through varied scenery, running in place can mean a real adjustment. This might mean it's time to set up the DVD player or add thumping new tunes to your iPod. Runners who relish the ever-changing scenery of the urban or rural landscape tend to find the treadmill's limited vistas lack appeal and offer little sense of adventure.

PACING If you stay at one pace for an entire workout, you can feel unbalanced. Make use of the many options for interval training to mix things up, varying your pace and incline to better mimic an outdoor workout.

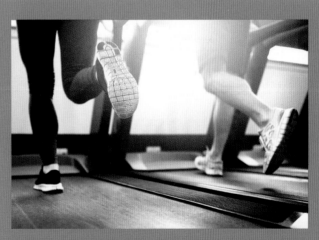

GAIT Some treadmill users who return to outdoor running feel like they've developed a short, upright, bouncy gait—possibly as a result of having no wind resistance indoors. This is another case where mixing up speed and incline can help.

COMPETITION If you're training for serious track and field events, the treadmill isn't the optimal training idea. You'll probably want to look for a good indoor or outdoor track.

147 GO FOR A RUN

Running and jogging are some of the most popular recreational sports in the world. This is not surprising, because scientists believe that our bodies evolved, quite literally, to run. Today, people run for a variety of reasons—to lose weight, lower blood pressure, and strengthen the heart, as a way to tone the body, and to increase fitness and endurance for a specific sport. The benefits are impressive: running burns an average of 135 to 150 calories per mile, increases lean body mass and bone density, regulates cholesterol, and improves your psychological state by boosting endorphins (see #153).

Running allows great freedom—you can run at any time of day or night and find a track, trail, or sidewalk in most places. And because you don't need health club memberships or sports trainers, it is also relatively low-cost. A good pair of running shoes, some comfortable clothing, and a portable water bottle, and you're good to go. Still, as is the case with any athletic discipline, there is a right—and a wrong—way to run.

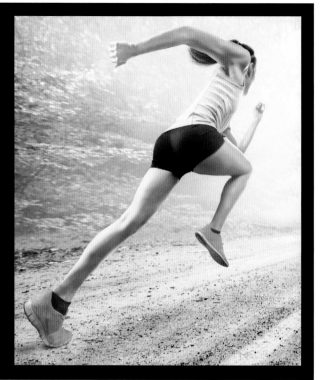

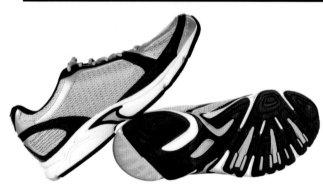

149 GET THE SUPPORT YOU NEED

Many female runners need added bust support in the form of a sports bra that minimizes movement but is not uncomfortably restrictive. Quality bras should be relatively seam-free, offer comfort, uplift, and have nonslip straps. They are typically made of a wicking synthetic fabric and come in sporty colors. If your sports bras are no longer doing the job, try wearing two at a time until you can find a workable replacement.

148 CHOOSE THE PROPER SNEAKERS

As a runner, buying a pair of quality shoes will be your main expense. Because these shoes are meant to support your feet, calves, and knees, and protect your body from injury, their workmanship and fit count big time. If possible, get measured at a store that specializes in sports footwear. The clerk should determine your arch shape—if you are flat-footed, or if you have a tendency to over- or underpronate the foot—and then suggest shoes that compensate. This person should also factor in your level of experience, how much you intend to run, and your average pace. Once you've gotten the proper shoes, break them in slowly. And bear in mind that most running shoes will last between 300 to 500 miles (500–800 km).

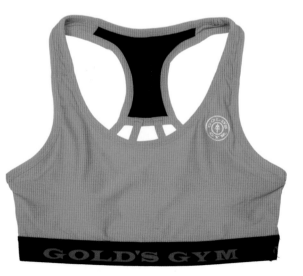

150 START OUT SLOW

All runners need to prepare for their sessions with a warm up, following each run with a similar cool-down period (see #158 and #159). If you are new to running, start out slowly so that your body can adjust to the new demands you'll be placing on it. Begin your regimen by walking 20 minutes three times a week. The second week, combine walking and running for 20 minutes over three nonconsecutive days. Pace yourself by alternating walking with running. During the third week, jog or run for 20 minutes for three nonconsecutive days. (A jog is trotting at a leisurely pace.) Pause or walk if you need to—but never stop moving. During subsequent weeks, gradually increase the duration, intensity, and frequency of your runs. If your body complains that you're doing too much, ease back.

GYM *etiquette*

151 FIND YOUR LANE

There are protocols to running on any track, but it is more critical to follow these rules on narrower, more confining indoor tracks. Faster runners traditionally keep to the inside track, and slower runners stay in the middle lanes, with walkers on the far outside. If two running buddies are moving abreast and hear someone coming from behind, the inner one should shift to the slower lane behind his or her friend. And if you are passing someone, call out "On your right!" to signal that you are approaching. Note that in most gyms the track direction changes every other day.

152 UNDERSTAND THE TERRAIN

When you are running on different surfaces, your body reacts to the impact in different ways. Switching surfaces is actually a smart tactic to strengthen your internal frame and lower the risk of repetitive-strain injuries and muscle imbalances.

GRASS One of the best surfaces to run on, grass is soft, low-impact, and great for speed work. It is often uneven, however, and long grass may hide animal holes, rocks, or other hazards. Grass also turns slippery when wet.

WOODLAND TRAILS Many parks and state forests offer well-maintained, level trails with soft, well-drained peat or wood chips underfoot. These materials are easy on the legs, and will help you develop your muscles and joints. Watch out for tree roots or slippery mud.

DIRT TRAILS The consistency of dirt can range from dry, sandy soil to moist, clay earth. Dry dirt is usually medium to soft underfoot, reducing your risk of training injuries and the impact of downhill runs. Avoid dirt trails in wet weather.

SYNTHETIC TRACK Outdoor tracks, with their flat, forgiving surfaces, are ideal for speed work and interval training. Tracks can become boring, however, and they may increase your risk of injury if you land hard on your inside leg, or if you roll your ankle and turn your foot outward negotiating the curves.

ASPHALT This common paving material is one of the fastest surfaces for running. It provides an even footing that will not stress your Achilles tendon. Unfortunately, there are traffic, potholes, and a hard unyielding surface to contend with.

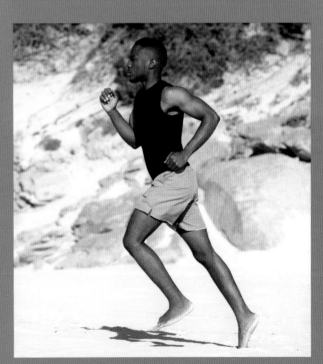

SAND Flat and firm sand offers a forgiving, low-impact surface. Running up and down sand dunes provides effective resistance training, strengthening the legs. Running in soft sand gives your calf muscles a good workout, yet is easy on your joints. It also allows you to shed your shoes and go barefoot, which many experts believe is the best way to run.

CONCRETE City runners quickly learn to handle concrete, which is often the only surface available for them. It is the hardest material to run on and takes a toll on the legs; it also comes with curbs, pedestrians, and traffic signals.

153 KNOW WHY YOU FEEL SO GOOD

As you perform your regular running workout, jogging on the pavement or sprinting along a trail, you may find yourself overcome by a glowing sense of euphoria—this is the celebrated "runner's high" that track and field athletes and marathoners frequently experience. Running, along with other cardiovascular exercise, can actually change your hormonal profile, triggering the release of "feel good" hormones, such as endorphins. These can elevate your mood, ease depression, and block pain. Serotonin, another pleasure-producing chemical, works with endorphins to make exercise almost addictive; it also provides energy and promotes clear thinking. Another benefit of cardio: other released hormones, like peptide YY, can act as appetite suppressants.

154 STAY HYDRATED FOR RUNNING

Keeping the body hydrated is paramount for runners. In addition to the water you carry on the trail, try the following problem solvers before or after your run.

SLUGGISHNESS Drink a cup of green tea 20 to 30 minutes before you set out. The caffeine will power you and pep you up, and the antioxidants may increase endurance.

SIDE STITCH Coconut water contains 15 times more cramp-preventing potassium than sports drinks. Drink eight ounces (240 ml) before or during your run.

SORENESS To prevent next-day aches and pain, try chocolate milk with its perfect ratio of carbs to protein and high calcium content. Drink a cup 30 minutes after a long run.

EXCESS SWEAT Sports drinks replenish sugars and electrolytes lost by sweating. Find one with no artificial colors, flavors, or preservatives, and sip six ounces (175 ml) every 15 minutes.

RUNNING APPS

Runners have access to a wide range of multifunction apps to monitor their workouts and nutrition, map their routes, and track their progress. RunKeeper, MapMyRun, Fitbit, Runtastic, and Pact all share info; Zombies Run doesn't share, but it's a great motivator for the reluctant runner. Competitive runners should check out RaceJoy or iRace, or download Motigo so that friends and family can cheer you on, or Strava to join in challenges.

- Couch to 5K
- Endomondo
- iRace
- MapMyRun
- Motigo
- Pacejamek
- Pact
- RaceJoy
- RunKeeper
- Runtastic
- SmartRunner
- Strava
- Wahoo
- Zombies Run

155 COMPETE ON THE STREET

Once you feel comfortable running over distances, you should consider entering an organized event. Anyone, at any age, can race if they are willing to compete—plus, race training is a great motivator that can boost your running to the next level. First, determine what race type appeals to you—there are short charity and fun runs, themed runs, trail races, team obstacle races, qualifying runs, marathons, and half marathons. You also need to consider the terrain (if you run on flat urban streets, a hilly off-road race is likely not for you), how far you are willing to travel, the climate and temperatures you prefer, and what kind of experience you hope to gain. The cost of races vary: charity races may require you to find sponsorship; other races may charge a fee—from as low as $5 to $20 for a 5K to hundreds for a marathon.

156 PREPARE TO RACE

If you are considering competitive running, Team USA duathlete Lindsey Torgerson has some tips for distance runners that can also be applied to other types of racing.

GIVE YOURSELF TIME Plan for a 5K race at least 6 to 8 weeks out—12 to 14 weeks for a half marathon—but don't rush training, because it can cause injury. Start by running three days a week: ideally a slow long-distance run, a tempo run, and a speed/interval training day.

GET STRONG Strength training is critical to becoming a strong, healthy runner. Incorporate two to three strength-training sessions per week.

TAKE TIME OUT If you are feeling tired, hungrier than usual, and stiff or sore, take the day off to allow your body to recover.

CHECK YOURSELF Ask a friend to film you running, then assess your foot strike and upper-body movements. If you are heel striking, this can cause lower back, hip, and knee issues. Midfoot should be your initial contact with the pavement, and your elbows should be sliding close to your sides, hands relaxed.

RUN OUTSIDE Do at least one of your weekly training runs outside on the street. You will be running your race outside, and you need to be comfortable on pavement.

FIND YOUR FUEL You should usually eat one hour before any physical activity. Use your training weeks to determine your best pre- and post-run fuels.

157 KNOW YOUR...
HIP FLEXORS

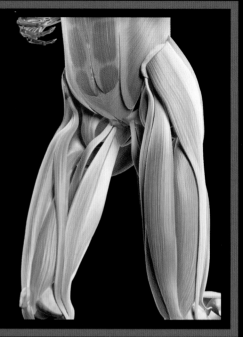

The hip flexors are a powerful group of muscles that you rely on whenever you walk, jog or sprint. These muscles are attached to the hip joint to allow your knee to pull upward. The hip itself is a large ball-and-socket joint that joins many ligaments, tendons, and muscles. The main hip flexor is the iliopsoas group, which consists of two muscles: the psoas and the iliac. These deep, hidden muscles are crucial to good posture, helping to stabilize your spine. Weak iliopsoas muscles may lead to lower-back and pelvic pain (running commonly triggers hip flexor problems). The rectus femoris and the sartorius are the other two major hip flexors. The sartorius aids in the flexion of your knee and hip and the rotation of your thigh and tibia bone. The rectus femoris—one of the four quadriceps muscles (see #110)—is the only muscle that crosses over the hip joint, which enables it to work as both a hip flexor and a knee extender. Other hip flexors are the tensor fasciae latae, along your outer thigh, and the gracilis, pectineus, adductor longus, and adductor brevis on the inner thigh. At the back is the adductor magnus, which acts as a hip extensor.

158 WARM UP AND COOL DOWN

It may seem as simple as dragging yourself out of bed and hitting the pavement, but a smart running regimen means warming up before you sprint at top speed and cooling down at the end of your run. Follow these tips to run at your best and avoid possible injury.

WALK BEFORE YOU RUN Start off with a gentle walk for a few minutes to ease your body into the intense workout to come. Walking will get the range of motion of your muscles, tendons, and joints up to speed and raise the temperature of your muscles and core, increasing the blood flow to your running muscles.

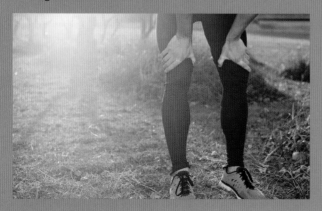

PICK UP YOUR PACE To transition from walking to running mode, move into a slow jog for two minutes. Then gradually pick up your pace, accelerating your speed over 200 to 300 feet (60–100 m), and then just as gradually decelerate. Next, walk a bit more, shaking out your legs for a couple of minutes. Repeat the whole sequence in the opposite direction.

STRETCH YOUR RUNNING MUSCLES Forget static, fixed stretches—although once a regular part of a running regimen, they can actually make you more susceptible to injury. Instead, perform a series of dynamic stretches. These controlled movements improve range of motion, loosen up muscles, and increase your heart rate, body temperature, and blood flow. Focus on dynamic stretches aimed at your running muscles, like your legs, glutes, and hip flexors (see #159).

COOL YOURSELF DOWN You may be tempted to just flop into a chair, but a proper cool-down will bring your body back to a resting state, just as the warm-up brought it to an active state. A proper cool-down should gently slow your elevated heart rate and help clear your muscles of metabolic waste. To cool-down, drop to a jog and then a walk. Your next step is to perform a series of dynamic stretches—you can march or skip with high knees and shuffle with straight legs, for example, or perform the same kind of stretches you did for your warm-up.

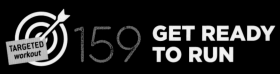

159 GET READY TO RUN

Dynamic stretches will warm your muscles and prepare them for a run. There are many dynamic stretches, but be sure to include in your warm-up those that target key running muscle groups: the ones that control flexion and extension of the legs and lateral movements. Always include exercises that warm up your hips—this is where the hip flexors, quads, and hamstrings come together.

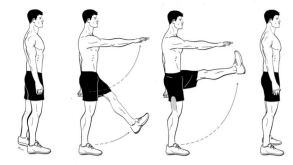

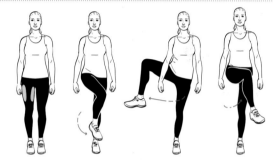

⊙ MONSTER WALK This walking exercise will stretch your hamstrings.

HOW While walking a distance of 20 yards (18.2 m), kick one leg up in the air to a comfortable height while trying to touch the toe with the opposite arm. Repeat for the full distance, alternating legs and arms.

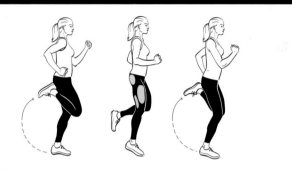

Ⓐ BUTT KICKS Butt kicks will warm up the muscles in your legs and increase your core body temperature. Start slowly, and work up to a faster speed.

HOW Stand tall with a tight core and flat back, and bring your left foot back and up to your glutes. Return your foot to the ground, and repeat with the right. Continue alternating legs, keeping your knees slightly bent at all times and pumping your arms to run in place for two minutes.

Ⓓ OPEN AND CLOSE THE GATE This move combines hip adduction and abduction to warm up your hip flexors and groin muscles.

HOW Walking a distance of 20 yards (18.2 m), every three steps march one knee up and then out to the side, and then circle inward across your body, and return to the ground. Alternate legs, and repeat for the full distance.

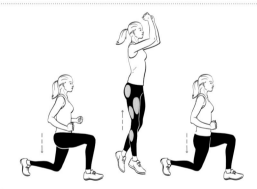

Ⓑ PLYO LUNGE This is a great plyometric move to warm up your entire lower body—including the quadriceps, glutes, hamstrings, and calves—and activate the stabilizer muscles in your legs and hips.

HOW Stand in a wide lunge with your right leg forward and your arms at your sides. Bend your knees, and then explode upward, switching your legs midair so that you land with your left leg forward and right foot back. Land softly, compressing right into another lunge, and then alternate sides for 10 reps.

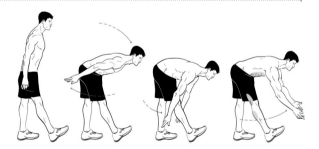

Ⓔ GROUND SWEEPS This exercise will activate your core and stretch your calf muscles and hamstrings.

HOW Walking a distance of 20 yards (18.2 m), step forward on the right foot, swing your arms back, and then slowly sweep your arms forward, trying to brush the ground with your fingertips. Return to standing, and then repeat, leading with the left foot. Alternate legs for the full distance.

160 LEARN ABOUT THE LUNGE

Lunges have long been valuable components of a runner's strength-training and stretching regimen. They help you improve your coordination and balance, while working your quadriceps, hamstrings, glutes, and hip flexors. Strengthening these muscles is crucial because strong legs and hips can help protect your knees from the pounding placed on these vulnerable joints while you run. These muscles also work together to pull the body in a forward motion to increase sprinting speed, and because they are asymmetrical standing exercises (meaning you shift your body weight from one leg to the other), they challenge your balance, proprioception, and dynamic flexibility. This makes them more effective for improving your running stride compared to bilateral moves that distribute the load between both legs—such as squats, which target a similar group of muscles.

Another plus is that lunges require no equipment, and you can perform them anywhere. There are many variations, too, so you never have to get bored doing the same moves all the time. If you want to add resistance, you can perform them with resistance bands or holding a barbell, dumbbell, medicine ball, or other free weight.

Ⓐ FORWARD LUNGE

WHY Targets the hips, glutes, core, and inner thighs

HOW Stand with your feet together and your hands on your hips or clasped behind your head. Lunge forward with on one leg, focusing on a downward movement of your hips until your front thigh is parallel with the floor. Firmly push off with the front leg to return to your upright, starting position. Repeat by alternating lunges with each leg leading.

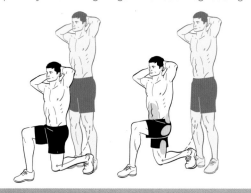

Ⓑ CURTSY LUNGE

WHY Adds some torso and hip rotation while working your hips, glutes, core, and inner thighs

HOW Stand with feet together, hands on your hips or down at your sides. Take a big step back with your right leg, crossing it behind your left leg. Bend both knees and lower your body until your front thigh is parallel with the floor. Return to the starting position, and repeat on the other side.

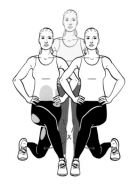

C SKATER LUNGE

WHY Offers the usual benefits of a lunge while adding an effective cardio component

HOW Stand with your feet shoulder-width apart and your arms at your sides. Take a large step backward with your left leg, and cross it diagonally behind the right as you extend your right arm out to the side and swing the left across your hips. Hop to the left, then return to your starting position. Repeat with the other leg, and continue alternating sides.

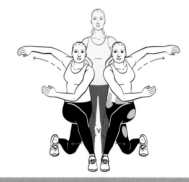

D WALKING LUNGE

WHY Offers the benefits of a forward lunge, while it activates your core and stretches your hip flexors

HOW Stand tall with your arms at your sides. Step far forward with your right leg while simultaneously lifting up onto the ball of your left foot. With your chest high and shoulders back, bend your knees, and drop your hips downward. Press up with your right leg, and bring your left foot forward. Take another step forward, and continue alternating sides.

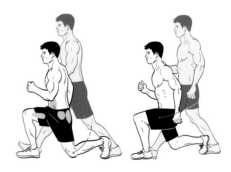

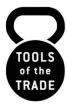

TOOLS of the TRADE

161 EXPLORE THE ELLIPTICAL

The elliptical trainer has become the go-to piece of equipment for those who want a thorough cardio workout that places limited stress on the joints. Also known as the cross-trainer or X-trainer, the elliptical is used to simulate stair climbing, running or walking. Simple models are self-propelled, while more deluxe models have motorized pedals with adjustable resistance and electronic consoles with readouts. The three basic types of elliptical trainers are categorized by the location of the motor, or "drive." The rear drive is the oldest design, the front-drive was a second-generation design, and the center drive incorporates the latest design technology.

To use an elliptical, adopt a comfortable standing position with your spine in a neutral position (straight back), align your knees, hips, and ankles, then distribute your weight between your heels and the balls of your feet. You then grip the handrails and move your arms with an even, controlled motion, and stride in either a forward or reverse motion, moving smoothly and continuously.

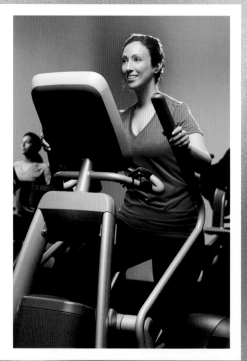

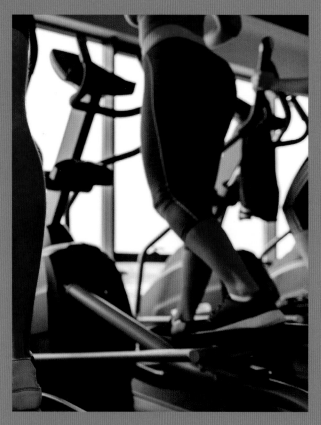

162 GAIN MULTIPLE BENEFITS

Depending on the speed and the resistance settings, your elliptical workout can range from light intensity to high cardio demand. Most ellipticals work the upper body (with the use of handle levers), and the lower body (via the foot pedals). Ellipticals produce an intermediate range of leg motion that is somewhere between a treadmill and a stationary bicycle, and they burn calories similar to the spin bike. In addition to offering a brisk cardio workout, the machine has other advantages.

LOW IMPACT By keeping the users' heels flat on the pedals, the machine reduces muscle and tendon stress.

FLUID MOVEMENT Users move so freely that they will experience a low relative perceived exertion (RPE), meaning they don't feel like they are working as hard as they really are.

VARIABLE STRIDES Studies have shown that the ability to vary the length of stride, a feature of late-model machines, works a larger variety of muscle groups and burns more calories—all without the user being aware of any extra work.

INEXPENSIVE HOME VERSIONS Commercial gym models might cost in the thousands of dollars, but home models can start as low as a few hundred.

163 TAKE IT IN INTERVALS

Interval training is one way to get the most out of your time at the gym—providing an effective cardio session that can also transform your physique. It involves alternating intense bursts of exercise with slowed-down recovery segments. You can implement it using two machines that require different rates of speed or degrees of effort or, more typically, you can work at differing levels—altering speed, incline, direction, and so on—on the same machine.

The benefits of interval training include burning more calories—even just by raising intensity for a short time—and improving aerobic capacity by increasing cardiovascular fitness, which then allows you to work longer or with more intensity. These routines alleviate the boredom of those "same old-same old" workouts, plus you can perform them on your usual equipment simply by modifying your routine.

Most up-to-date cardio machines feature a setting for interval training so you don't even have to think about configuring your session. Here are some alternative workouts on four popular machines.

ELLIPTICAL INTERVALS Adjust the workout setting to "interval," and follow the routine through periods of high and low activity with varying levels of resistance for 10 or 15 minutes. Halfway through, change the direction so you are pedalling backward.

STATIONARY BIKE INTERVALS These machines should also have an "interval" setting. Once it is set in motion, assume a "spinning" position—butt off the seat, arms braced on the handles, and your weight forward. For increased results, find a comfortable position on the seat while holding a dumbbell in each hand, and perform two sets of 10 to 12 reps of lateral raises (see #093C). Or start in the same position, but this time perform two sets of 10 to 12 reps of bicep curls (see #096A).

TREADMILL INTERVALS If your treadmill has an "interval" setting, activate it. Enhance your upper-body workout with punches: Hold your arms close to your body, bent at about 90 degrees, and jab outward with rotation, so that at the end of the motion your knuckles face away from your body. Alternate hands with a steady rhythm; perform for 10 to 15 minutes. Another challenging motion is the side shuffle: set the speed for two to four miles per hour, and pivot to the side, holding on to one of the handles for support, shuffling along sideways as the tread moves for 3 to 5 minutes. Or face away from the console, hold both handles, and walk or run backward.

STAIR CLIMBER INTERVALS Adjust the setting to "interval," and try one of these variations, each for 3 to 5 minutes. As you raise your left leg, swing you right leg behind you, and then alternate. Or try taking the steps two at a time. Finally, try the sidestep. Stand sideways on the machine, holding the stability bar, and carefully step up, placing one foot over the other. Midway through, pivot 180 degrees to switch directions, and lead with the opposite foot.

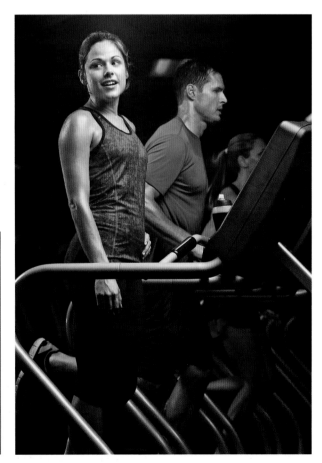

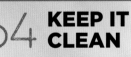

GYM *etiquette*

164 KEEP IT CLEAN

One of the reasons gym-goers carry a small towel is to dry off after a taxing workout. But don't forget to wipe down any machines or equipment you might have perspired upon. Few things in the gym experience are more distasteful than sliding onto damp seats or gripping sweaty handles—left by the previous user. Some people even carry two towels—one for personal hygiene and one to swipe over equipment before and after they use it.

165 WALK THIS WAY

It might surprise you to know that walking at a brisk pace burns roughly two-thirds of the calories that outright running does—113 calories per mile walked versus 151 per mile run. Once those large muscles in your limbs and core get set in motion calories get incinerated. So don't feel you have to hit the treadmill at the highest setting or pound the pavement to get a good cardio workout. Walking is a low-impact activity, which makes it ideal for seniors or those with joint issues, plus it can be a great gateway activity to running.

Trainers recommend mixing up your walking workout to avoid getting into a rut. Push yourself on the treadmill by trying programs that vary the speed and incline, and add in days on the elliptical or stair climber—or take it outdoors every do often if the weather permits.

Walking—or power walking, which also includes exaggerated arm swinging—helps you maintain a proper weight and prevent or manage heart disease, high blood pressure, and type 2 diabetes. It strengthens bones and muscles and even improves your mood. Even on days when you can't make it to the gym you can get in some steps—you don't need extra equipment or special clothing, and it's something you likely do every day already. You simply need to increase your volume of steps and build your intensity to aerobic levels.

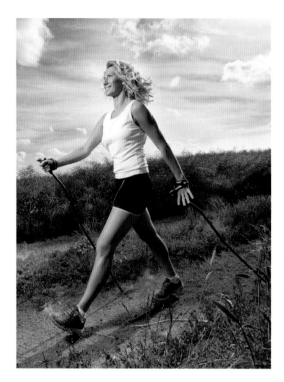

166 TWEAK YOUR TECHNIQUE

"Tweak what?" you think. "It's only walking!" But the truth is, just as with any form of exercise, to benefit most, you need to perform it properly. As you walk, aim for good posture, an easy stride, a tight core, and purposeful movements.

WARM UP Always walk slowly for the first 5 or 10 minutes.

LOOK AHEAD Keep your head up, so that you are gazing forward, not at the ground.

GO EASY Relax your neck, shoulders, and back, so that you are not standing stiffly upright.

STAY LOOSE As you walk, swing your arms freely, with a slight bend in the elbows. A little arm pumping is also okay.

TIGHTEN UP As you move forward, tighten your stomach muscles, and make sure your back is straight, not arched forward or backward.

SMOOTH OUT Make sure you are walking with a smooth gait, rolling your foot from heel to toe.

COOL DOWN Every brisk walk needs a period of cooling down—try five minutes of slow walking followed, perhaps, by some dynamic muscle stretches.

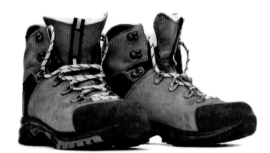

167 CHOOSE YOUR SHOES

For walking on a track, sidewalk, or street, shoes need to have proper arch support; firm, thick heels; and thick, flexible soles to cushion your feet and act as shock absorbers. Some makers of athletic gear offer walking shoes with more techie features—orthotic footbed inserts, gel pads in the heels, or reflective panels for walking at night.

If hiking is your thing, it's critical to invest in good quality footwear. Hiking shoes, usually worn for day hikes, are low-cut with flexible midsoles. Mid- or high-cut flexible hiking boots are used for both day hikes and weekend backpacking. High-cut backpacking boots are the sturdy, supportive option, designed for carrying heavy loads through back country on trips of multiple days.

168 HIKE FOR HEALTH

Hiking—walking outdoors across varied terrain, especially woodlands or hills—can supply a great cardio-respiratory session. Hiking works nearly every part of the body: legs, knees, ankles, arms, hips, glutes, abs, shoulders, and neck. And like any weight-bearing activity, it lowers your risk of heart disease, improves blood sugar and blood pressure levels, and boosts bone density. A person weighing 155 pounds (70 kg) burns an average of 370 calories for every hour of hiking. And you needn't be in tip-top shape to begin—start with easy routes through relatively level areas, and work your way up to steeper, more demanding terrain.

You can map new treks and share your favorite routes with other hikers online or on your phone with apps such as MapMyHike. To get detailed terrain maps, try offline GPS apps like BackCountry Navigator or MotionX GPS.

And while of course the whole point of hiking is to get out in the great outdoors, you can greatly benefit by using your gym time to improve your hiking experience. Step classes or time on the elliptical build endurance, while squats, lunges, and core exercises make it easier to scramble up steep trails. Speak to a personal trainer about building a resistance program geared to your outdoor-fitness plans and goals.

169 BRING THE KIDS

Hiking can be a great family wellness activity. Children get many of the same benefits as adults, as well as lowering their risk factors for heart disease, high blood pressure, type 2 diabetes, depression, and sleep disorders. Decreased levels of stress can make children more ready to learn in school. And just think of the good example you're setting—for many kids who are encouraged to be active during their formative years, fitness becomes a lifelong habit.

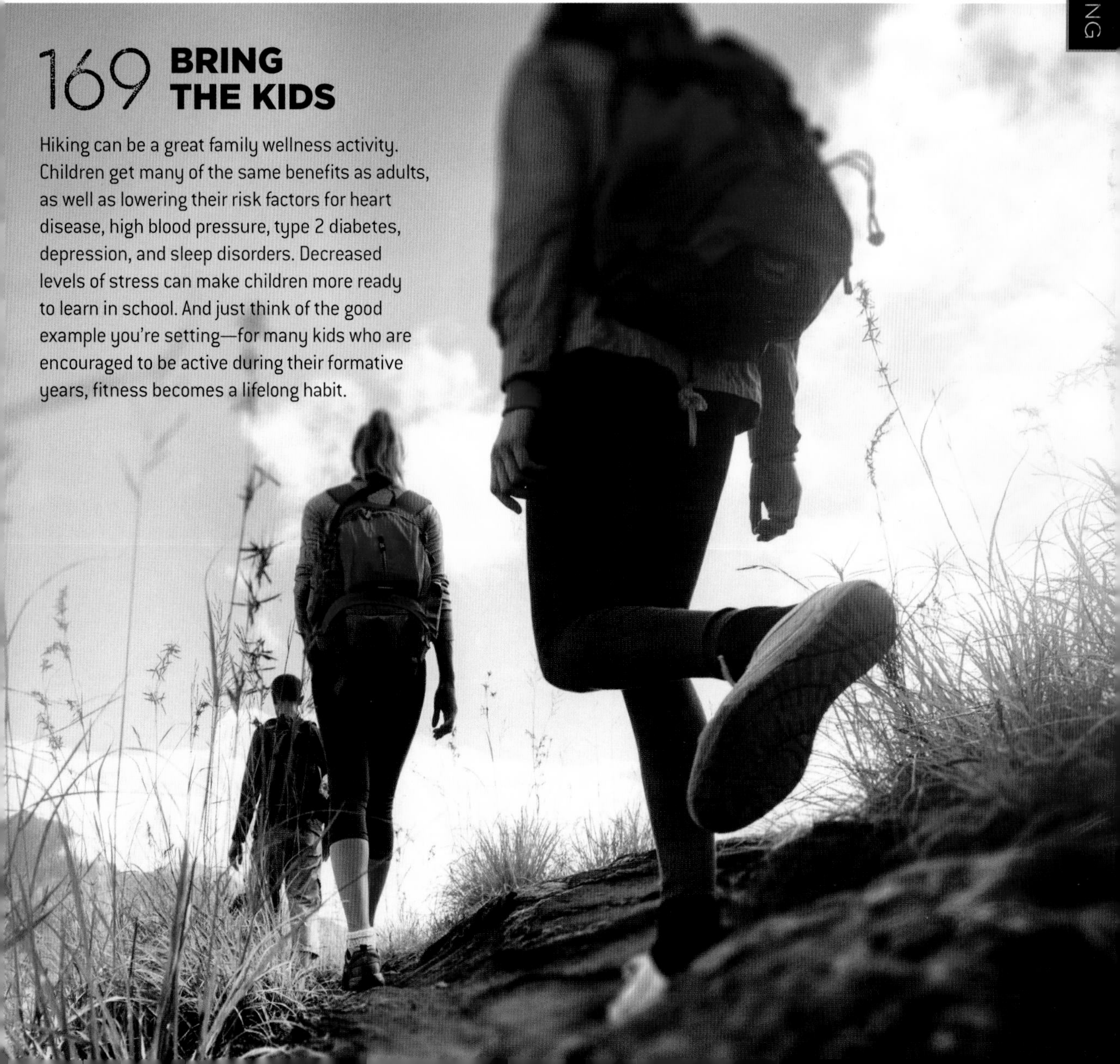

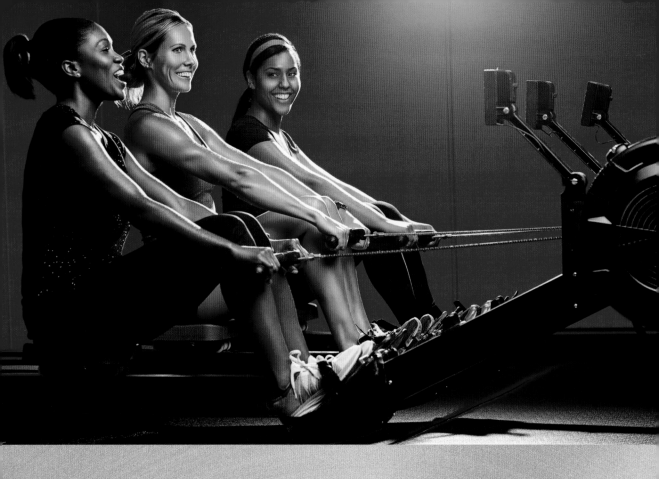

170 CLIMB ABOARD THE ROWER

The rowing machine, also called the indoor rower or ergometer, simulates the movement of oars propelling a watercraft. It can be used for exercise or as a training tool for competitive (crew) rowers. The machine typically consists of a seat, a foot stretcher, a handle or handles, and a mechanism to create resistance, using a flywheel, pistons, magnets, water, or air. There are three machine configurations: rowers upon which the foot stretcher and flywheel are fixed and only the seat moves, ones with both the seat and foot stretcher on a rail, and versions upon which the seat is fixed and only the foot stretcher slides backward and away from the rower.

Rowing steadily for 20 to 30 minutes provides the cardiovascular system with an intensive workout that really burns calories. Rowing is considered a low-impact activity—although there may be some risk to the lower back, it can be avoided by using the proper form. Rowing also works many muscle groups; as such it is often referred to as a strength-endurance activity.

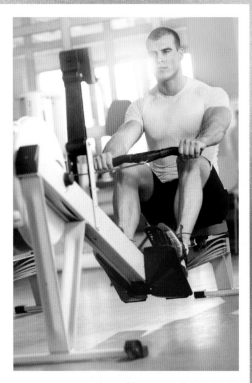

171 GET A WORKOUT IN NINE MINUTES

On a tight schedule? Then this "lightning" workout from Gold's Gym Fitness Institute specialist Robert Reames might be perfect for you. "With the Nine-Minute Express Cardio Rower," Reames explains, "you have an opportunity for a fast-action, heart-pumping workout that is time efficient and will challenge you, while delivering benefits afterward as well." You can also perform this five-step workout on a stationary bike, treadmill, elliptical trainer, or stair climber.

Because individual fitness levels vary so much, Reames devised a 1 to 5 perceived effort zone system for cardio workouts. Zone 1 is a light warm-up, and Zone 5 is nearly maximum effort—in other words, in Zone 1 you should barely break a sweat. In Zone 5, you'll be grabbing for the gym towel.

STEP 1 Warm up for 1 minute (Zone 1)

STEP 2 Warm up for 2 minutes (Zone 2)

STEP 3 High-intensity 3-minute blast (Zone 5)

STEP 4 Cool down for 2 minutes (Zone 2)

STEP 5 Cool down for 1 minute (Zone 1)

ZONE 1 ◌		**ZONE 4** ◌◌◌◌	
ZONE 2 ◌◌		**ZONE 5** ◌◌◌◌◌	
ZONE 3 ◌◌◌			

172 KEEP UP THE PACE

Endurance refers to your body's ability to exert itself and remain active over time, as well as withstand fatigue, stress, and pain. Endurance training helps you improve cardiovascular, respiratory, and muscular stamina when performing both aerobic and anaerobic exercises. It is most closely associated with swimming, bicycling, and running (the three events of triathlon competitions), yet team sports such as basketball, soccer, and lacrosse, as well as activities like hiking, skiing, and snowshoeing, also require endurance.

To build endurance the right way, Gold's Gym fitness experts suggest these training guidelines. Always schedule at least one day of recovery time per week.

TARGET A GOAL Research a charity race or a competition (or try for a personal best) that is three to six months away and train for it.

ADD 10 PERCENT Build stamina by gradually increasing your mileage; the rule of thumb is no more than 10 percent per week.

VARY THE PACE Interval training will raise your endurance to the next level. Aim for your fastest times at the end of your workout—so you learn pacing and how to finish strong.

TREAT FOOD AS FUEL Eat clean as you build staying power; check the nutrition guidelines in Chapter 1 of this book for more specific recommendations to suit your goals.

TRAIN FOR STRENGTH Building strength will help keep you injury free and ensure good form during workouts and competitions. Try timed circuits that simulate intervals, high weights with lower reps, and plyometrics.

173 GAUGE YOUR EXERTION

Here is another handy rule of thumb for measuring the degree of effort in an exercise: if the instructions call for "moderate" intensity, that means you should have the ability to talk but not sing during the activity. Moderate intensity allows you to continue on with the exercise, breathing at an even pace. If "vigorous" intensity is required, it means you can't say more than a few words without pausing for breath—this pace may only allow you to work for a few minutes at a time.

GYM etiquette

174 SPACE OUT

As we all know, the gym floor can get pretty crowded during peak hours. Common courtesy, as well as safety concerns, requires that we don't invade anyone else's space. Don't linger near areas or equipment, like the free weight section or cable crossover machine, where members need room to perform. If you are lifting, don't crowd others. Never exercise in high-traffic areas or by doorways where people need to walk. Don't park yourself so close to a weight rack that you prevent access. Before exercising in front of a mirror, make sure you aren't blocking someone else's view. And don't place your personal things on the equipment or set it down where people might be walking.

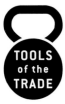

175 RIDE A STATIONARY BIKE

Also known as the exercise bike or exercycle, the stationary bicycle is a special-purpose exercise machine with a saddle, pedals, and handlebars—but no actual wheels—that offers outstanding cardio benefits. The pedals provide adjustable resistance to increase the intensity of the exercise; some models even allow the user to pedal backward to work the antagonist muscles. These bikes typically have a crankshaft and bottom bracket that powers a flywheel by means of a belt or chain. Specialized models that use weighted flywheels at the front are known as spinners. While spinners and stationary bikes imitate the form of a regular bike, recumbent bikes provide back support with low, chairlike seats.

Stationary bicycles are not only great for improving cardio fitness and achieving weight loss, they are also a long-valued tool of physical therapists, primarily because of the safe, low-impact, and effective workouts they provide. Exercise bikes are even used on the International Space Station; called veloergometers, they counter the cardiovascular de-conditioning that can occur in a microgravity environment.

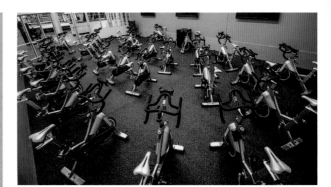

WHICH BIKE POSITION IS BEST?

Ask the EXPERT

Your goal when performing stationary bike cardio is to accelerate your metabolism, and there is little difference between cycling upright and pedaling in the recumbent position. A recumbent bike does, however, allow you to rest your lower-back muscles, while cycling without this feature forces you to use your core muscles to support your torso. For those with back pain, the recumbent style is probably the better choice—upright models can put too much stress on vulnerable lower-back muscles.

176 TRY A CYCLING CLASS

Gold's Gym, along with many others, offer intense cycle classes, where members on stationary bikes follow an instructor—often with the added bonus of lively music and lighting effects. These classes typically focus on metabolic intervals—from light to heavy resistance that challenges but rarely fatigue the muscles—making them ideal for most age groups. Cycle classes burn calories, improve cardiovascular health, offer an effective yet low-impact workout, and help you achieve tighter abs and toned, attractive legs. And if you can't always keep up, simply progress at your own pace. Cycling aficionados say they often leave class with high energy and a feeling of euphoria.

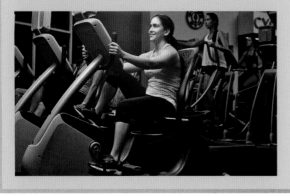

177 STAY HEALTHY

On any given day in the average gym, dozens of people will end up using a particular piece of equipment, whether it's a barbell or dumbbells, squat rack or bench press, treadmill or stationary bike—and a lot of those people are going to work up a sweat. With this in mind, bring a small hand towel with you and be sure to wipe down the area you've used. It's not only polite, but it also helps prevent the spread of colds or other communicable illnesses. Once again, courtesy and consideration are primary in the close confines of the gym floor.

178 HIT HIGH INTENSITY ON THE STATIONARY BIKE

The experts at Gold's Gym developed these four high-intensity interval (HIIT) workouts for the stationary bike. To perform this regimen, first determine your MHR, or maximum heart rate (see #137), and then add a new HIIT set to your cardio routine each week for four weeks, but avoid doing them on consecutive days.

WEEK 1: 30-MINUTE WORKOUTS

WORKOUT 1
- 10-minute warm-up at 65 percent MHR
- 30-second sprint at 75 percent MHR, then 60 seconds recovery at 65 percent MHR
- Repeat for 15 minutes
- 5-minute cool-down at 65 percent MHR

WORKOUT 2
- 10-minute warm-up at 65 percent MHR
- 30-second sprint at 75 percent MHR, then 90 seconds recovery at 65 percent MHR
- Repeat the above intervals for 15 minutes
- 5-minute cool-down at 65 percent MHR

WEEK 2: 35-MINUTE WORKOUTS

WORKOUT 1
- 10-minute warm-up at 65 percent MHR
- 30-second sprint at 80 percent MHR, then 60 seconds recovery at 65 percent MHR
- Repeat for 15 minutes
- 10-minute cool-down at 65 percent MHR

WORKOUT 2
- 10-minute warm-up at 65 percent MHR
- 30-second sprint at 80 percent MHR, then 90 seconds recovery at 65 percent MHR
- Repeat the above intervals for 15 minutes
- 10-minute cool-down at 65 percent MHR

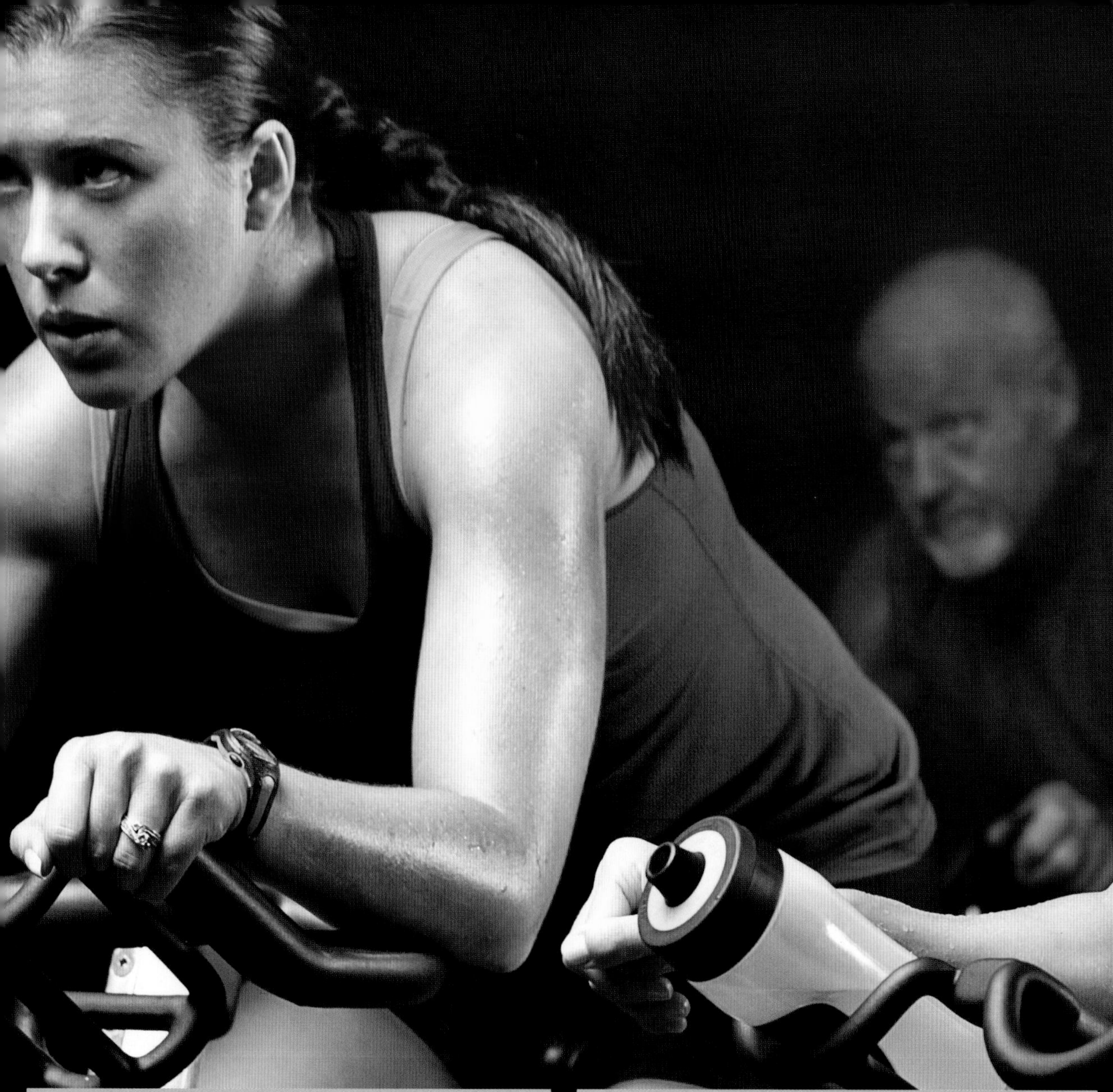

WEEK 3: 40-MINUTE WORKOUTS

WORKOUT 1
- 10-minute warm-up at 65 percent MHR
- 30-second sprint at 85 percent MHR, then 60 seconds recovery at 65 percent MHR
- Repeat for 15 minutes
- 15-minute cool-down at 65 percent MHR

WORKOUT 2
- 10-minute warm-up at 65 percent MHR
- 30-second sprint at 85 percent MHR, then 90 seconds recovery at 65 percent MHR
- Repeat for 15 minutes
- 15-minute cool-down at 65 percent MHR

WEEK 4: 45-MINUTE WORKOUTS

WORKOUT 1
- 10-minute warm-up at 65 percent MHR
- 45-second sprint at 85 percent MHR, then 90 seconds recovery at 65 percent MHR
- Repeat for 15 minutes
- 20-minute cool-down at 65 percent MHR

WORKOUT 2
- 10-minute warm-up at 65 percent MHR
- 45-second sprint at 85 percent MHR, then 120 seconds recovery at 65 percent MHR
- Repeat for 15 minutes
- 20-minute cool-down at 65 percent MHR

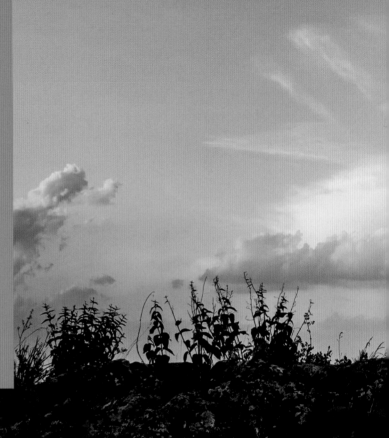

179 FREEWHEEL FOR FITNESS

Riding a traditional bicycle outdoors offers the same health benefits as using a stationary bike in the gym: a great cardio workout, effective body toning, increased weight loss, and low-impact exercise, but has the additional pluses of diverse scenery, variable terrain, and changing elevations. And then there is the longevity factor—many bike enthusiasts are able to keep riding well into their golden years.

A bicycle is also legitimate transportation. Try using your bike to commute to work, visit friends, head over to the library, or to do some shopping. Once you make bike-riding a regular part of your life, you will anticipate that rush of exhilaration whenever you pedal out into the street—a throwback, perhaps, to your childhood, when hopping onto a bicycle meant complete freedom.

If you want to track your biking action, try apps like Cyclemeter and Strava.

180 CHOOSE THE RIGHT WHEELS

There are currently a number of bicycle styles on the market. Before you decide on a model, ask yourself these questions: Where do you intend to ride, and will you ride for pleasure or for utility? Who do you normally ride with, and what sort of bikes do they use? (You'll want a bike that can keep up.) What was it that you like or dislike about previous bikes you've owned? To help you make the right choice, the following chart lists the most popular bike models and covers their features and uses.

TYPE	FEATURES	USAGE
ROAD BIKE	Lightweight frame; skinny tires; drop handlebars; multiple gears	Made to be ridden fast on smooth pavement; also called a "racer"
TOURING BIKE	More sturdy than a road bike; drop handlebars; low gear range	Made for distance riding; rider sits more upright than on a road bike; good for commuting
MOUNTAIN BIKE	Shock absorbers; rugged tires; flat or upright handlebars; very low gear range	Meant for off-road terrain and unpaved trails
HYBRID BIKE	Large padded seat; upright handlebars; medium tires with semi-smooth tread	Offers advantages of both a road and mountain bike; meant for casual riding around town or on bike paths
CRUISER BIKE	Large, comfortable seat; wide balloon tires; upright/swept-back handlebars; single speed/three speed; coaster brake	Made for casual riding and running errands in a high, upright position

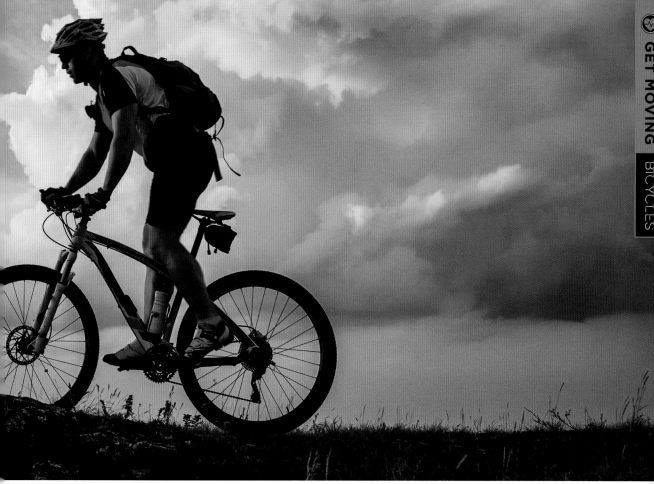

181 CRUISE IN COMFORT

Clothing for serious cyclists is form fitting and aerodynamic, typically made of fabrics that wick away moisture and keep you cool. Tops and shorts are also available in compression fabrics. Bike jerseys come in many patterns and colors—opt for the brighter ones that make you more visible to automobile and truck drivers. In winter, try a cold-weather jersey or a cycling jacket that allows your body to air out.

If you are planning a long ride or just intend to ride often, invest in bicycle shorts that feature a padded seat—your butt will thank you. For colder weather, try donning cycling tights over your shorts. You should also consider purchasing fingerless riding gloves, biking shoes that allow you to clip your feet into the bike pedals, and biking socks that wick moisture away and keep your feet aired out. Face masks made from compression material that keep your face warm and protected from the elements are another cold-weather option.

Always check the weather report before a ride to make sure you dress appropriately. And after your ride, wash your clothes immediately to prevent the growth of bacteria.

182 PROTECT YOUR HEAD

Always wear a helmet when cycling, even if you are just "going down the street." A minor fall could still cause serious brain injury. And don't cheap out at a discount store—buy a quality helmet from a reputable bike shop. If it's cold outside, you can use a helmet cover or wear an approved head covering under it—or both (it's dangerous to just add a beanie or bandana, as this may change the helmet's fit).

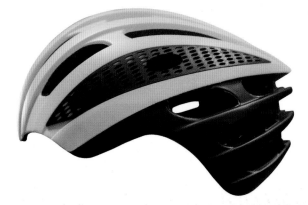

183 FUEL UP AND PEDAL

Make sure to eat breakfast before a morning ride—even if it's just instant oatmeal or a fruit smoothie—to replenish your liver's glycogen stores. During long rides, refuelling can be tricky; try filling your water bottle with a sports beverage, or stash healthy snacks in your jersey. Also make sure to eat some "recovery food," say, a sandwich and a salad, within 30 to 60 minutes of ending your ride. Needless to say, staying hydrated throughout your ride is key—take a sip at least every 15 minutes—then refill your bottle at ride's end, and drink it within an hour.

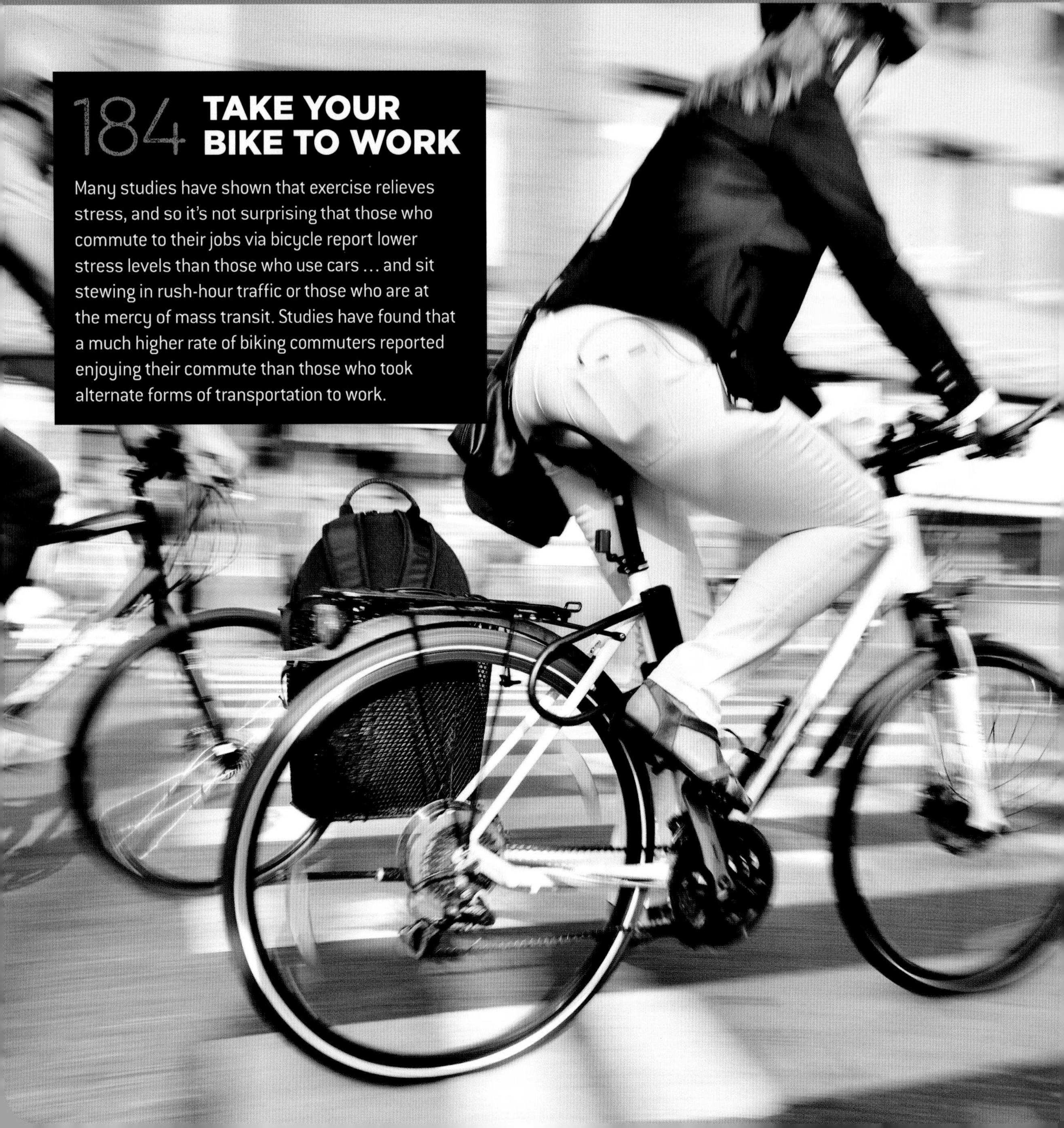

184 TAKE YOUR BIKE TO WORK

Many studies have shown that exercise relieves stress, and so it's not surprising that those who commute to their jobs via bicycle report lower stress levels than those who use cars … and sit stewing in rush-hour traffic or those who are at the mercy of mass transit. Studies have found that a much higher rate of biking commuters reported enjoying their commute than those who took alternate forms of transportation to work.

Every year, Gold's Gym teams up with the American Diabetes Association to sponsor Tour de Cure, a series of fund-raising cycling events held nationwide. If you participate in this kind of event, hours in the saddle can fatigue your abs and lower back, making it difficult for your to maintain strong cycling form.

Below are exercises that will help keep your core stabilized and solid. Cycling is a non-weight-bearing activity, so it's smart to also strength train your lower body. The more strength you build in your glutes, quads, and hamstrings, the easier it will be to power up hills and maintain an efficient pedal stroke.

Whether you plan to take part in a competitive cycling event or just want to be in shape for rides around town, incorporate the following exercises into your training program to improve your cycling efficiency and decrease your risk of injury.

For each exercise, aim for three sets of 20 reps each, with a 60-second rest between sets.

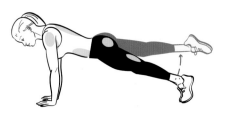

Ⓐ PLANK WITH GLUTE RAISE Combining the classic core-strengthening plank with a glute raise will target your abs, pecs, delts, back, glutes, and hamstrings.

HOW Get into plank position with arms extended as if you were about to do a push-up. (Too hard? Modify it by supporting your weight on your forearms.) With your glutes, lift your right leg off the floor until it's in line with your back, then pause. Lower, and keep alternating legs.

Ⓒ STABILITY BALL BRIDGE A bridge is another classic core stabilizer—and adding the stability ball amps up the stabilizing effect to work your abs, hips, quads, and glutes.

HOW Lie flat on the floor with your heels resting on a stability ball. Lift your hips off the floor as you pull the ball toward your butt with your feet. Roll the ball away from you, and lower your hips.

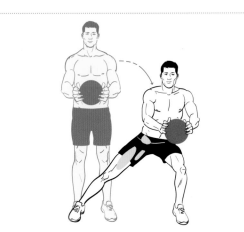

Ⓑ SIDE LUNGE This lunge adds emphasis to your hip adductors as it works your quads.

HOW Start with your feet together and your arms at your sides. Step sideways into a long lunge, keeping your planted leg straight. Bend your knee to form a 90-degree angle. Press back up with your bended leg, and return to the starting position. For an advanced version, hold a medicine ball.

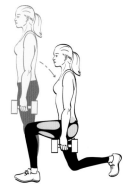

Ⓓ REVERSE LUNGE A reverse lunge will give you a thorough lower-body workout, targeting your hamstrings, quads, glutes, and hips.

HOW Start with feet shoulder-width apart. Lunge behind you with your right leg as if you were about to take a big step backward. Pause there for a moment, before returning to the starting position. Repeat with your left leg. For an advanced version, hold a pair of dumbbells at your sides.

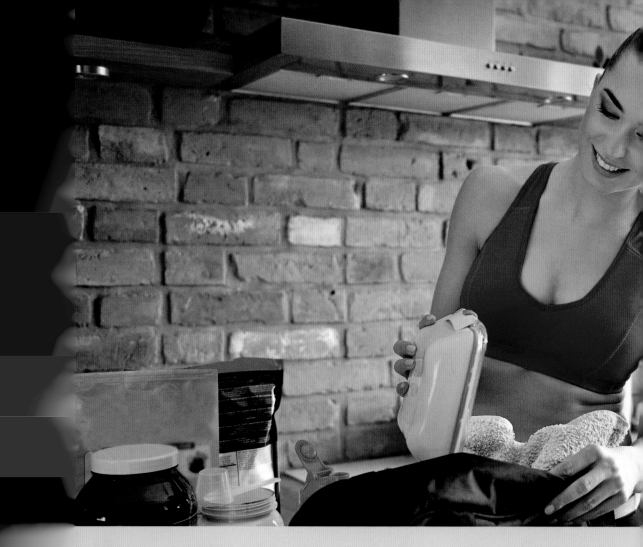

 PREPARE PROPER MEALS Now that you've begun to eliminate unhealthy eating habits, it's time to make sure that your meals are properly nutritious and geared to the increased caloric burn as you work your way through the escalating physical demands of the Challenge. Most gym members are trying to burn calories, but during an intense workout program such as the Challenge, you need to refuel your muscles, so that you can come back and do it again. Choosing the right foods is therefore just as vital as jettisoning the wrong foods.

It's especially important to eat within 30 to 90 minutes after a workout. This "meal" should replace roughly half the calories you burned off, with 60 percent of the calories coming from carbs, 25 percent from protein, and the final 15 percent from fats. This will replenish glycogen stores and shorten recovery time. For regular meals, stick with the 60 percent carbs guideline, but switch both the protein and fat to 15 or 20 percent.

SWAP UP TO HEALTHY CHOICES There are many alternatives to the unhealthy or high-calorie foods we commonly consume. For example, try swapping high-sodium salt with savory herbs and spices (some spices can actually speed up your metabolism). Or go for an English muffin in place of a hamburger bun and save 120 calories. Olive oil or mashed avocado are heart-healthy options to replace saturated fats like butter or margarine, and adding ground zucchini, mushrooms, or other veggies to ground-meat recipes adds fiber and vitamins. For dessert, skip the frozen yogurt, and toss a partially thawed frozen banana into the blender—add cocoa powder for a chocolaty delight.

Paula Castano
Female Winner, Ages 40-49

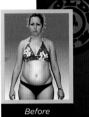
Before

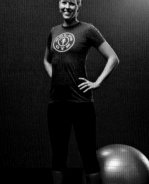

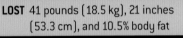

LOST 41 pounds (18.5 kg), 21 inches (53.3 cm), and 10.5% body fat

Paula was going through a number of family crises. "I lost my mom," Castano explains, "and my husband's job moved us to Missouri, which took me away from all of our friends and family." She found herself eating junk food as an emotional response. "I turned 40 extremely overweight and depressed." Then she discovered that her neighbor had done the Challenge the year before. He said he would support her if she decided to go for it.

"The day I signed up," she recalls, "I started eating clean. I went to the gym seven days a week and switched up my training methods to keep my body on its toes." Friends noticed the changes in her and asked if she was working out all the time. "No, I was only at the gym for an hour or so a day," she responded.

"It just comes down to commitment," she adds, "clean eating and consistent exercise. My neighbor, and my trainer Lindsay, who helped with my diet—I think of them as angels sent from God because they transformed my life."

DITCH THE PACKAGE
To upgrade your nutritional intake, avoid consuming anything that comes from a box, a bag, a can or a package—at least for a time. If a food item is processed, chances are it contains sugars, salt, thickeners, by-products, and chemical additives to ensure shelf life. Prepare your own meals from scratch using fresh, wholesome ingredients—you'll not only burn calories in the kitchen, you'll also control exactly what goes into each dish. Let the clerk at an organic grocery store guide you toward more nutritious options.

WINNER'S WORDS

"Nighttime was when I really liked to binge, so instead of eating, I drank flavored teas like peach or wild berry."

~ Paula Castano

8 TOOLS of the TRADE

186 CLIMB ABOARD

The stair climber, also known as the stair machine, stair stepper, tread-climber, or step machine, is a relatively recent addition to the fitness industry. It was introduced in 1983 and quickly became one of the most popular cardio machines in the gym. (For at-home use, Gold's Gym offers mini steppers.) If you are looking for a high-intensity workout that targets multiple fitness goals, there are few machines that can beat it.

By simulating the resistance movement of climbing stairs—which automatically raises your heart rate—the stair climber gives you a highly efficient cardiovascular workout. This machine also increases strength and body tone by engaging your major muscle groups, which boosts metabolism, burns calories, and aids in weight loss. Stair climbing engages your entire lower body, including the glutes, hamstrings, quadriceps, and calves. The stair climber also allows you to ascend indefinitely, thus avoiding any descent, which can be hard on your knees. It also helps to improve your balance, engaging your core muscles with every step, which will build core strength and endurance.

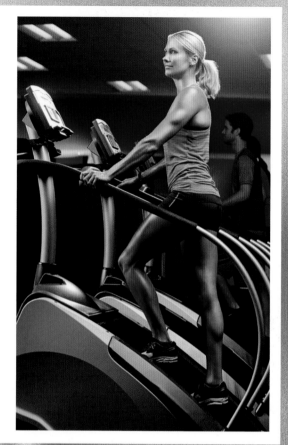

187 STEP LIVELY

If you take the right approach to utilizing the stair climber, you can reap maximum benefits.

USE CORRECT FORM Use the side handrails to maintain balance only; never rest your weight on them or, worse yet, cling to them so that you can move faster. Stand upright with your head up—don't lean forward as you ascend—and try not to swing your arms.

BEGIN SLOWLY Start at a gentle pace for five minutes, then slightly increase the speed or steps per minute. Work at this pace for 25 to 30 minutes. Cool down with another slow five minutes.

INTRODUCE INTERVALS Varying the speed on the climber can increase the calories you expend and your aerobic capacity. Simply alternate between bouts of high and low intensity after your warm-up: 60 seconds of fast short steps, 60 seconds at lower speed, 60 high, 60 low—for a total of 10 times. Finish with a cool-down.

VARY YOUR STEPS There are a number of ways you can alter your stepping motion. Try stepping up every two steps instead of one, relying on the handrail to maintain balance. Or set the machine at a low speed, and try walking backward, also holding the handrails.

MIX IT UP If you get bored working on the stair climber, try doing a HIIT routine combining the stepper with other cardio work. Start with a five-minute treadmill warm-up, then switch to the climber for 60 seconds, hop on a stationary bike for 60 seconds, jump rope for 60 seconds, get on the rowing machine, and row for 60 seconds, then return to the treadmill, and run for 60 seconds. Follow this procedure 10 times; finish with a five-minute cool-down on the treadmill.

INCREASE YOUR EFFORT Once your stair-climbing speed begins to feel comfortable, increase the number of steps per minute and/or your exercise duration to avoid a fitness plateau.

188 COMPLETE THE CIRCUIT

One way to avoid boredom at the gym is to explore circuit training—a mixed regimen of cardio workouts and strength exercises. You will typically perform from 10 to 25 reps, lasting from 30 seconds to three minutes, on a given machine or piece of equipment before moving to the next modality.

You can work out at a comfortable pace, or increase the number of reps or level of intensity. Whether you have athletic aspirations or simply want a comprehensive workout, circuit training is a great tool for engaging your major muscle groups. Include exercises that improve flexibility, such as stretches;

increase cardiovascular conditioning by running or jumping rope; and build your strength with activities such as lifting weights or using other resistance equipment.

In her 3-2-1 Method, Gold's Gym Fitness Institute member Ramona Braganza mixes short bursts of cardio with three sets of strength training to keep the workout interesting and the muscles guessing. This particular workout focuses on the triceps and legs, but you can easily sub in alternate exercises. Follow the chart below for cardio and strength circuit phases, and finish the workout with 5 to 10 minutes of stretching.

PHASE	EXERCISE	TIME/REPS	NOTES
CARDIO	Recumbent bike	10 minutes	Begin at a moderate pace for the first three minutes, then gradually increase pace and resistance for the remaining seven minutes.
CIRCUIT 1 (Perform three times, with one minute of rest between exercises.)	Incline bench press (#077D)	20 reps	Use a challenging but liftable weight.
	Reverse lunge (#185D)	20 reps for each leg	Don't drop so low that your knee touches the ground, it's too stressful for the joint.
	Bench dip (#102)	20 to 30 reps	For a more challenging variation, place your feet on a bench in front of you.
CARDIO	Treadmill	10 minutes	Jog at a moderate pace for one minute, then switch to intervals: Every 30 seconds, increase pace to a sprint, then return to normal speed. For the final five minutes, gradually increase the incline.
CIRCUIT 2 (Perform three times, with one minute of rest between exercises.)	Dumbbell fly (#077A)	20 reps	Use a challenging but liftable weight.
	Squat thrust (#124D)	15 reps	Want to make it more challenging? Add a pushup at the bottom at a jump at the top.
	Overhead triceps extension (#100A)	30 reps	Perform 10 reps for each arm, plus 10 reps for both arms together
CARDIO	Stair climber or elliptical trainer	10 minutes	Gradually increase resistance every 30 seconds until you are at about 80 percent heart rate.
CIRCUIT 3 (Perform once, with one minute of rest between exercises)	Basic crunch (#108A)	30 reps	Add a stability ball, BOSU ball or incline to crank up the intensity.
	Reverse crunch (#108B)	30 reps	Control your legs throughout the motion, don't just drop quickly back to starting position.
	Elbow plank (#109C)	Hold for 30 seconds to one minute	As long as your elbows are kept directly beneath your shoulders, your forearms can be positioned at whatever angle is most comfortable for you.
STRETCHING	Chapter 4 has a wide range of stretches.	5 to 10 minutes	Let the way you body feels guide which stretches you do, but be sure you do a full range.

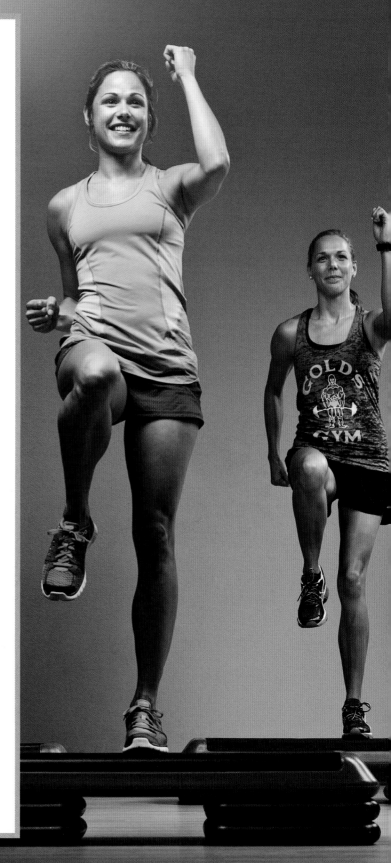

189 GET PHYSICAL

The allure of the aerobics class, popularized by the press and Hollywood in the 1980s (especially those iconic Jane Fonda exercise videos), has never faded. This kind of fitness class, which features rhythmic, strength and stretching moves performed to music, gives you high cardio value and can be a whole lot of fun. Instructors lead class members in routines composed of dancelike exercises that are geared to different levels of intensity and complexity. Most gyms offer a range of aerobics options designed for specific levels of experience, including seniors. A well-balanced class typically consists of 5 to 10 minutes of warming up, followed by 25 to 30 for cardio conditioning, 10 to 15 minutes of strength conditioning, followed by 5 to 8 minutes of cooling down, and then finally, 5 to 8 more for stretching and flexibility moves.

190 STEP IT UP!

Step aerobics adds an elevated platform, which you mount and dismount in tempo. Some platforms feature adjustable heights for varying levels of intensity. The basic 4-beat step calls for you to place one foot on the platform, followed by the other, and then removing them in the same order. Variations include the corner kick, repeater knee, T-step, lunge, straddle down, and many more. The class instructor combines these moves, typically timing them to 32 beats per set. More advanced choreography may include turns, mambos, and stomps. Class members learn the various steps during class and then perform two or three complete routines at the end.

Steps aerobics classes can help you burn fat and calories, reduce stress, foster good sleep habits, strengthen muscles, and create a sleek, streamlined physique. As with regular aerobics classes—or most any class—you can proceed at a comfortable pace until you feel strong enough to complete the entire routine.

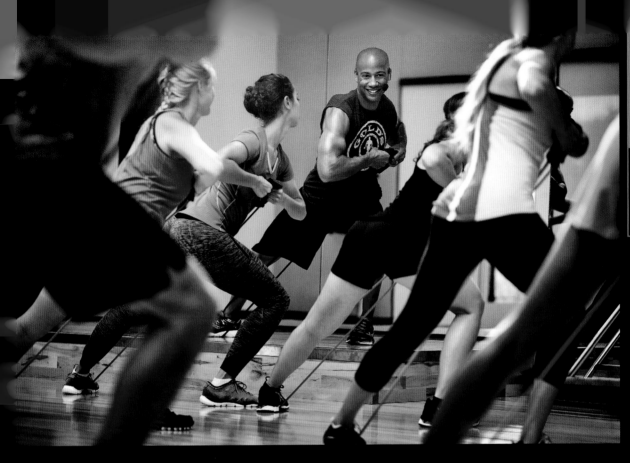

191 BE A CLASS ACT

Taking classes is a great way to tone up and have fun. Classes are perfect for beginners and those returning to the gym: you'll find motivation, accountability, and structure in a group that solo workouts lack. But with so many choices, which classes are right for you? Gold's Gym recommends first determining which fitness issues you want to tackle. To improve overall well-being, cardio classes—including fast-paced interval training—are the best way to go. Gold's Gym's BODYATTACK classes are high-energy interval training, sports-inspired cardio workouts for building strength and stamina. To give your physique a long, lean look with excellent flexibility, try yoga or Pilates classes, or try a dance-based class like BODYJAM. To burn calories, increase endurance, and build leg strength, take a cycling class. For a powerful full-body workout that lets you "unleash the beast," mixed martial arts could be the answer.

Once you decide to sample a class or two, you might need some guidance on how to get the most out of the experience. Here are some of the insights from the fitness experts at Gold's Gym for doing just that in any exercise class.

ARRIVE PREPARED Get to class early, bring a towel and a water bottle, and wear supportive sneakers and comfortable clothing that allows you to move easily. If you're new, introduce yourself to the instructor, and mention any injuries or medical conditions that could affect how you exercise.

FIND YOUR SPOT Try to position yourself near the front of the class with a good view of the instructor. If you have questions, ask them after class.

SEEK YOUR LEVEL During class, the instructor may show you how to modify an exercise to make it easier or more challenging. Do the version that you're more comfortable with.

TAKE A BREAK Some classes, like weight lifting, should not be taken two days in a row. Allow a cardio day or rest day in between—and try to add some yoga or stretching to the mix.

RESERVE JUDGMENT Attend at least three sessions of a new class before you decide whether or not it's for you. By the third session, you'll be familiar with the movements and exercises and can make an informed decision.

STAY FOR STRETCHING Don't bolt as soon as the heart-thumping action ends. Remember, you will burn more calories post workout if you allow yourself time to stretch.

192 LET THE MUSIC DRIVE YOU

As anyone who dances for a living can tell you, dancing takes a lot of hard work. Yet the many benefits of this activity make it worth all the effort—dancing offers a total-body workout that conditions the heart and lungs, strengthens your muscles and skeletal system, reduces bone loss, increases flexibility and joint mobility, and improves coordination and balance. There is also evidence that dancing can heighten your brainpower and improve your mental outlook. In research studies that compared dancers to non-dancers, there was evidence that dancing preserves both perceptual abilities and motor skills. What's not to love?

The rhythmic response we have to the beat of throbbing music is hard-wired into our brains. Musical vibrations actually light up timing circuits within our brains that prompt us to start moving in tempo. These same circuits are entwined with our communication and memory systems—which is why certain songs can evoke such a strong emotional response. This is also why working out to music can feel so fulfilling: it satisfies us on several levels. And the more time we spend dancing, the more our brains learn to release those pleasurable feelings, eventually leaving us with a more positive outlook and a strong sense of well-being.

193 SIGN UP FOR A DANCE CLASS

For years, fans of dance who wanted to learn ballet, jazz, tap, Latin, or ballroom dance had to go to specialized studios and pay for expensive classes—and rarely get a real cardio workout. Within the last few decades, gyms have begun offering "dancercise" classes that incorporate dance moves into fitness routines. Today, many gyms allow you to choose from a number of traditional dance classes—salsa, ballet or barre work, and swing. Or, if you're feeling particularly adventurous, you can find a workout based on pole dancing, jazz moves, or even acrobatics, to let your inner circus performer come out to play.

Gold's Gym offers a number of dance-inspired cardio classes that take inspiration from jazz, ballet, salsa, hip hop and other sources to create cardio routines that are fun and easy to follow. If you want to dance in your living room, you can also try Gold's Gym Dance Workout for the Nintendo Wii game system.

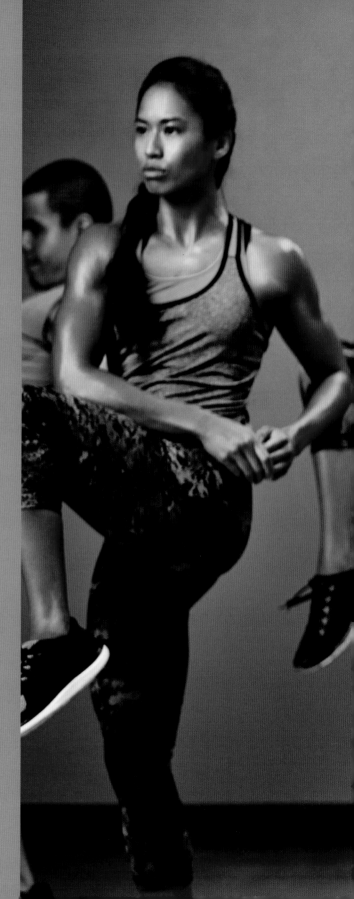

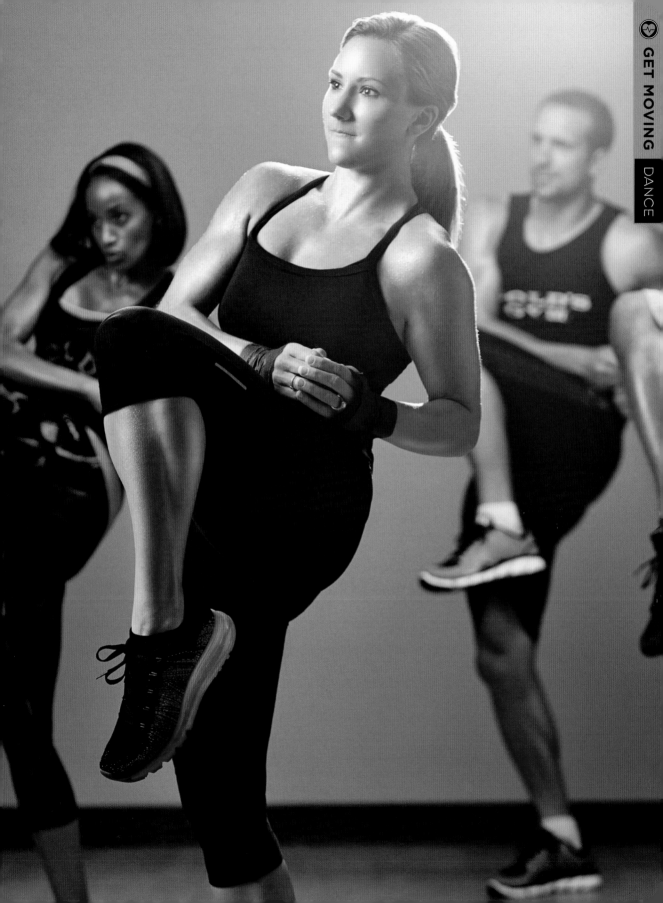

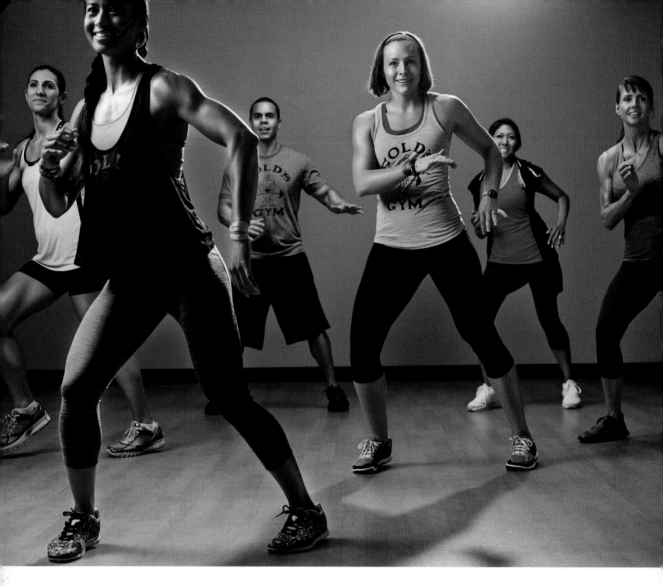

194 GET YOUR GROOVE ON

In addition to traditional dance classes, a new generation of dance-exercise has arisen, which incorporates choreographed dance moves with fitness routines and a fun atmosphere that feels more like a dance party than a traditional cardio class—while still burning hundreds of calories an hour.

Classes feature dance-based exercises to get your heart pumping and your body moving to the beat while often also incorporating some bodyweight-based resistance work for a full-body workout. If you're recovering from an injury, or just enjoy a different set of challenges, look for dance-based "aquarobics" classes that take place in a pool.

Whether you're trying out a class based on world music, old-school disco, or the latest club moves, be assured that you'll have fun whether or not you have any dance experience.

Popular classes are often crowded and heat up, so wear layers of clothing you can shed, and wear supportive shoes that allow you to easily pivot. And don't forget your heart-rate monitor to keep track of how hard you're working.

THINK about it

In a recent study, cardiac patients who danced three times a week for 20 minutes saw their heart health improve significantly more than patients who stuck to traditional cardio routines.

195 TUNE IN AND TONE

In conjunction with the annual March Music Madness contest, when gym members vote on their favorite workout tunes in a bracket-style competition, Gold's Gym has come up with four dance moves guaranteed to work your groove thing.

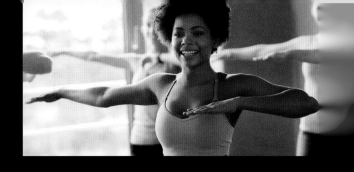

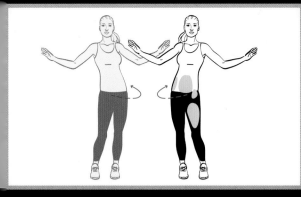

A BELLY DANCE This undulating Middle Eastern move works the abs, hips, and thighs. Repeat for two counts of eight.

HOW Stand with your feet hip-width apart, your knees slightly bent, and your arms extended to the sides. Create a figure 8 with your hips, swaying to the left front, side, and back,, and then sway to the right front, side, and back.

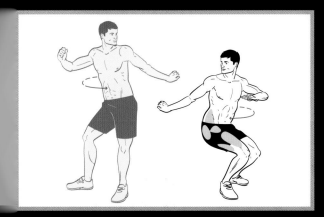

B THE TWIST Chubby Checker's dance sensation is still a great way to sculpt abs, thighs, and glutes. Perform one count of eight standing, and then lower to the floor twisting for one count of eight.

HOW Begin with your feet shoulder-width apart and your arms extended out to the sides. Stand on the balls of your feet, and rotate your hips, torso, and legs as a single unit while keeping your arms stationary. As you twist, lower yourself with knees bent and back straight until the backs of your quads hit your calves. Repeat, alternating directions.

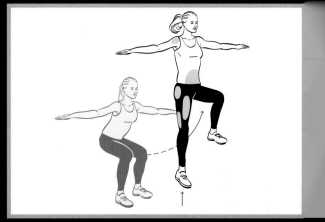

C KNEE KICKS These lively chorus line moves shape your legs, abs, and shoulders. Repeat with each leg four times.

HOW Stand tall, with your feet together and your arms out to the sides. Hop on both feet, and then lift your left leg with your knee bent to 90 degrees. Hop on both feet again, and then raise your right leg. You can also kick with a straight leg on each side, or alternate bent leg and straight leg.

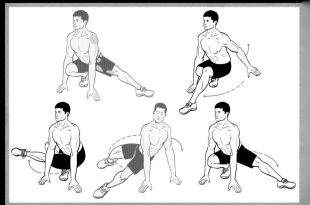

D PINWHEEL This old-school break dance move tones the upper body and works the core. Do eight sets on each side.

HOW Lower into a squat, with the back of your thighs touching your calves. Place both hands on the floor in front of you, and extend your left leg straight to the side. Move your left leg in a forward circle all the way around your body, lifting first your left arm, then the right arm, then the right foot (hopping over the leg.)

196 FUNCTION FLAWLESSLY

Functional training is a fairly recent trend, but it has a swarm of devotees, including personal trainers and athletic coaches. It teaches your muscles to work together to prepare them for daily tasks by simulating the movements you do at home, at work, and during sports, and can play a key role in rehabilitation after stroke or other brain trauma. The training emphasizes both upper- and lower-body muscles, as well as core stability. Think of functional training as a continuum of movement—humans run, jump, lift, pivot, push, pull, stand, climb, lunge—each activity incorporating smooth, rhythmic motions in the three cardinal planes of movement: sagittal (left and right), frontal (front and back) and transverse (upper and lower).

Improving functional strength means more than increasing the force produced by a group of muscles: it means improving coordination between the nervous and muscular systems. The goal is to transfer improvements in strength achieved in one movement so that the performance of another movement is enhanced by involving the whole neuromuscular system. This way, the brain learns to think in terms of whole motions rather than individual muscles. Here are some basic guidelines for beginning functional training.

EQUIPMENT Workout tools include: barbells, dumbbells, kettlebells, cable machines, medicine balls, body weight, stability balls, resistance bands, rocker and wobble boards, plyometric boxes, balance disks, sandbags, suspension straps, clubbells, macebells, and more.

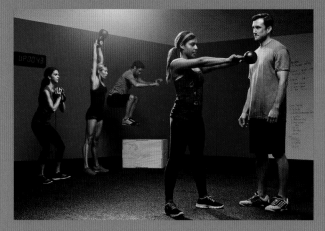

WORKOUT COMPONENTS You can customize functional training to fit your needs and goals. It should also integrate exercises that work on flexibility, core stability, balance, strength, and power. These exercises, in turn, need to be varied and become progressively more difficult. The manipulation of real-life objects should also factor into workouts, as should context-specific environments. Be sure to incorporate self-feedback, trainer, and/or therapist feedback.

RELATED REGIMENS You can find a range of programs out there that incorporate aspects of gymnastics, weight lifting, running, rowing, and other activities performed with relatively high intensity with the goal of improving both strength and cardiovascular health. Look into boot camp programs or other group classes at your gym to see what's available, or work with a personal trainer to develop your own personalized routine to suit your specific needs.

TOOLS of the TRADE

197 TAKE HOLD OF BATTLE ROPES

Battle ropes are thick, heavy, woven cables that are anchored to a wall or beam and used in pairs to provide intense cardio exercise while challenging your core. A stable core will keep your spine in line while you move your extremities, and by working each arm independently, these ropes eliminate strength imbalances while sculpting muscle. Rope workouts are relatively low impact and strengthen the abs, arms, shoulder, and legs. Other benefits include ease of use for a wide age and fitness range, speed (a vigorous workout takes 10 minutes), and effectiveness (burning about 10 calories a minute).

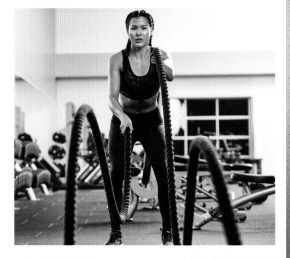

TARGETED
workout

198 GRAB A ROPE

Head to the gym, and grab a rope for a full-body workout that can build muscle, burn fat, and strengthen your entire frame.

Before you take hold of the rope, however, ask your Gold's Gym trainer for assistance. A consultation with a pro can help you to work safely. Without learning the proper form—if you aren't breathing properly or performing a move correctly—you may risk pain in your shoulders or other joints.

Once you know the basics, you can try these five battle rope exercises. For each, aim for three 30-second sets with a 30-second rest between sets.

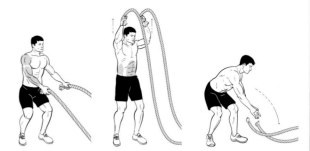

C CHOP AND LIFT This is a great core move, working the external obliques, in addition to your arms and shoulders.

HOW Start in a half-squat position, holding one rope in each hand pulled nearly taut. Bring the ropes above your head, and then slam them down to the floor on your right side, and release. Lift the ropes up again, pause for the briefest moment to ensure a straight spine, then slam them down on your left.

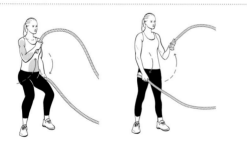

A DOUBLE WAVE Keep your body stable, focusing on an even tempo, as if you were beating a drum. This will work your forearms and shoulders, as well as your core.

HOW Start by standing in a half-squat position with your spine straight and your feet a little more than shoulder-width apart and your toes pointed forward. Take one rope in each hand, then move both arms up and down to create an even wave in the ropes.

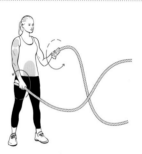

D DOUBLE DUTCH This is double Dutch for adults. It will work your forearms in addition to your shoulders and core.

HOW Take one rope in each hand, then make circles, your right arm going counter-clockwise and your left going clockwise. After each set, switch the direction.

B ALTERNATING WAVE This one emphasizes your arms and shoulders, with the benefit of being a full-body workout as well. The waves can be small if your arms are pumping faster or bigger to work your shoulders a little bit more.

HOW Stand in a half-squat position with your spine straight and your feet a little more than shoulder-width apart with your toes pointed forward. Take one rope in each hand and move one up while the other one is going down to create a wave, and then switch.

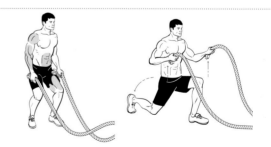

E DOUBLE WAVE WITH ALTERNATING STEP-BACK LUNGE This advanced move combines the double wave with a second exercise to give a total-body workout.

HOW Stand in a half-squat position with your spine straight and your feet a little more than shoulder-width apart, your toes pointed forward. Take one rope in each hand, and move both arms up and down to create a wave. At the same time, step back with your right foot, and bring your knee to the floor. Rise, and then repeat the sequence with your left leg.

199 TRAIN LIKE A NAVY SEAL

It might be hard to believe that a hard-core workout for elite military groups could be adapted for the masses, but that is exactly what a former Navy SEAL did when he developed TRX training, which stands for total body resistance exercise. These suspension-based workouts help you to develop flexibility, power, balance, and core stability. This form of functional training increases the body's capacity to take on the stresses of life by improving performance and preventing injuries. With practice, your body will be more balanced and have better motor skills. All that's needed for TRX training is a simple strap system that hooks on to an anchor point strong enough to hold your weight.

The best introduction to this workout is to take a group TRX class at a Gold's Gym so that a licensed instructor can show you the proper form and provide a guided session designed to help you progress at your own pace. With more than 300 different exercises to choose from, you can put together a TRX workout that can help you achieve a full-body workout in 30 minutes. And you don't need to be in peak shape to try out TRX—it can be adapted to any fitness level or exercise group.

NEW USER Quickly develops power and endurance.
POST-REHAB USER Allows for control that can help stabilize the body and provide support when you resume training.
SENIOR USER Strengthens muscles and increases balance and coordination.
ADVANCED USER Challenges you with unusual patterns that force the body to train in a multidimensional way.

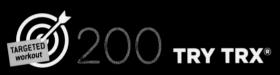

TARGETED workout 200 **TRY TRX®**

This six-move TRX® workout will benefit your entire body, and once you have the prerequisite strength and muscle endurance to maintain proper posture safely during the applied movements, you can take TRX anywhere. The straps are highly mobile and easy to set up. Bring them with you to the gym, or throw them in a suitcase for a work trip. Just attach them to any secure anchor point overhead. The ideal height is about nine feet (2.7 m). You can secure a strap to equipment such as a pull-bar, cable crossover piece, low supporting rafters, or basketball hoop, as long as there is enough ground space beneath your anchor point. You can even secure it to a door if you're working out at home.

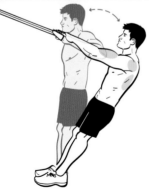

Ⓐ SUSPENDED HIGH ROW The row targets your upper back, lats, biceps, and deltoids. Perform two sets of 12 reps.

HOW Stand with your feet hip-width apart. Face the anchor point. Grab the handles of the straps. Your elbows should be raised and parallel with your shoulders. Lean back, and straighten your arms out, and then pull yourself up into an upright standing position with your upper back muscles. Your back should be straight, shoulders down, and elbows out.

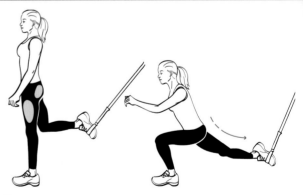

Ⓑ SUSPENDED REVERSE LUNGE This lunge targets your glutes and quads. Perform two set of 12 to 15 reps on each leg.

HOW Stand facing away from the anchor point. Place one foot in the strap. You may need to hold on to a trainer or bar to maintain balance. Bend your front knee to lower your body into a lunge position, and straighten the back leg while you move. Extend your arms forward; keep your chin up and eyes looking straight ahead.

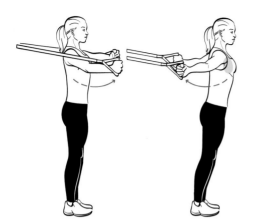

C SUSPENDED CHEST FLY This version of a fly targets your chest muscles. Perform two sets of 15 to 20 reps.

HOW If you can't do a push-up, this is a good place to start training your pecs. Begin facing away from the anchor point. Place one hand on each handle. Extend both arms out to the sides. Lean forward. Keep your arms straight or slightly bent at the elbow. Allow the straps to pull your arms back slightly, and then use your chest muscles to pull your arms together slightly. Challenge yourself by taking a small step or two forward before the next set, deepening the angle and increasing the resistance.

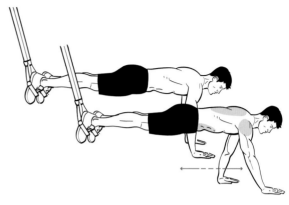

E SUSPENDED ALLIGATOR CRAWL This crawl will stabilize your rotator cuffs, back, and core muscles. Perform two to three sets, moving continuously for 15 to 20 seconds.

HOW Start by placing your feet in the straps. Lie facedown with your hands on the floor by your shoulders. Press into a push-up position. Walk four steps forward on your hands, then return by walking the same number of steps back to your starting position. Your goal is to maintain core stability with your body straight and aligned with no sway for 15 to 20 seconds without dropping. Do not let your lower-back arch or sag during the movements.

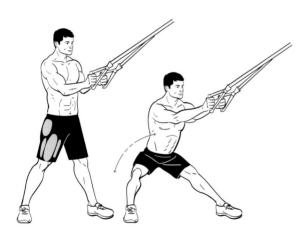

D SUSPENDED LATERAL LUNGE This lunge variation strengthens your glutes, quadriceps, and inner and outer thighs. Perform three sets of 10 to 12 reps on each side.

HOW Place your feet shoulder-width apart, and face the anchor point. Grab the handles, keeping your arms extended in front of you. Take one step to your right, and bend that knee. Try to control your motion as well as the depth of the knee bend. Your body should be aligned and straight. Squeeze your inner thighs, glutes, and quadriceps to push back up to a starting position. Alternate sides.

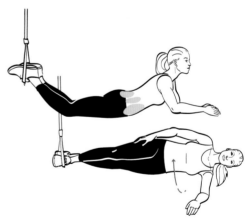

F SUSPENDED SIDE PLANK This plank exercise strengthens your abdominals, lower-back muscles, and obliques. Perform two sets, 30 seconds for each side

HOW Begin facedown on the floor with both feet in the straps and your elbows resting on the floor or a mat. Rotate to one side. Rest on your elbow, and hold that position as long as possible. Try to maintain the position for 30 seconds, lifting your body off the floor—hips and back in alignment. Use your internal and external obliques to keep your body held in a long, straight line.

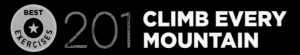

BEST EXERCISES 201 CLIMB EVERY MOUNTAIN

Long a favorite with military special forces and functional training devotees, the mountain climber exercise gives you a full-body workout. Its inspiration is real mountain climbing, which calls for impressive amounts of core strength and muscle endurance. Performing mountain climbers will work a long list of muscles: your delts, biceps, triceps, pecs, obliques, rectus abdominis, lower trapezius, lats, quadriceps, hamstrings, hip adductors, and hip abductors. It's also an effective cardio move that can improve circulation and burn calories, while helping you develop better flexibility, coordination, and range of motion. This is also a highly versatile exercise with scores of variations that you can include in your warm-up, cardio, or strength sessions. Here are just a few versions.

Ⓐ MOUNTAIN CLIMBER

WHY The key to proper form is keeping your core tight. To place less strain on your back, bring your knee up using your lower ab muscles.

HOW Start in a plank position, with your hands just wider than shoulder-width apart, body straight out, core tight. While balancing on your toes, bring your right knee toward your chest, and then quickly alternate legs as if you were running continuously.

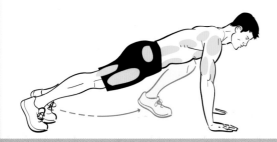

Ⓑ CROSS-BODY MOUNTAIN CLIMBER

WHY This version adds a leg and torso rotation that will add some emphasis to your obliques and increase your hip flexibility.

HOW Start in a plank position, with your hands just wider than shoulder-width apart, body straight out, and core tight. Raise up your right foot, and bring your right knee toward your left shoulder. Return to the starting position, and then quickly alternate legs.

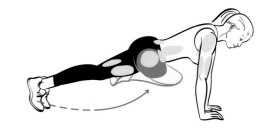

Ⓒ BOSU MOUNTAIN CLIMBER

WHY The instability of the BOSU ball adds a greater challenge to the basic mountain climber, forcing you to up the engagement of your core muscles.

HOW Place a BOSU ball dome-side down, and then get into a plank position with your shoulders directly over your wrists. Keeping your hips in place and your core tight, bring your right knee toward your chest, and then quickly alternate legs.

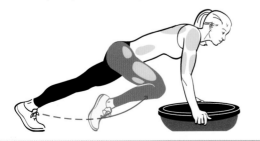

Ⓓ SLIDING MOUNTAIN CLIMBER

WHY This variation forces you to work against the friction of a glider, increasing the challenge to your core and leg muscles.

HOW Place a sliding disc, paper plate or small towel under each foot. Move into a plank position, with your hands just wider than shoulder-width apart. Bring your right knee toward your chest, pulling the sliding disc, and then quickly alternate legs.

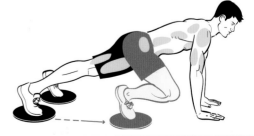

202 GO TO BOOT CAMP

Boot camp–style resistance training (in other words, nonstop, heart-pounding workouts that employ a mix of medicine balls, kettlebells, and your own body weight) is at the heart of the functional fitness craze. These kinds of workouts have a history of real results and can help you get in show-off shape. The key to these workouts is to keep your heart rate high by moving constantly, but make sure to rest as instructed between sets. To make the training more fun and motivating, get a partner to join you.

To get you started with functional training, here's a six-move workout that can be done at the gym. Do the six activities in a circuit, meaning you perform one set of an exercise, and then move on to the next, in the order shown. Follow the guidelines for each level on the chart to the right.

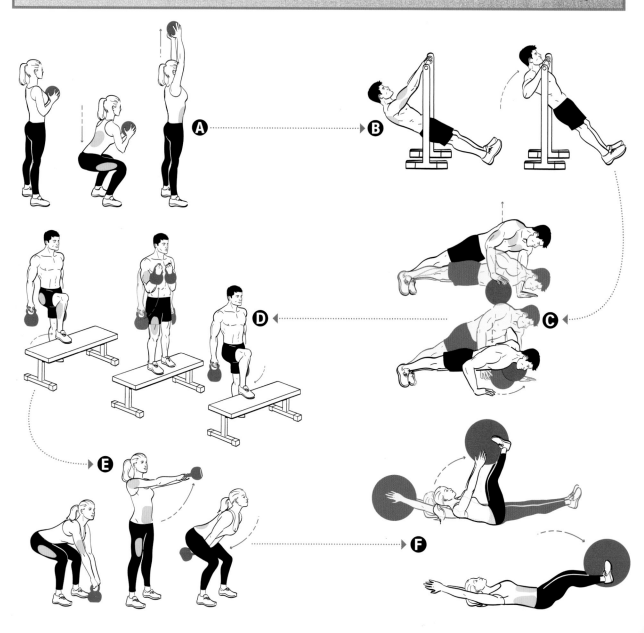

Ⓐ SQUAT PRESS WITH MEDICINE BALL Squat with a medicine ball held in front of your chest. Stand, and then press the medicine ball above your head until your arms are fully extended. Bring the ball back to your chest.

Ⓑ INVERTED BACK ROW Sit under a bar set just above where you can reach it from the floor, and grab it with an overhand grip. Walk your feet forward until you can lean back with your heels on the floor with your neck and chest above the bar. Slowly lower, and then pull back up.

Ⓒ ALTERNATING PUSH-UP WITH MEDICINE BALL Get in a push-up position. Place the medicine ball under your right hand. Lower your torso toward the floor; as you push back up, roll the medicine ball from your right hand to your left.

Ⓓ STEP-UPS WITH KETTLEBELLS Stand facing a bench with a kettlebell in each hand. Step onto the bench with your right foot, and then bring your left up to meet it. Curl the kettlebells up to your chest, and then lower them. Return your left foot to the floor, keeping your right foot on the bench. Repeat with your left foot, then switch sides, stepping up with your left foot to begin.

Ⓔ KETTLEBELL SWINGS Place a kettlebell between your feet. Bend down as if sitting, pick it up, snap your hips, and swing it up to chest level.

Ⓕ BALL PASS CRUNCH Lie on your back holding a stability ball above your head. In one motion, lift your legs, arms, and upper body off the floor, and place the ball between your legs. Lower your arms and legs, and then repeat the motion, passing the ball from your legs back to your hands.

GET IT DONE Boot camp–style training lets you go through a total-body workout in a short time. People want to get in their exercise and then get out of the gym. And you don't get bored: you have a set of exercises, and you go quickly from one to the next, so it keeps you engaged. Classic strength training is more start, stop—like lift a weight, put it down, stop, wait, start again—and is normally aimed at one major muscle group at a time. That takes a great deal more time and dedication. With this kind of training you don't stop, so it's a quicker workout, and many of the exercises work the entire body.

GEAR UP Your best resistance tool is just your own body weight—using only that is really intense. Then, you also use kettlebells, medicine balls, resistance bands, battle ropes, and box steps.

START SLOW Make sure you can comfortably lift a weight. After you've done eight or nine reps, you should still be able to lift the weight, even though your body is telling you not to.

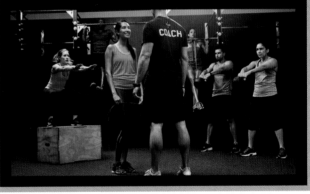

LEVEL/TIME	ROUND 1	ROUND 2	ROUND 3	ROUND 4	ROUND 5
BEGINNER 20 minutes	10 reps of each **Rest** 1 to 3 minutes until you get your breath back.	10 reps of each (Try to work up to 15 reps this round.)	Once you can perform 15 reps of each, move up to Intermediate.	—	—
INTERMEDIATE 45 minutes	15 reps of each **Rest** 30 to 90 seconds, depending on how you feel.	20 reps of each **Rest** 30 to 90 seconds, depending on how you feel	25 reps	Once you can perform 25 reps, move up to Advanced.	—
ADVANCED 45 minutes	15 reps of each **Rest** 30 seconds if you need to—if not, keep going.	20 reps of each **Rest** 30 seconds if you need to—if not, keep going.	25 reps of each **Rest** 30 seconds if you need to—if not, keep going.	20 reps of each **Rest** 30 seconds if you need to—if not, keep going.	15 reps of each

203 PRACTICE MARTIAL ARTS

Although hand-to-hand martial arts, such as wrestling and grappling—which simulated combat situations—were practiced for millennia, in the late 19th century Asian-style martial arts began to spread beyond their national borders. Adults and youngsters in many parts of the globe eventually embraced disciplines such as jiu jitsu and judo from Japan, kung fu from China, and taekwondo from Korea. The TV series *Kung Fu* and the movie *The Karate Kid,* plus a host of Asian martial arts films, helped broaden the appeal during the 1960s and '70s. Soon dojos (training facilities—the Japanese term actually translates as "place of the way") began to crop up in many cities. The practice of these martial arts disciplines not only provides a useful fitness tool for adults, many behaviorists discovered that they help children release much of their pent-up energy.

Today, people of all ages pursue a range of martial arts. Enlightened martial artists like to point out that the study of any style will ultimately benefit the student. Some of the most popular options are listed below.

AIKIDO Practitioners of this Japanese grappling art learn to flow with the motion of the attacker.

JUDO The goal of this relatively modern Japanese defensive art is to throw the opponent to the ground or grapple with them until they are immobile. Judo and taekwondo are the only Asian martial arts sanctioned by the Olympic Games.

JIU JITSU This Japanese discipline is aimed at defeating an armed or armored opponent with no weapon or only a short weapon. The Brazilian version, with its throws, takedowns, and sweeps, provides a good method of self-defense for women.

KARATE Developed in Okinawa, Japan, karate stresses striking techniques such as punching, kicking, knee and elbow strikes, and open-hand techniques.

KRAV MAGA Developed in Israel, this form of hand-to-hand combat, which combines wrestling, grappling, and striking techniques, is known for its lack of rules and its variety of brutal counterattacks.

KUNG FU OR WUSHU These are the umbrella terms for the hundreds of defensive arts of China. There are scores of styles or schools, and some mimic animal movements, such as Eagle Claw, Five Animals (Shaolin), Monkey, Praying Mantis, and Wing Chun. The Shaolin form of kung fu is regarded as one of the first codified styles of Chinese martial arts.

MUAY THAI (THAI BOXING) This tough Thailand discipline uses stand-up striking and clinching techniques incorporating punching, kicking, and knee and elbow strikes—involving eight points of contact—as well as fight strategies.

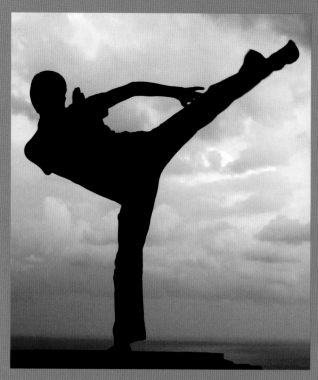

TAEKWONDO The popular Korean art of self-defense dates back by more than 2,000 years. It utilizes punches, blocks, takedowns, throws, and open-hand strikes, and it emphasizes high kicks requiring explosive action, speed, and agility.

WRESTLING While wrestling offers a great cardio workout, it also features dangerous takedowns and body manipulations, and so is not for the injury prone.

204 MIX IT UP WITH MMA

Mixed martial arts (MMA) is a full-contact sport that combines several martial- and nonmartial-arts disciplines that, over time, have morphed into one cohesive style. This is a demanding pursuit, requiring familiarity with many skills and positions, as well as speed, endurance, strength, and agility. Practitioners typically have to master Brazilian jiu jitsu, wrestling, muay Thai, and aspects of taekwondo. As a result, MMA athletes are among the fittest in the world. Most gyms support the study of MMA without the actual fighting matches, although light sparring is allowed. Many Gold's Gyms offer classes in MMA—check their website for a gym near you, and click on the class schedule to check for days and times.

205 TRY OUT KICKBOXING

Karate, a striking art incorporating punching, kicking, knee and elbow strikes, and karate-chop "knife hands," is one of the most popular martial arts. Karate became widely known in North America after World War II servicemen studied it in Asia and opened karate schools back home.

In the 1960s, a new discipline arose in Japan, dubbed kickboxing. This concept encompassed stand-up combat sports that incorporate both kicking and punching, and developed from karate as well as Muay Thai and Western boxing. At first, kickboxing was practiced as a form of self-defense and a competitive sport, then as a fitness regimen. In the 1990s, a more aerobics-friendly version was developed called Tae Bo.

As a fitness tool, kickboxing with a heavy bag provides a terrific workout that increases heart rate, burns fat, and builds muscle. Punches employed include the jab, cross, hook, and uppercut, and kicks include the front, side, and roundhouse. The average person will expend 800 to 1,200 calories per class. No wonder trainers warn newbies that they are likely to feel exhausted after their first few workouts, and, meanwhile, their metabolism will hum along 10 to 15 percent higher than normal for the next 18 hours.

Gold's Gym offers kickboxing classes in some locations; check their website for days and times. Here are some tips for starting out (and don't forget to bring a towel).

GATHER YOUR GEAR Wear loose workout clothing and shoes that allow you to move from side to side.

WARM UP Before approaching the weight bag, perform a few minutes of light calisthenics, some stretching, and body-weight exercises.

ADOPT A FIGHTING STANCE Before you land a punch, practice the basic stance in the mirror until you get it right. Start with feet shoulder-width apart, knees slightly bent. Hold your right hand up near your ear, and keep your left hand in front of your face with elbows down, near your body.

LEARN TO PUNCH A jab is quick surprise punch aimed at an imaginary nose. A cross is a straight punch thrown from the rear hand. A hook is a circular punch from the lead hand, with a cheek or ear being the imaginary target. An uppercut is a thrusting punch to the chin delivered from the rear hand, fist pointing at the ceiling.

KICK UP YOUR HEELS The basic front kick is delivered with the heel—imagine kicking a door closed using your raised foot. The roundhouse kick is circular, with your leg moving in an arc, as if you were slapping the target with your shoelaces. The intimidating side kick is powered by the glutes; think of it as kicking through a target with your heel.

206 DE-STRESS WITH TAI CHI

T'ai chi ch'uan is one of more than 300 Chinese martial arts. There are many forms of tai chi, both traditional and modern, but the five most practiced, Yang, Chen, Wu, Sun, and Woo, were derived from the original Chen family style. Initially tai chi was performed as defensive training, with an emphasis on strength, speed, flexibility, and balance—in Mandarin, the name literally translates as "supreme ultimate boxing." Over time, it evolved into a slow, soft, gentle form of exercise, with flowing motions, that can be practiced by those of all ages. Advocates call it the "ultimate low-impact workout."

Tai chi's health benefits include the ability to elevate heart rate, ease stress levels, lower blood pressure, improve balance, posture, and circulation, and even increase longevity. According to gait and balance experts, tai chi offers the best biomechanical scenarios for keeping a person stable. Perhaps the nicest benefit, users (even seniors) tend to leave their sessions feeling empowered.

Some Gold's Gym locations offer classes in tai chi; check their website for places and dates.

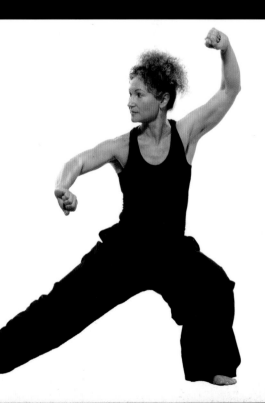

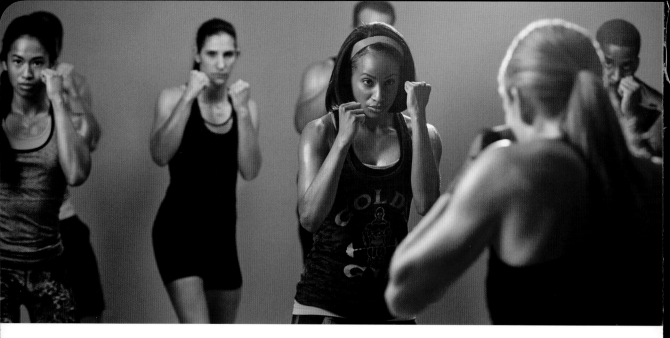

207 PUNCH IT OUT

Boxing—it's not just for pugilists anymore. Nope, not since gymgoers of all kinds discovered that learning basic boxing moves in a class or taking repeated shots at the heavy bag is a great way to tone up, increase cardiovascular fitness and coordination, and build muscle—not to mention that they also get to work off a ton of aggression and stress.

The sport of boxing, which is roughly 80 percent anaerobic and 20 percent aerobic, targets the entire body and furnishes what might just be the ultimate HIIT workout. It is a demanding pursuit that requires strong endurance, hand-eye coordination, power, and a certain amount of nerve—even if you don't ever actually climb into a ring.

Here are some basic tips to follow to make sure you are "fighting in the proper weight class."

GET TONED The toning effects of boxing comes from the way in which you punch—your lower-back and abdominal muscles provide power by initiating an explosive hip turn, while your arms and shoulders bear the brunt of the muscle recruitment that's needed to strike hard and fast. A consistent boxing regimen can add significant definition to these areas and even create mass.

TAKE A CLASS If the thought of boxing intimidates you, try learning the basic moves—punches, footwork, and defensive maneuvers—in a class with a qualified instructor. And don't be afraid: there is no contact between you and other participants in the class: these sessions are meant to hone your technique, but they can also be a great body workout and a ton of fun.

FIND A TRAINER Even if you aren't scheduling any Golden Gloves matches, consider visiting a boxing gym and booking a few hours with a real trainer, someone who can teach you how to strike properly. Boxing can be a jarring, contact-heavy activity, and you shouldn't just find a heavy bag and start whaling on it. A good coach can help you develop the right technique, teach you to pace yourself, cut down your risk of injury, and help keep you from developing bad habits.

DO YOUR RESEARCH If you can't hire a pro trainer, research technique as much as you can. Remember that the average human body is not geared to repeatedly generate these types of forces. Furthermore, maintaining the proper technique allows you to benefit from a sport that provides multiple levels of fitness.

DANCE AND JAB Begin by dancing around the bag and applying the basic punches—the hook, the cross, and the uppercut—and incorporating the jab (see #205). After three rounds or so, spend one round just using the jab, making sure to perfect your strike. (This is the most important punch in boxing because it sets up everything else you do.)

SWITCH SIDES After your jab-only round, try switching hands. If you are right-handed, now lead with your left. This is beneficial to your body and your central nervous system, and teaches you how to deploy your jab and power punches with both hands.

PICK UP THE PACE Once you have mastered the rhythm you need to complete your individual rounds, increase the intensity during the last 30 seconds of each round. Stay in place instead of dancing, and use punishing power punches on the bag.

208 THINK INSIDE THE BOXING RING

Suppose you decide you actually want to engage in some sparring with a partner to experience the thrill of taking a punch and returning one. How would you go about arranging it? The good news is that some gyms—including the Gold's Gym facility in Los Angeles, California—feature a boxing ring. Another alternative is to contact a boxing gym, and ask if they know of other amateur boxers who are looking to spar. (There are two types of boxing gyms, those that cater to boxers-in-training and those that offer boxing to other athletes as a way to get in shape. You want the former, although some gyms do both.) Obviously, you don't want to get into the ring with a prizefighter, but there are bound to be other boxers at your level who are also looking for ring experience. Or contact a pro trainer, if you used one, and ask him to check around for potential partners.

There are also new boxing franchises opening up that are moving away from the gritty, sweaty, old-school boxing facilities of the *Rocky* films and creating fresh athletic environments that are welcoming to almost everyone.

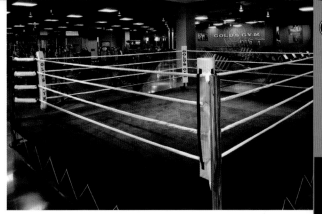

209 BOX YOUR SHADOW

Shadow boxing enables you to practice the boxing techniques that you've learned, as well as allow you to try out various combinations of punches. You simply box in front of a mirror, imagining your reflection as your opponent. It's great as a warm-up or a way to fill your time if the heavy bag is in use. It also let you check your stance and footwork and to make sure you are properly keeping your guard up.

210 BECOME BOXER FIT

Boxing itself is a type of exercise, but it is a taxing and demanding one, so it may make sense to train yourself up to it with other forms of exercise. Consider a combination of upper-body resistance work and skipping, running, jumping rope, calisthenics, and wind sprints.

211 TAKE THE PLUNGE

Like biking and rowing, swimming is an athletic discipline that gives the whole body a workout, benefiting the cardiovascular and respiratory system, the core, arms, shoulders, legs, glutes, and back. And because humans are buoyant in water, aquatic workouts—whether done swimming or standing—tend to be low impact, even gentle on the body. This makes swimming ideal for exercising when recovering from injury. On the other hand, the weight of water offers resistance as you move through it, creating an opportunity for building strength. Another plus is that even though you are raising your heart rate, the water keeps your body cool, so you can perform longer than, say, running on a hot, humid day. Fans of swimming also point out that it is fun and relaxing.

If you make swimming part of your fitness regimen, plan on spending two and half hours in the water each week. Warm up with some light cardio and stretches, then start with a low-to medium-intensity workout of laps. Gradually build up the impact by swimming faster or by doing more laps. Ideally, you want to swim in a pool, where you can monitor your mileage, but if you go for a swim in the ocean or a lake, plot the distance between two landmarks on shore, and swim between them. In open water, never swim alone, and make sure you know how to stay safe when dealing with currents.

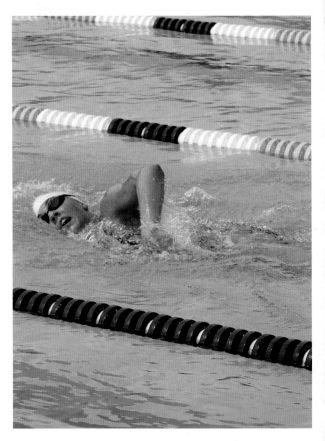

212 LEARN BASIC SWIM STROKES

If you crave the benefits of swimming, but don't know how or never mastered a proper stroke beyond a dog paddle, you can take classes at community pools and many gyms. It's important to know how to swim, if only for the sake of your safety, even if you never use it for exercise.

There are a number of different competitive strokes—which most of us see during the summer Olympics—but the most common ones for recreational swimming are the speedy freestyle (or front crawl), the fluid backstroke, and the calm, relaxed breaststroke.

STROKE	DESCRIPTION	BENEFITS
FREESTYLE	Arms alternately stroke with a windmill motion; face is down in the water, head turns to one side to breathe as that arm rises; knees together; legs kick powerfully	As you gain speed, laps fly by; works the chest muscles, the lats, and other back muscles.
BACKSTROKE	Start by floating on your back with hands at your sides. Your arms alternately stroke up and back over your head as you simultaneously flutter kick your legs.	Great for recovery swims between intense workouts; engages the lats and hamstrings.
BREASTSTROKE	Feet together; bend knees, bring feet up to butt, then kick out to sides with froglike whip kick; at same time, arms push forward from chest, separate, move in a circular stroke, return to chest.	Perform with face in or out of water; easy on the body, therefore good for beginners.

213 SYNCHRONIZE YOUR MOVES

Water aerobics classes, or aqua fitness, offer the benefit of low-impact exercise while getting your heart pumping and your body moving. Because they are easy on the joints, these classes are favorites of seniors, but they are great for anyone who wants to increase fitness levels. Classes may include work with buoyant hand weights or noodles, dancing, or Zumba. Some of the basic moves are listed below.

JOG IN PLACE Show great energy; keep your knees high.

TICK-TOCK HOP Quickly jump from side to side with your feet together.

KNEE TWIST Cross your right elbow toward your left knee at your waist. Alternate sides.

SQUAT JUMP Squat down with arms extended at shoulder height; jump as high as possible while raising arms overhead.

OUTER-THIGH LIFT Stand with left side at wall, feet together, holding edge with left hand. Lift right leg out to side.

214 GET STRONG IN THE SHALLOW END

There are a number of strength and endurance moves you can do in the water, taking advantage of your natural buoyancy to elevate your heart rate and sculpt your legs and core. Perform these in a shallow portion of the pool

BICYCLE Lean back against the side of pool, with your arms outstretched at the edge. "Pedal" your legs at the surface.

PENDULUM SWING Lean back on the pool's edge with your arms resting on the sides. Extend your legs in front of you. Swing them over to the right, then to the left, keeping them together and underwater.

CRUNCH IN THE WATER Start as in the pendulum swing. Then extend your legs, feet together. Pull both knees into your chest. Return to the starting position.

FLUTTER KICK Hold on to the edge of the pool with your arms extended and body at water level; kick legs quickly.

215 GET THE BEST AQUA GEAR

Here are several handy helpers that might be perfect for your water workouts.

WATERPROOF FITNESS TRACKER A waterproof fitness tracker allows you to time yourself in the pool as well as monitor your heart rate and calorie burn.

SUBMERSIBLE SNEAKERS These super light shoes dry quickly. They also offer nonslip soles and ankle support.

FOAM HAND BUOYS If you want to take your aerobic aquatics to the next level, try foam hand buoys (barbells), which range in size from 2.5 to 9 pounds (1–4 kg).

WEBBED GLOVES Emulate Aquaman with webbed gloves that increase resistance when your hands cut through the water.

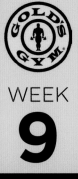

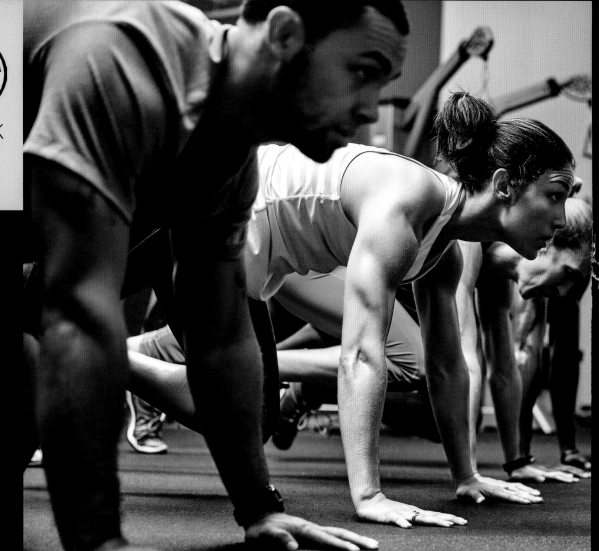

OVERCOME THE PLATEAU At some point during the Gold's Gym Challenge you will probably hit a plateau, when you stop losing weight or cease gaining muscle and tone. It's now time to up the intensity—the rigorousness—of your workouts. By increasing the demands of your routine, you can bypass the sameness of what might have become ho-hum sessions and really make the most of your time in the gym. And, as any trainer will tell you, workouts need frequent updating for you to see continual results. Your body soon adapts to even the toughest fitness challenges you throw at it—some experts claim it only takes two weeks.

KEEP IT SHORT Short, intense training offers multiple benefits for your strength and toning. Try taking just a 60-second break between exercises to add a fat-burning boost. Include genuine cardio intervals to your strength training: for example, you can jump rope or hop on the stationary bike, and sprint for 20 seconds between lifts. You can also add in some fast, powerful explosive movements, such as box jumps, kettlebell swings, burpees, or squat thrusts. Just remember, though, in order for these intensity builders to work, you must avoid interruptions. Don't stop to chat or stroll to the water fountain during your strength-training session.

PASS ON THE MACHINES User-friendly exercise machines certainly have a legitimate place in fitness

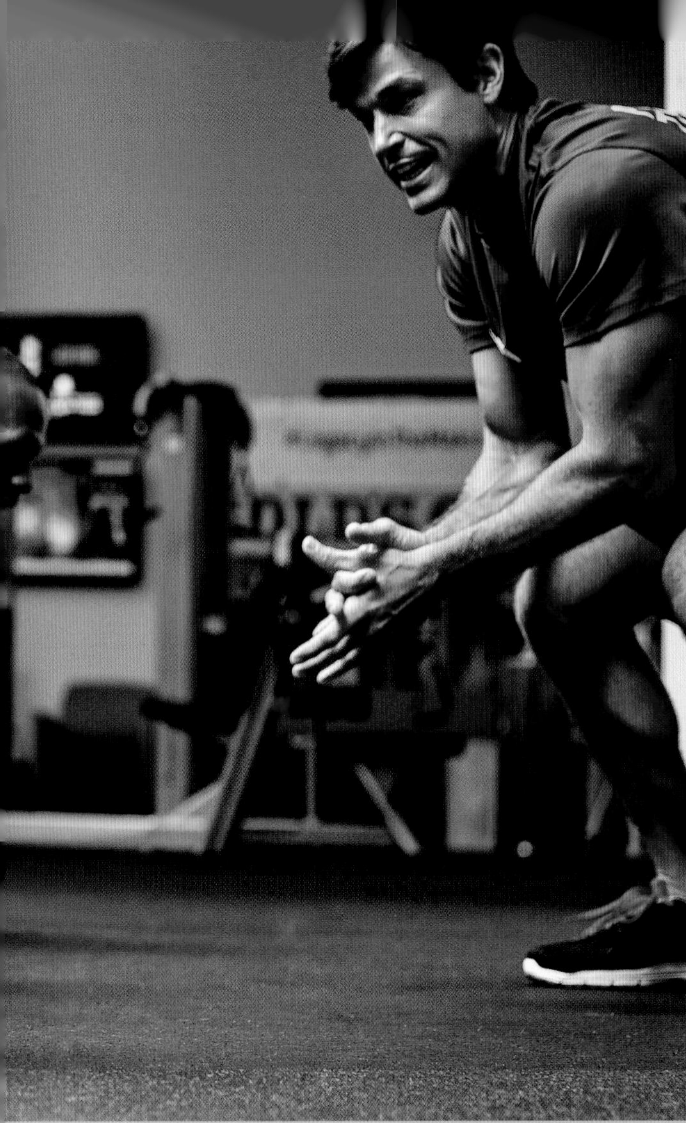

FOLLOW A WINNER'S JOURNEY
Dominique Brooks
Male Winner, Ages 18–29

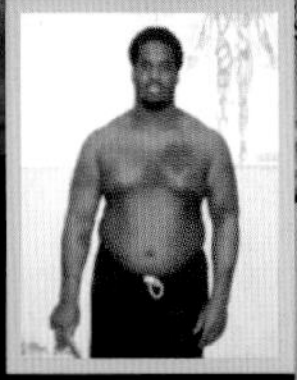

Before

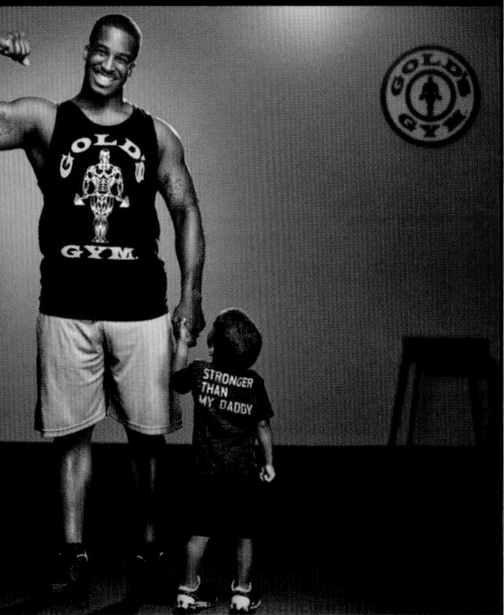

LOST 55.4 pounds (24 kg), 20.8 inches (52.8 cm), and 2.9% body fat

In 2010, Dominique met the "love of his life." Despite his happy circumstances, he gained 40 pounds the following year. In 2012, he met "the joy of his life"—his new baby. But he'd gained another 20 pounds while his wife was pregnant, and his weight soon hit 261. He started practicing jiu jitsu and lost 30 pounds over six months, but after he stopped his martial arts studies to focus on school, he gained back 20 of those pounds.

When his father died of cancer at age 47, Dominique knew he really had to take control of his life. "So I could be here for my family," he explains. He started going to the gym regularly and stopped eating meat, and after hearing about the Gold's Gym Challenge, he jumped right in.

He began a routine that combined cardio training, like jumping rope, with exercise machines and weight lifting. Even a severe, work-related laceration to his forearm did not stop him from competing. "Every single day you have to master your craft," he says, "and don't let anybody tell you what you can and can't do."

centers, but to get the biggest bang for your gym "buck," choose free weights. Barbell and dumbbell lifts incorporate more stabilizing muscles into your movement, so they burn more calories than a similar machine exercise. Even body-weight routines, which will use your own weight for resistance, are more effective at stabilizing your core and using up calories than any machine workouts. Instability work using BOSU balls, Xerdiscs, stability balls, or wobble boards can also aid muscular development and equalize strength.

WINNER'S WORDS

"When the alarm clock goes off ... don't let it be the only thing that wakes you up. Don't ever let a day go by that you waste."

~ Dominique Brooks

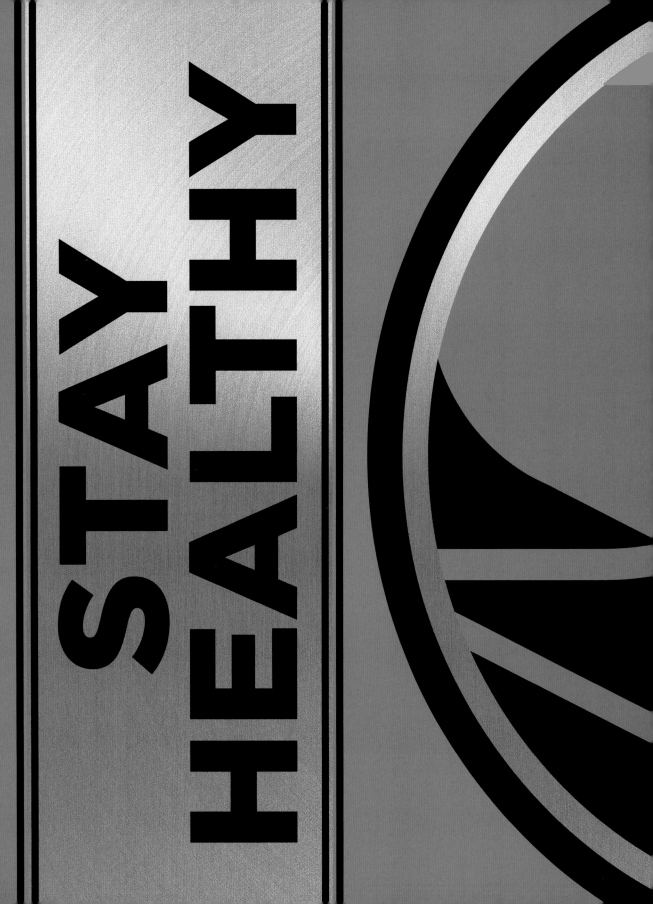

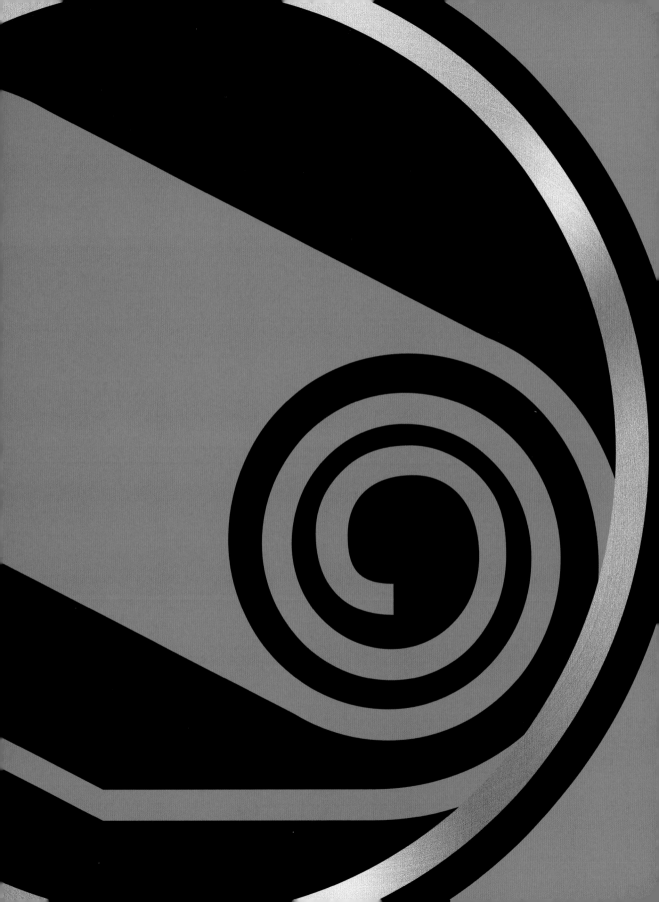

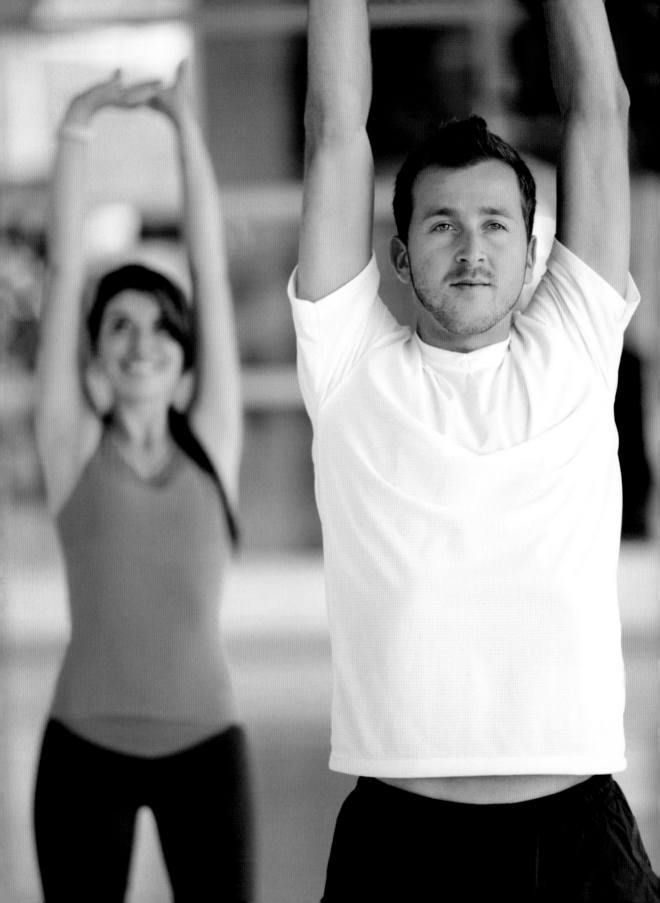

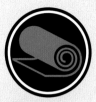 Congratulations! You have begun an exercise regimen, including both resistance and cardio work, and have started watching what you eat. Yet, there are other measures you can also take to ensure continued good heath.

Increasing your flexibility—with stretching exercises, massage, and various exercise classes—becomes another piece of the fitness puzzle that can keep you moving comfortably and exercising robustly throughout your life.

WORK OUT ON THE GO

In order to extend your fitness plan, consider adding workouts to areas of your life beyond the gym. While on vacation or a business trip, seek out the hotel fitness room or swimming pool—or turn your room into a mini gym with a toolkit of lightweight workout aids. Perform stretches or resistance training exercises while at the office or even while commuting to and from work. And don't forget to involve important people in your life, like friends, spouses, or children. Kids, especially, can benefit from the discipline and structure of regular exercise sessions.

UNDERSTAND INJURIES

Injuries to muscles or joints are always potential threats for an exercise regimen, especially if you're broadening your scope or increasing your lifting load. Learn to recognize minor injuries (and the difference between treating them with heat versus ice packs) and how to determine if

a visit to a doctor is in order. Understand how to apply the stretching and limbering techniques that will allow you to recuperate swiftly and resume your workouts.

STAY FIT AT ANY STAGE OF LIFE

No matter where you are in life you should always be able to get a workout. Pregnancy shouldn't derail your fitness goals. There are effective, gentle ways to help you prepare for the birthing process and equally effective ways to return to pre-baby shape. Seniors, perhaps more than anyone, benefit from keeping active and flexible. Studies have shown that arthritis pain and stiffness can be reduced through exercises or classes, like yoga, that focus on mobility.

MAKE IT A FITNESS LIFESTYLE

Getting fit is not just about reaching a strength or endurance goal or a desired weight; it's also about retaining that conditioned physique and adhering to the lifestyle changes you made. You will find that mental attitude is just as critical for maintaining fitness as it is for achieving it. Yet, once you find yourself looking and feeling strong and confident, those gains will reinforce your will to stick to your fitness plan for years to come.

216 STAY LOOSE

Limberness, is the ability to move flexibly—to stretch up, down, or sideways, and bend, squat, and twist—with fluid ease. In fitness terms, flexibility means more than simply being able to touch your toes. Flexibility helps prevent injury during exercise, loosens you up so that your muscles and joints can move through their full range of motion during weight work, such as lifts and squats, and it improves your overall posture. This latter benefit is especially important to the large portion of the workforce that hunches over a computer keyboard all day.

Flexibility also means an increased blood flow to your muscles, and it can even help ward off occasional or chronic back pain. Staying active and stretching are both simple ways to improve your flexibility and prevent the loss of mobility that often affects people as they age.

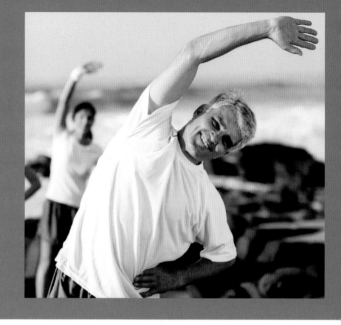

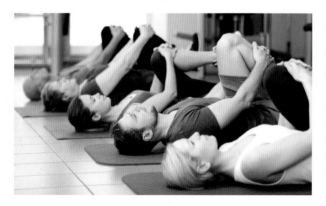

Ask the EXPERT
WHEN DO I STRETCH?

One thing trainers generally agree on is that stretching, which offers so many benefits to the body, needs to be included in a fitness plan. But its placement, duration, type, and intensity are often debated, and different trainers have differing answers. You can stretch both during and after strength exercises, but beforehand, the muscles must be first thawed out and thoroughly warm prior to stretching. Although some general light stretching when "cold" probably won't result in a muscle tear, it is best to ease into stretching when the body is warm and properly up to speed. It is good to stretch the working muscles between your sets to keep them warm and pliable.

217 STRETCH IT OUT

What most people traditionally think of stretching is holding your body in an extended posture for a few seconds, like thrusting your arms over your head as you yawn. There are three basic types of stretches: static, dynamic, and ballistic. Other advanced techniques that combine passive and active stretching are often employed by physical therapists.

STATIC STRETCHING Static stretching consists of holding a joint in a stretched position for a designated length of time, typically 10 to 30 seconds. This stretch allows a muscle to slowly adapt to a new range of motion; it is considered passive because the muscle remains relaxed the entire time.

DYNAMIC STRETCHING Dynamic stretching utilizes an increased range of motion, through the use of body-weight exercises such as squats or lunges. As the body moves in multiple planes of motion, the muscles both contract and relax. These active stretches help prepare the muscles for a hard training session, such as running or cycling.

BALLISTIC STRETCHING Ballistic stretching forces the body into a deeper stretch by using powerful movements—such as bobbing up and down to touch the toes. Ballistic stretches increase risk of injury and don't improve flexibility, and, in some cases, they actually cause muscles to tighten up.

218 STAY STILL

An isometric, or static, contraction is a type of stretch that creates tension in a muscle without changing its length. Stretching out your leg on a chair is a passive stretch. If you contract your hamstrings—by trying to bend your knee by putting pressure on your heel, for example—the stretch becomes isometric. This, in turn, increases the range of motion. You can use the floor, a wall, a chair or a partner to create the resistance needed to achieve the static contraction of an isometric stretch.

Isometrics also allow you to increase your strength in stretched positions so that, during a lunge for instance, your legs do not slide out of control. Muscle strength is increased during isometrics because, in a stretched muscle, not all fibers will elongate, whereas when a contraction occurs in a stretched muscle, more of those resting fibers will react—and those already stretched will elongate to an even greater extent.

Typically, for most general fitness goals and weight loss, it is best to include as many muscles of the body as possible in an exercise session to get the most out of your isometric work and provide a full-body effect. Isometrics are not recommended for those under 18, nor are they advised for warm-ups—they are considered too intense.

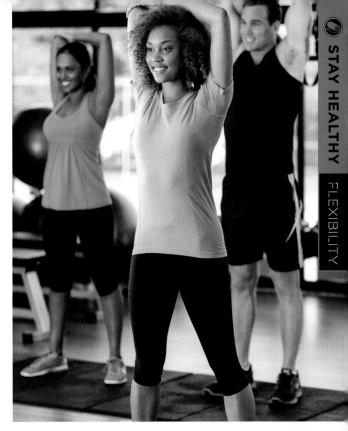

219 INCREASE YOUR FLEXIBILITY

Increased flexibility can enhance performance during aerobic training and muscular conditioning, as well as in sports. As such, it should be an ongoing goal of your fitness plan. Stretching not only benefits muscles and joints, it also prepares you for strenuous exercise. Massage and relaxation therapy can help you ease those knots of tension and loosen up.

START WITH DYNAMIC WARM-UPS Begin your cardio workout with dynamic stretches such as squats, lunges, side lunges, push-ups, and jumping jacks. Perform at least two of these—three sets of 20 reps will get your body ready for a serious workout.

END WITH STATIC STRETCHING Post-workout, try long-duration static stretches to lengthen muscles made tight by weight lifting. Your chest, lats, or hip flexors may also need work due to daily stresses on posture.

APPLY FULL RANGE OF MOTION Partial range-of-motion workouts may increase strength, but using a full range of motion will boost your limberness. Full-depth squats, for instance, improve hip flexibility. When lifting, first perform full-range exercises with lighter weights.

UTILIZE MASSAGE This hands-on approach boosts flexibility by breaking up the knots in muscles and tissues that restrict motion. Applying foam rollers pre-workout will prepare you for exercise; afterwards, they can flush away waste products. Focus on the key players: calves, quads, upper back, and lats. Visiting a massage therapist several times a month can also ensures that you get muscular relief.

TAKE TIME TO RELAX Nothing tightens up the body like stress, which can occur when the mental pressures of home and work combine with the physical demands of the gym. To counteract stress, seek out a relaxing activity like walking, light yoga, or a recreational dance class a few times a week to help your mind—and joints—open up.

BE AWARE The issue of whether or not you should stretch before you exercise is still disputed. Based on various studies, some trainers advise stretching beforehand, while others say to avoid it. For instance, weight lifters may find themselves weakened by warm-up stretches. The best course is to discuss when and how to stretch with your trainer, someone who understands your specific fitness requirements.

220 LIMBER UP

Begin your day with this quick full-body stretch routine. When performing these moves, focus on isolating the targeted muscles and moving with control. The more you practice, the easier it will become for you to move with fluid grace. Be sure to hold each stretch for 30 seconds, using whatever form of timekeeping that works best for you.

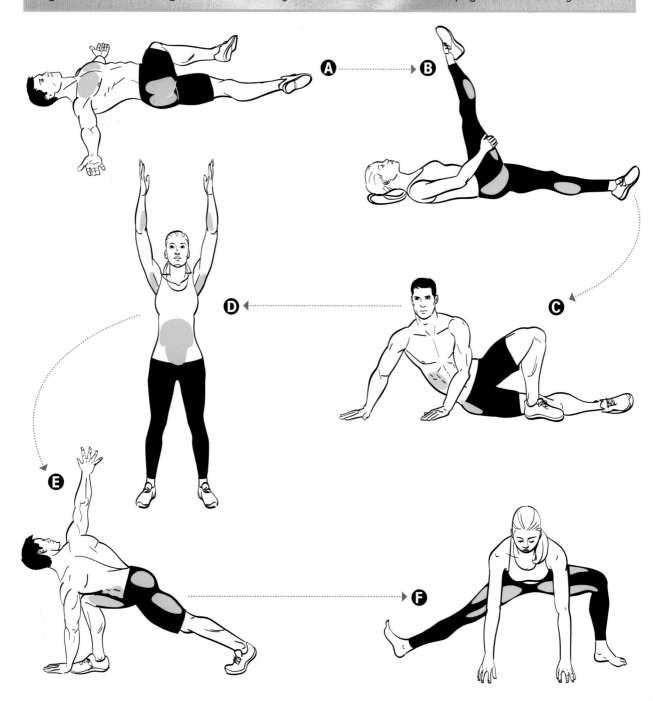

Ⓐ LYING-DOWN PRETZEL STRETCH Lie on your back, with both legs elongated and parallel and your arms extended away from your torso, palms facing up. Bend your right leg and place the sole of your foot on the floor. Lift your butt off the floor, tilting your torso slightly to your left, and cross your right leg over to your left side, with your knee bent at a right angle. Hold, and then return to the starting position. Repeat on the other side.

Ⓑ UNILATERAL LEG RAISE Place your hands on your right hamstring just below your knee, and then extend your right leg toward the ceiling, pointing your toes. Hold, and then lower your leg. Repeat on the other side.

Ⓒ SIDE-LYING RIB STRETCH Lie on your right side with your legs together and extended. Place both palms on the floor, your right arm supporting you and your left arm positioned in front of your body. Your upper body should be slightly lifted. Bend your left leg, and rest your foot just in front of your right thigh, knee pointing up toward the ceiling. Keeping your legs in place, press down with your hands as you raise your body upward, feeling a stretch around your right rib cage.

Ⓓ GOOD MORNING STRETCH Stand tall with your legs and feet parallel, shoulder-width apart. Keep your knees soft, and tuck your pelvis slightly forward. Reach your arms fully up toward the ceiling, keeping them long and parallel with your body. Focus your energy on the middle of your palms, which should be facing inward. Turn your gaze upward as you stretch. You should feel a stretch from your toes to the tips of your fingers.

Ⓔ FORWARD LUNGE WITH TWIST Stand with your feet together, hands on your hips. Lunge forward on the right leg, focusing on a downward movement of your hips, until your thigh is parallel with the floor. Bend forward to place your hands on the floor on either side of your right foot. Balance your weight on your left hand, and carefully and slowly guide your right arm up toward the ceiling, twisting your torso. Return to the starting position, and repeat on the other side.

Ⓕ SIDE LUNGE STRETCH Stand with your feet wide, toes facing outward. Bend your knees and hips to slowly lower into a sumo squat. Once you feel the stretch in your glutes and hamstrings, drop your hands onto the floor in front of you, transferring some of your weight onto your arms. Staying as low as possible, slowly shift your body to the right, bending your right knee while extending and straightening your left leg. Rise to the sumo squat position, and then stretch to the other side.

EXERCISE	TIME/SETS/REST	TARGET
LYING-DOWN PRETZEL STRETCH	Hold for 30 seconds for two sets on each side with a 10-second rest between sets.	Rotator muscles, chest, and glutes
UNILATERAL LEG RAISE	Hold for 30 seconds for two sets on each side with a 10-second rest between sets.	Lower back groin, glutes, and hamstrings
SIDE-LYING RIB STRETCH	Hold for 30 seconds for two sets on each side with a 10-second rest between sets.	Rib cage, lower back, obliques, and outer thighs
GOOD MORNING STRETCH	Hold for 30 seconds for two sets with a 10-second rest between sets.	Back, neck, abs, obliques, palms, forearms, and upper arms
FORWARD LUNGE WITH TWIST	Hold for 5 seconds for four sets on each side with a 10-second rest between sets.	Quads, glutes, hip adductors, hamstrings, obliques, rib cage, shoulders, and chest
SIDE LUNGE STRETCH	Hold for 5 seconds for four sets on each side with a 10-second rest between sets.	Hip adductors, hip flexors, hamstrings, inner thighs, and glutes

BREATHE DEEP Don't forget to breathe as you stretch: proper breathing helps your body to relax, and it increases blood flow to your internal organs. Exhale as you move into the stretch, and then once you are in the stretch, inhale deeply. To relax the muscles in the back of your neck and your diaphragm (which lets oxygen in to feed your muscles), relax your jaw, letting your mouth hang just slightly open.

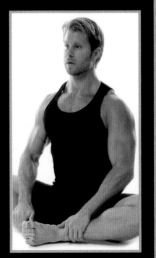

221 STRETCH WITH A BUDDY

You don't need any equipment to stretch effectively, however, working with another person offering resistance can enhance your routine. Perks include a greater degree of flexibility and an increased range of motion. Some Olympic athletes even use partner stretches to get in shape for their events. As with any shared fitness activity, your buddy will help keep you accountable—so you meet up at the agreed times.

Among the many ways to stretch with a partner is PNF, or proprioceptive neuromuscular facilitation. One version of PNF is contract-relax stretching, by which you contract a muscle isometrically against resistance provided by your partner. You rest for several seconds, and then your partner helps you move that same muscle into a passive stretch. The typical duration is six reps before you switch places. Another version, known as hold-relax stretching, calls for a passive stretch followed by an isometric one (see #223). Any form of PNF can purportedly increase limberness even more than regular stretching.

When it's your turn to be the helper, you will use your body to provide leverage. To lower the risk of injury, use the major muscles of your legs and trunk to resist your partner's movements. Avoid unnecessary twisting or bending, and stop if you feel pain in either role.

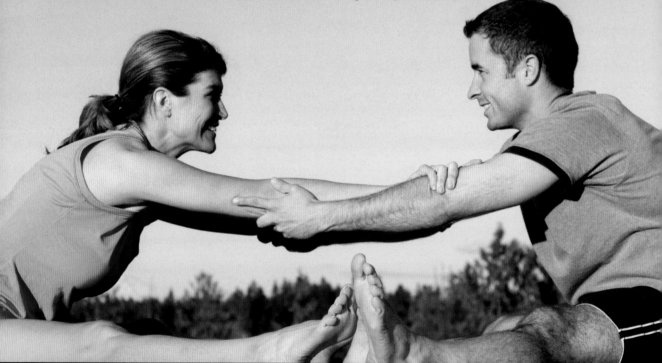

222 CHOOSE YOUR PARTNER

If you are interested in partner stretches, it's wise to first work out with a personal trainer or physical therapist familiar with the movements. Once you have mastered the various techniques, try them out with a gym buddy, friend, co-worker, or family member. There is a theory in the fitness community that romantic couples who stretch together can increase their bond—forging a strong sense of connection and trust. To amplify this effect, stretches that involve facing each other should also include lots of held eye contact. Imagine an exercise regimen that not only gets you in shape, but also

Here are some tips to follow when working with a partner, to focus on safely and properly helping each other stretch.

DO Let the desire to keep up with your partner motivate you to work past performance plateaus.

DON'T Avoid continuing with any stretches in either role if you begin to feel pain. Stretching should never hurt.

DO Combine social time with fitness by stretching with a friend with whom you rarely spend one-on-one time.

DON'T If your partner corrects your form, don't be offended.

The following quick stretch routine offers you and your partner an introduction to the hold-relax method of PNF stretching. For each of these exercises, the helper should move the stretcher to the point of being in a comfortable yet challenging stretch. The stretcher then isometrically contracts those targeted muscles by gently pushing against the force of the helper's movement. For example, during this phase of the assisted, unilateral leg raise, as the helper pushes the elevated leg back, the stretcher pushes it forward with the same force so that the leg remains static. After holding this passive stretch for 10 seconds, both helper and stretcher relax before repeating all steps, this time holding the passive portion for 30 seconds.

A ASSISTED UNILATERAL LEG RAISE This stretch targets the hamstrings, calves, and glutes.

HOW Assuming the role of helper, stand to the right, and face the stretcher, while the stretcher lies faceup on the floor. Take hold of the stretcher's right leg as the stretcher lifts it toward the ceiling, positioning yourself so that the lower calf rests comfortably on your right shoulder. Place your other hand on the thigh just above the kneecap. The stretcher then leans in toward you, providing a comfortable stretch and holding this position for 10 seconds before relaxing. Then, while you provide resistance, the stretcher pushes the leg against your shoulder, holding for 6 seconds, and then relaxing. Repeat again, this time holding the stretch for 30 seconds. Perform a second set, and then switch your roles.

B ASSISTED CHEST STRETCH This stretch targets the chest and shoulders.

HOW The stretcher sits on the floor with legs slightly bent, heels together, and hands clasped behind the head. As the helper, stand behind the stretcher with your knees bent and slightly knocked inward, so your knees are at the sides of the stretcher's middle back. Place the inside of your forearms on the inside of the stretcher's upper forearms and inside of the biceps. Pull the stretcher's arms in toward yourself, while providing stability with your knees on the middle back. Hold for 10 seconds, relax, and then repeat, this time with the stretcher pushing against your resistance. Hold for 6 seconds, and then relax. Repeat again, this time holding the stretch for 30 seconds. Repeat for a second set, and then switch your roles.

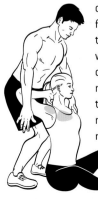

C ASSISTED SEATED FORWARD BEND This stretch targets the hamstrings, lower back, upper back, and calves.

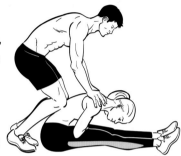

HOW The stretcher sits on the floor with both legs extended, feet in a relaxed, flexed position. The stretcher then relaxes the weight of the upper body over the thighs. As the helper, stand behind the stretcher, and bend your legs so that your shins lightly rest on the stretcher's lower back. Put your palms on the stretcher's shoulder blades. Apply gentle pressure with your hands and your shins to create a comfortable stretch for your partner. Hold the stretch for 20 to 30 seconds. Relax, and repeat for a second set, and then switch your roles.

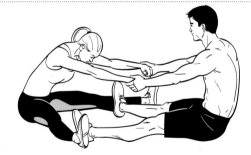

D RUSSIAN SPLIT SWITCH This stretch targets the hamstrings and hip adductors.

HOW Sit upright facing each other with your legs spread as widely as is comfortable, with your feet slightly flexed and legs turned out from the hips so that your toes point upward. The soles of your feet should rest above each other's inner ankles. Reach out, and clasp hands. You then lean back slightly, moving your partner forward. Hold for 20 to 30 seconds. Relax, and repeat for a second set, and then switch roles so that your partner brings you forward.

224 KNOW YOUR...
IT BAND AND TFL

The iliotibial band, usually just called the ITB or IT band, is a thick band of fibrous tissue that runs down the lateral or outside part of the thigh, beginning at the iliac crest (the border of the most prominent bone of the pelvis) and extending to the outer side of the tibia (the shinbone), just below the knee joint. The ITB also attaches to the gluteal muscles and the tensor fascia latae (often called the TFL). The tensor fasciae latae is the muscle on the outside of your hip that moves your leg outward. The ITB functions in coordination with several of the thigh muscles to provide stability to the outside of the knee joint.

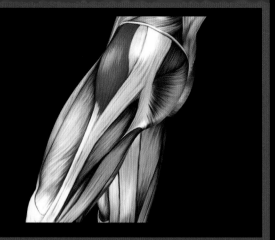

225 RECOGNIZE THE SIGNS

Many runners, cyclists, hikers, dancers, and other athletes experience a common injury called iliotibial band syndrome, or ITBS. In these activities, the IT band, which helps stabilize the knee, continually rubs over the lower extremity of the femur while it moves from behind the bone to in front of it. This friction, along with the repeated flexion and extension of the knee that all of these activities demand may cause the iliotibial band area to become inflamed, producing hip and knee tightness and pain.

ITBS, one of the leading causes of lateral knee pain in runners, is sometimes caused by physical abnormalities, such as high or low arches, pronation or supination of the foot, bow legs, or uneven leg length. Another culprit could be muscular imbalance—weak hip abductor muscles or uneven left/right stretching of the band, possibly caused by sitting cross-legged. Foam roller massage may be helpful in preventing and relieving the discomfort ITBS produces.

SYMPTOMS Signs of ITBS include a stinging sensation above and outside the knee joint or along the whole band, tightness of the band, or swelling of the tissue where the band rubs over the femur. Most often, when ITBS occurs, an individual will no longer be able to run, but can continue to walk and perform other activities.

DIAGNOSIS Pain may not always be present during activity, but it is usually felt as the foot strikes the ground or as you turn a corner when running, or, especially, as you walk down stairs. Some borderline sufferers choose not to see a doctor, but the pain can intensify over time if not treated.

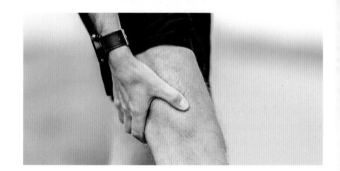

CAUSES ITBS often results from certain training methods—habitually running on a banked track or cambered surface, requiring the downhill leg to bend inward, excessively stretching the band against the femur; not warming up properly; a pounding foot strike; or too much up-and-down hill or stair work. Long-distance running, as well as other athletic pursuits, such as cycling with angled-in toes, hiking long distances, rowing, swimming the breast stroke, and water polo, can sometimes be at fault. Even a change of footgear, perhaps made to address another problem, can cause a flare-up.

TREATMENT Rest, icing, compression, and elevation (RICE) are initially essential for healing. Some form of massage therapy, even self-massage, can also help offer relief. Early treatment is key—research has shown that three days of immobility (through bracing the affected knee) and use of crutches cured a majority of acute ITBS cases. Once you are back on the road, limit the frequency, duration, and intensity of runs, always warm up first, and place an ice pack on your leg afterward. In future, avoid any potentially painful stimuli, like running downhill.

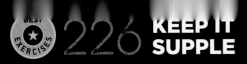

226 KEEP IT SUPPLE

If you are prone to ITBS, a fitness plan that includes stretching the IT band is the best way to alleviate any inflammation or irritation. Pay careful attention to how long you hold each stretch. For these kind of stretches to be effective, you must remain in the pose for 30 to 60 seconds, and repeat two or three times. To start, try these three stretches, which might help to keep your IT band supple and pain-free.

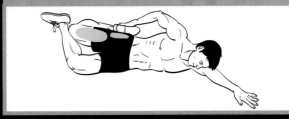

Ⓑ SIDE-LYING IT BAND STRETCH This stretch can help keep your IT band flexible, while also stretching your quads.

HOW Lie on your side. Kick your top leg back, and grasp your foot. Bend your bottom leg, and tuck the ankle over the knee of your top leg. Repeat on the other side.

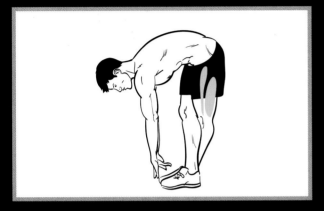

Ⓐ CROSSOVER TOE TOUCH Crossing one foot over the other helps to keep the focus of this stretch on the outside of your thigh. Like any toe touch, it will also stretch your back and hamstrings muscles.

HOW Start standing. Cross one leg over the other. Bend at the waist with the goal of touching your hands to your toes.

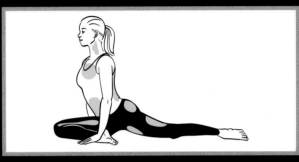

Ⓒ PIGEON STRETCH Try this yoga-inspired seated stretch to target your IT band.

HOW Start in a push-up position. Bend one knee, and move your leg forward until you can rest the outside of your knee and foot on the floor. Gently press down on your hip, while distributing the weight between your hands and your bent leg.

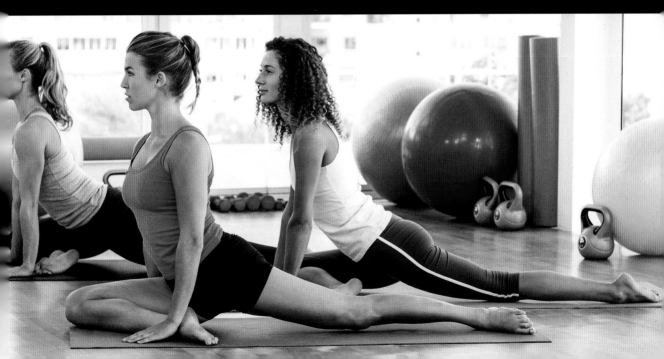

227 RELEASE THOSE KNOTS

When stretching a muscle with painful knots in it, you only end up stretching the healthy muscle tissue—the knot remains intact. In most cases, massage is needed to relieve these knotted muscles. If you don't have your own masseuse, consider hands-on massage using a ball or foam roller, a process known as self-myofascial release, or SMFR. In this technique, gentle pressure slowly loosens the painful myofascial tissue restrictions that can be caused by injury, inflammation or surgical procedures—and which often do not show up on x-rays or scans. SMFR can reduce the risk of injuries, and it can also help you to achieve long, lean muscles, while improving flexibility, functionality, and athletic performance. Although it's considered a form of alternative medicine, many physical therapists rely on SMFR.

Myofascial therapy administered with a small flexible ball, such as a massage ball or even a tennis ball, may offer the greatest reward for the smallest price. A ball this size can travel with you anywhere—you can even use it for a discreet massage at work or on an airplane. This kind of massage relieves pain and physical stress and helps the body become more limber, as well as easing foot and calf muscle cramps (especially those caused by high heels). Try it on your calves, hamstrings, glutes, quadriceps, and back.

228 SERVE IT UP

To give yourself a relaxing foot massage, try this form of SMFR using nothing more complicated than a simple and readily available tennis ball. Just sit comfortably on a chair in your bare feet. Place a tennis ball under the arch of one foot, and roll it back and forth, going all the way from the ball of your foot to the heel. Then carefully return it to the arch position. If any areas feel tight or crampy, apply some extra pressure. Continue the process for 60 seconds, rest, and then repeat. Switch feet, and repeat the sequence.

229 FIND RELEASE WITH A FOAM ROLLER

TOOLS of the TRADE

The tool most often used to apply SMFR is a roller, usually made of dense foam or knobbly rubber and shaped like a bolster pillow. You simply roll your body over the roller, and when you find a tender spot or trigger point, you keep pressure on that area until the pain lessens by half or more. Eventually, you will be able to roll over that spot without pain.

Make sure you control your body weight on the roller to generate the pressure necessary to break up problematic spots. Roll back and forth across any stiff, painful areas for approximately 60 seconds, rest for 10 seconds, and repeat. Maintain a slight contraction in your abdominal muscles to stabilize and protect your core (lower back, pelvis, and hips) during the rolling process. Keep your breathing slow and natural to reduce any tension caused by the

discomfort the roller sometimes produces. Be careful not to roll over bony areas, such as elbows or knees. Follow up with stretches that target the muscles you just focused on. Remember, you can treat your specific trigger points before they knot up.

In addition to their therapeutic effectiveness, these foam rollers offer other benefits.

ADAPTABILITY The roller lets you control the amount of pressure placed on the trouble spots.

COST These rollers make a relatively inexpensive fitness tool.

PORTABILITY A small foam roller can travel with you to work or on vacation.

CONVENIENCE You can experience a customized massage any time you wish.

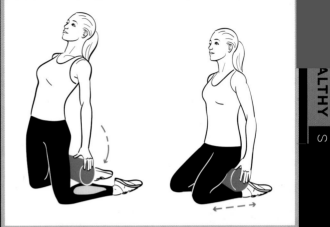

230 ROLL WITH IT

Practicing self-myofascial release with a foam roller can help you relieve the muscle aches and knots that can develop after vigorous strength workouts or intense cardio sessions. This kind of massage will also aid in the removal of metabolic waste, such as lactic acid, from the muscle. These exercises target four common areas of post-workout soreness: the IT band, calves, hamstrings, and back. Perform foam roller stretches three times a week to prevent stiffness and injury, and feel free to roll over any tense or knotted areas two to three times a day.

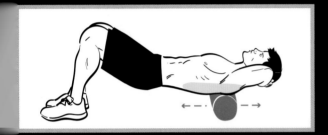

B FOAM ROLLER BACK STRETCH This stretch targets your back muscles, including the lats and erector spinae.

HOW Sit with your knees bent and your feet flat on the floor, shoulder-width apart. Place the roller behind your lower-back region. Lean back carefully onto the roller. Raise your hips slightly off the floor, lifting your butt as you simultaneously take small steps forward, allowing you to begin rolling the foam roller upward on your back with your hands clasped behind your head or in front of you. Pause over uncomfortable areas before rolling back and forth over them until you feel relief. Continue rolling for 60 seconds. Rest, and then repeat.

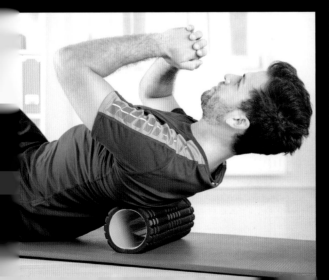

C FOAM ROLLER CALF AND HAMSTRINGS STRETCH
This exercise targets your gastrocnemius and hamstrings.

HOW Kneel upright, and place the foam roller behind your knees. Carefully rock your pelvis slightly forward, just enough to place the foam roller deep behind your kneecaps. Lower your body weight by sitting gently on the foam roller. As you begin to sit, you will find that the foam roller naturally moves over your calf muscle. Guide the roller with your hands, moving the roller slowly down toward your heels.

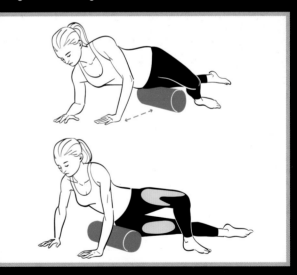

A ITB ROLL This stretch will target your IT band and quads.

HOW Rest your right upper thigh against the roller, bend your left knee up toward your right knee, and then place as much of your foot on the floor as possible. Tilt your body slightly to the right, adjusting your body weight to achieve the desired pressure on your upper thigh, rolling slowly down to just above your knee. Pause over uncomfortable areas before rolling back and forth over them until you feel some relief. Continue rolling for 60 seconds. Rest, and then repeat. Switch sides, and repeat.

231 COMBINE BALANCE AND COORDINATION

Balance and coordination are two additional components of the fitness equation, as well as major factors in many competitive sports. Balance is the ability to remain upright and stay in control of your movements. Humans use their eyes, ears, and proprioception or "body sense" to help stay balanced. There are two types of balance: static and dynamic—maintaining equilibrium while staying still, and while moving, respectively.

As we age, the ability to balance well can deteriorate— sometimes as early as in our twenties. Retaining a strong sense of balance can help to ensure personal independence as we enter our golden years; statistically, more than a third of adults over 65 will suffer a fall, which is the number one cause of traumatic brain injury in this age group.

Simple actions like walking, climbing stairs, stretching, and resistance training can delay this deterioration, along with exercises that incorporate balance-challenging equipment such as stability balls, BOSU balls, and wobble boards. "Balance exercises speed up your reaction time and improve the brain-to-muscle connection," explains Gold's Gym Fitness Institute trainer Ramona Braganza.

Coordination, the ability to skillfully combine multiple actions, not only requires good balance, but also agility, sharp reflexes, and strength. As you raise the complexity of your workouts and place more demands on yourself physically, these two components become increasingly important. Fortunately, both can be improved through training and practice.

232 ACHIEVE PROPER ALIGNMENT

A fit athlete is an aligned athlete. This means that your load-bearing joints are in neutral alignment—where they are at their strongest, at the least odds with gravity, and are able to maximize the use of force, allowing you to use the least amount of energy to maintain a specific position and activate the correct muscles during exercise. Neutral alignment also optimizes breathing and the circulation of bodily fluids.

In neutral alignment, your pelvis is angled to create the optimum space between your vertebrae. There are three curves to your spine: the inward arch of the neck, the outward curve of the mid-back region, and the inward arch of the lower-back region. Neutral alignment helps these curves cushion the spine from excess stress or strain. This stance should be effortless, arising from a healthy and balanced musculature. Here are some guidelines for working toward neutral alignment.

STRADDLE THE SCALES Stand with each foot on a different scale: if they show different weights, your balance is off. This could strain your body during workouts, so talk to a trainer or physiotherapist about realigning your posture and spine.

LOCATE YOUR CENTER Nearly all bodily movements radiate from the central "power pack" of strong muscles around the lumbar spine. One way to improve alignment is to locate this "center," and perform movements that generate from this central core: your abdomen, lower back, hips, and buttocks.

STAND TALL Correct posture requires holding your head up, with chin in, and earlobes aligned with the middle of your shoulders, lengthening your neck, and keeping your shoulders back, knees straight, lower back slightly concave, and abs firm

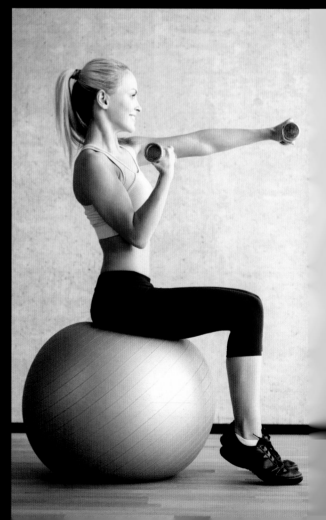

TOOLS of the TRADE

233 SAMPLE THE STABILITY BALL

Stability balls, also known as Swiss balls, exercise balls, body balls, fitness balls, and balance balls, are heavy-duty inflatable spheres originally developed to be used by physical therapy patients. They range in size so you can find one that works best for your height (see #234).

The stability ball has become a valued tool of the fitness trainer, the sports conditioner, and the physical therapist. Children, adults, and seniors can use these versatile balls to build strength, improve balance and coordination, work core muscles, and raise endurance. Stability balls are often incorporated into Pilates classes, weight training, and abdominal fitness routines, and their low cost and ease of use make them ideal for the home gym. Stability ball workouts can engage multiple muscle systems, especially those of your core, which challenges your whole body to maintain balance throughout an exercise.

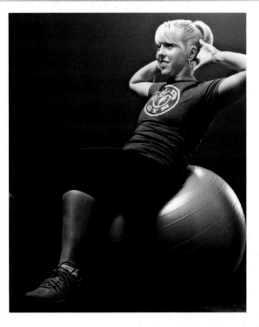

234 FIND YOUR SIZE

It's important to work with a ball suitable to your height. This chart will help you find the right size (note that size labels such as small, medium or large may vary between manufacturers). Look for one that comes with a pump, and fill it until it is firm and not squishy.

YOUR HEIGHT	BALL SIZE	BALL HEIGHT
Up to 4 feet 7 inches (140 cm)	Extra Small	14 inches (35 cm)
4 feet 7 inches to 5 feet (140 to 152 cm)	Small	18 inches (45 cm)
5 feet to 5 feet 6 inches (152 to 168 cm)	Medium	22 inches (55 cm)
5 feet 6 inches to 6 feet 1 inch (168 to 185 cm)	Large	26 inches (65 cm)
6 feet to 6 feet 8 inches (185 to 200 cm)	Extra Large	30 inches (75 cm)
Over 6 feet 8 inches (200 cm)	Extra, Extra Large	33 inches (85 cm)

235 TRAIN AND GAIN BALANCE

Balance training is sometimes overlooked as a vital element of fitness conditioning. Fortunately, there are plenty of tools on the market that provide the instability needed to improve your sense of balance. Most of them work by constantly shifting resistance, which challenges the body's center of mass, forcing the core to work harder.

Balance tools can also boost upper body strength. Try a push-up on a balance board—a skateboard-shaped deck that uses a single tubular roller as a fulcrum to simulate lateral and radial movements. Grasp the sides of the board to use as your base as you execute a push-up. The trick is keeping the board evenly balanced. Noting which side you tend to lean toward is a good way to check for your dominant side.

Below are a number of other popular balance aids.

XERDISC Stand on one of these or straddle two of these inflatable rubber balance discs to achieve unstable footing.

BALANCE BEAM This trapezoidal foam plank mimics a gymnast's balance beam and provides a wider or narrower surface for toe-to-heel walking.

ROCKER BOARD This seesaw-like board uses a tubular half circle to create one plane of instability.

WOBBLE BOARD The rounded base of a wobble board furnishes multiple planes of instability.

M-BOARD This board, atop a rounded ball, allows a wide range of movement. A support tripod is also available.

AQUA BOARD Perform normal gym exercises while balancing on a board floating in a pool for a great core workout.

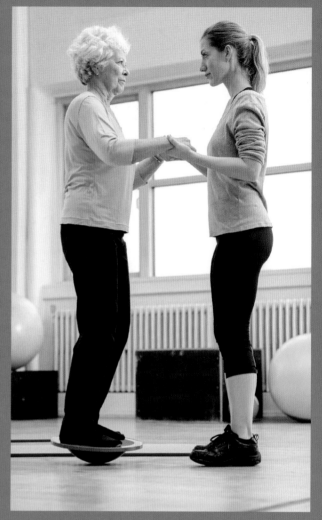

TOOLS of the TRADE

236 FLIP OVER A BOSU® BALL

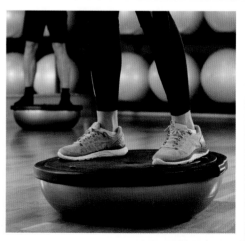

The BOSU ball is a balance-training device that was invented in 1999 by David Weck. This inflatable rubber hemisphere, with its rigid platform, can be used dome-side up, offering an unstable top surface with a stable base for athletic drills and aerobics. Dome-side down, it provides an unstable base for balance exercises. (The acronym originally meant Both Sides Up, but now refers to Both Side Utilized.) Some studies have indicated that the imbalance the half-ball provides does not significantly affect muscles, while other studies concluded that working on an unstable surface, at minimum, increases activation of the rectus abdominis muscles.

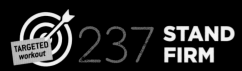

TARGETED workout

237 STAND FIRM

It's hard to believe, but starting as early as your twenties, your sense of balance begins to decrease. How rapidly it diminishes depends on your genes and on the natural process of aging. It also depends on how physically active you are and what kinds of activities you perform. The best exercises challenge your sense of balance by incorporating BOSU balls, wobble boards, and Xerdiscs into your leg workout. Incorporating this equipment not only makes for a more challenging routine, but also builds up your agility. Here are four moves to help you stay grounded.

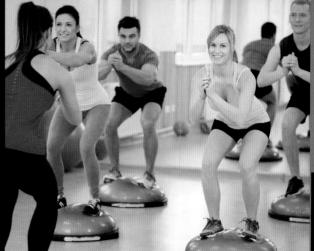

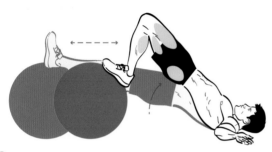

A SINGLE-LEG STABILITY BALL HAMSTRING CURL

This targets your glutes and hamstrings while stabilizing your core. Perform 10 reps.

HOW Lie on your back with your ankles and heels placed on top of a stability ball, toes pointing up. Raise your hips, contract your glutes, and keep your arms out from your sides to stabilize yourself. Roll the ball in toward your hips by rolling from your heels onto the flat part of your feet. Pause momentarily, and then roll the ball back out, making sure to keep your hips elevated.

B ROMANIAN DEADLIFT ON XERDISC
Performing this classic strength-building exercise on a Xerdisc targets your glutes, hamstrings, quadriceps, and inner thighs, while also improving your balance. Perform 20 reps.

HOW Place your left foot on one Xerdisc and your right foot on another. Hold a light dumbbell in each hand. Slowly lower from the waist down until your hands are almost to the floor. Then slowly rise back up.

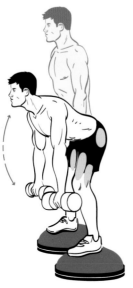

C SQUATS ON A BOSU BALL

This version of a body-weight squat targets your glutes, hamstrings, and quadriceps while improving your balance. Perform 10 to 15 reps.

HOW Begin standing on the BOSU ball, dome side up, with your feet spread as wide as possible and your arms extended forward or clasped in front of you for balance. Descend slowly into a squat until your thighs are parallel to the floor. Pause, then stand back up. To raise the difficulty, attempt the same squat with the dome side down.

D SINGLE-LEG LUNGE ON A WOBBLE BOARD

Performed on a wobble board, this version of a stationary lunge will target your glutes, quads, hamstrings, and calves while improving balance. Perform 10 reps on each side.

HOW Stand facing the smaller side of a wobble board. Place one foot on the board, shifting your weight to your heel. You will now be in somewhat of a lunge position. Lower and raise your body on the ball of your back foot and the heel of your front foot. Keep the board parallel to the floor. With your foot on the board, make sure that your knee doesn't tracking over your ankle.

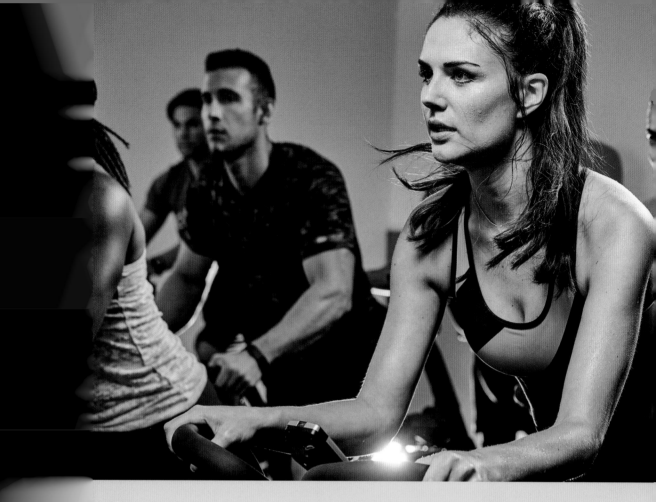

 JOIN IN To maintain your high level of dedication (and to help keep your enthusiasm soaring) try adding a group class or two to your Challenge regimen. The great sense of community you'll get from your classmates, and the motivation from instructors, can keep you going. The diversity in class schedules also allows for more accessibility, and the classes are individually adapted. An instructor will help you match the class to your own intensity level, be it expert or beginner. Whether you're trying to get lean, build muscle, or improve performance or overall health, classes can help you do all four. Gold's Gym offers several tempting options: weight and resistance sessions, cardio training on a stationary bike, and martial arts that demand concentration and focused strength. Combat daily stress, which leads to increased levels of cortisol and body fat, by participating in yoga or tai chi classes.

 SHAKE IT UP, BABY Don't forget to try dance—exercising to music can amp up your results, so get out on the floor! Gold's Gym offers fun, highly active, dance-based classes of all kinds. One of the most well-known and popular is Zumba, which combines high energy and motivating music with unique moves and combinations.

 TAKE A RIDE Whether you're already into cycling or new to the sport, give a stationary bike class a spin. Studio-based cycle training lets you learn proper cycling skills as an instructor guides you through simulated flat and incline rides in one of the many studios at Gold's Gym locations.

 POWER UP If you're looking for sleekness and strength along with flexibility, try Pilates. This mat workout, based on techniques developed by Joseph Pilates, includes concentrated work on core strength, body alignment, and muscular balance. PiYo® Strength is a combination of

FOLLOW A WINNER'S JOURNEY
Luis Collazo
Male Overall Challenge Winner

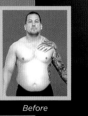

Before

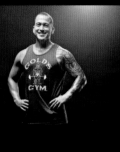

LOST 57 pounds (25 kg), 18 inches (45.7cm), and 27% body fat

Luis sustained multiple injuries while training as a Marine. Despite a number of surgeries, he never healed properly. After facing unemployment and a divorce, he moved to Texas to be near his family. There, he remarried and had another child, but during this time his weight ballooned to 275 pounds (125 kg). He regularly experienced pain in his back, knees, and hips and was now a borderline diabetic.

He found the solution to many of his health issues by joining the Gold's Gym Challenge in 2012. His trainer showed him how to do low-impact cardio and resistance exercises that allowed him to train around his injuries and also helped him plan a diet. Whenever he lost five pounds, he had permission to cheat. "A real motivator for this food lover!" Luis admits.

Today, he and his kids are healthier and more active than ever. Luis eats fresh foods more often and grills several times a week to prepare meals in bulk. "I haven't touched anything in a can for two years now," he says proudly. Another plus: he went from being a stay-at-home dad to managing a Gold's Gym in San Antonio.

Pilates and yoga that helps you build strength and gain flexibility; its choreographed moves flow together for a class that's fun and challenging—and will make you sweat. If you seek resistance training, BODYPUMP™ is a 60-minute calorie-burning barbell class that works the entire body by challenging all your major muscle groups. Great music and awesome instructors will inspire you to get the results that you came for—and fast! Gold's Gym also offers BODYCOMBAT™, an intense class with driving music and powerful instructors. Unleash yourself in this energetic program inspired by karate, boxing, taekwondo, tai chi, and Muay Thai.

WINNER'S WORDS

"It's an everyday struggle. If I slow down my workouts or stop eating correctly, my body lets me know I'm slacking off."

~ Luis Collazo

238 OPEN YOUR JOINTS WITH YOGA

The practice of yoga, which developed in India thousands of years ago, was originally meant to educate the body, mind, and spirit. Today, it has become one of the most popular paths to fitness around the world. Yoga promises active flexibility, as it's about full range of motion in your joints. Practicing yoga can help you to increase muscle strength and tone, maintain a more balanced metabolism, lose weight, and improve athletic performance. It can also relieve chronic lower-back pain, soothe inflammation, ease anxiety, boost heart health, and leave you with a euphoric sense of accomplishment.

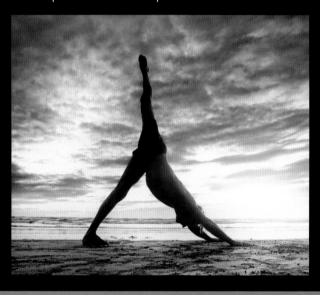

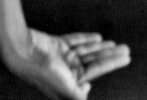

239 EASE YOUR CONCERNS

If you want to get started in this peaceful practice, here are suggestions compiled from several yoga pros for overcoming common newbie concerns, along with some additional guidelines.

TOUCH YOUR TOES You don't need to be a circus contortionist to study yoga. In fact, many first-time students are in their 50s or 60s. And if you can't touch you toes or complete certain poses, there are tools or props to aid you.

START WITH THE BASICS Even seasoned athletes who take up yoga need to start with beginner classes. Although yoga poses (called asanas) may look easy, they require a lot of control and attempting advanced movements could result in injury.

RAISE YOUR HAND If you have question, simply ask them during a lull or after class. If the instructor doesn't have an immediate answer, be assured that he or she will find one.

DON'T BE EMBARRASSED Never be afraid of looking silly. Remember, all eyes are on the instructor, not on the new folks who are just figuring things out. Everyone was a beginner at one time. Anyway, in yoga, students help each other: there is no competition.

FIND YOUR STYLE It pays to sample a number of different yoga disciplines, such as hatha, vinyasa, Iyengar, Bikram, kundalini, and ashtanga, and different instructors before making a commitment. Take two classes every week for at least a month.

RELAX AND DECOMPRESS In addition to increased flexibility, relaxation is another great benefit of yoga. Students report that they often leave class feeling like they just went to a spa.

CLEAR THE CLUTTER Yoga helps to clear mental chatter from your mind, by placing you into positions that result in being actively conscious of all your movements, and forcing you to slow down.

FEED BODY AND MIND Yoga's dual nature offers you a better body *and* mind. Many people who initially take yoga to improve their core and reduce body fat stick with it because it also increases confidence, reduces heart rate, and offers a more authentic way of being.

END WITH MINDFUL RELAXATION A yoga session typically ends with its own cool down period—a five-minute full-body relaxing pose called savasana (see #247). Some students insist that nothing matters in class as long as you have a great savasana.

240 PUMP IT UP WITH PIYO®

PiYo, a combination of Pilates and yoga, requires no weights or jumping, however, it can result in a sculpted body and improved flexibility by offering a program of continuous fluid movement. Instead of the sustained poses that are part of a normal yoga class, PiYo speeds things up, introducing dynamic, flowing sequences that burn calories and lengthen and tone your muscles. PiYo classes are not only designed to increase strength and flexibility and improve stability, they also do so with fun, energetic rhythmic choreography that will really get you moving.

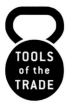
241 ASSEMBLE A YOGA KIT

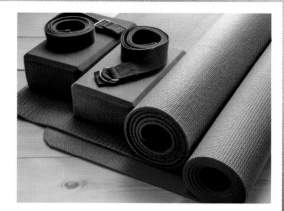

You will need only a few inexpensive accessories to make the most of your yoga experience.

YOGA MAT Yoga poses are performed on a special "sticky" mat. A yoga mat not only helps define your personal space during class, its tacky surface also creates traction so that you can hold poses, even when you're sweaty. Make sure you use one that is long enough for you to lie down on without your head or feet touching the floor. You can buy a decent mat for the cost of a few barista coffees. For purposes of hygiene, frequently cleanse your mat and other yoga tools with a mild detergent.

YOGA TOWEL "Thirsty" towels made of microfiber work best for absorbing sweat during your session.

YOGA BLOCK A yoga block, which is usually made from compressed foam or cork, can increase your flexibility, allow you to balance more steadily, and provide support so that you can maintain a pose longer and more comfortably. Most yoga studios and classes make these handy tools available to students.

YOGA STRAP These long, narrow straps are used as props to aid movement. They can help you align your posture and ease into poses, especially if you are new to yoga or have tense muscles. They are made of sturdy fabric webbing and have two D-rings on the end so that you can form them into a continuous loop.

YOGA BLANKET Another prop that you'll often see in a yoga studio is a blanket. You can fold or adjust these blankets in any way that you want to support your body in a yoga pose—rolling it up or folding it under your back, legs or neck, for example.

242 CHANNEL YOUR INNER GURU

The practice of yoga typically requires comfortable, breathable, and somewhat stretchable clothing. One of the beauties of yoga is that you don't need to be an athleisure fashion star to attend classes. On the other hand, there are some items of clothing you might want to avoid.

BOTTOMS Cropped or full-length leggings of a decent weight and in dark colors or yoga pants are fine. Avoid short shorts or loose shorts—these may not cover you properly during some poses. Also, to avoid embarrassment on both sides, ditch those old, thin pastel leggings with tears or holes in the seams.

TOPS Stick with T-shirts, fitted tanks, sports bras, or athletic tops. Avoid too-loose tops or cropped tops that can reveal too much skin during certain forward bends—look for long, sleek tops that stay put and stay comfortable throughout your entire yoga routine.

UNDERWEAR Cotton underwear may become saturated and heavy during a strenuous workout and dampen or discolor your clothing. Spend a little extra for moisture-wicking briefs or boxers.

FOOTWEAR Yoga is traditionally performed with bare feet, but some athletic manufacturers offer yoga socks, slippers, and shoes with open toes and slip-resistant soles.

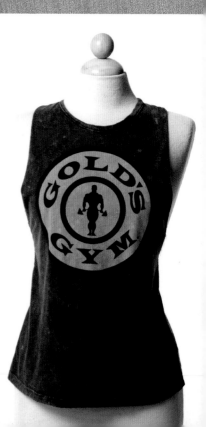

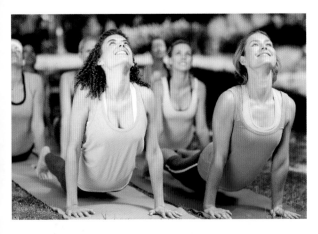

243 INHALE THE FRESH AIR

Nothing is as relaxing as taking an al fresco yoga class in a park or woodland, with the soothing sounds of birds, bees, and the breeze accompanying your asanas. The word *yoga* means "union," and outdoor yoga enables you to feel connected to nature and in harmony with the natural world—all without the artificial "calming" ambience of the indoor class.

Practicing yoga outside can intensify the experience—focusing your awareness, deepening your breathing, and helping to truly practice stillness. It also opens up the sense of smell … to pine trees, rivers, oceans, or wildflower meadows. And anything you do outdoors reminds the primitive "hunter-gatherer" part of your brain to become more alert (as a survival tactic) so open-air yoga sessions will likely elevate your energy levels. Conversely, natural settings lower your concentrations of the stress hormone cortisol.

Performing yoga on uneven surfaces, like grass, sand, or woodland trails, can also build up the muscles of your feet, hips, knees, spine, and shoulders.

Check your local gyms or neighborhood website to find where you can participate in outdoor yoga classes.

THINK *about it*

If you feel discomfort or need a break, assume the "time-out" child's pose: kneel on the mat, lower your chest to your thighs, and lower your forehead to the mat. Stretch out your arms or drop them at your sides.

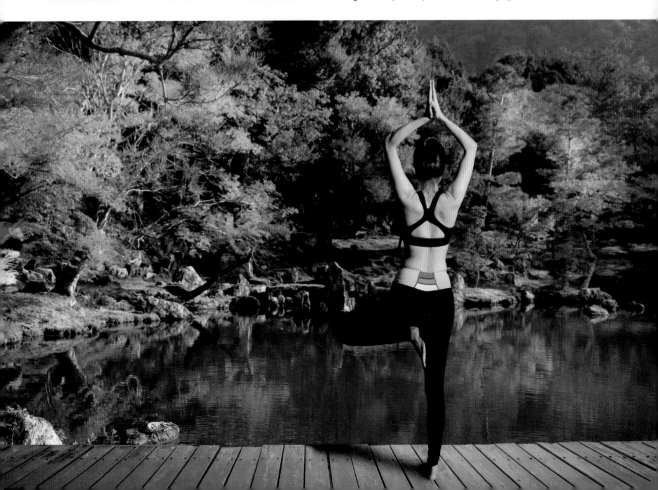

244 BREATHE DEEP

Yoga fosters both physical well-being and serenity—the positions you assume help to strengthen and elongate your muscles, while your body relaxes through a method of controlled breathing, which is called *pranayama* in Sanskrit. By using these deep, controlled-breathing techniques and by perfecting the various yoga poses, practitioners can refresh both body and spirit.

Breathing can be viewed as a link between the physical and mental aspects of human beings. As such, pranayama, which draws in sustaining oxygen and expels harmful carbon dioxide, should always be incorporated into the asanas that you practice.

Before practicing pranayama while seated, do it lying down in savasana, or corpse pose (see #246). Breathe evenly, and focus on filling every part of your lungs with oxygen from the bottom up. First, your diaphragm expands to fill your abdomen, then air fills the middle of your lungs, until it finally reaches the top of your lungs, indicated by the rising of your chest. Both sides of your chest should rise equally. When practicing pranayama while in a seated position, place one hand on your chest and the other on your abdominals to help you observe your breath. Some of the numerous pranayama exercises are listed below.

SAMAVRITTI (SAME ACTION) First, even out any breathing irregularities, and then inhale for four counts, and exhale for four counts. Samavritti calms your mind and creates a sense of balance and stability.

UJJAYI (THE VICTORIOUS BREATH) Maintain samavritti, and then constrict your epiglottis in the back of your throat. Keep your mouth closed, and listen for the *hisssss.* Ujjayi improves concentration.

KUMBHAKA (RETAINING THE BREATH) Begin with ujjayi or samavritti. After four successive breaths, hold your breath for four to eight counts. Then reduce the counts in between held breaths, and increase the number in your inhale. Kumbhaka restores energy.

ANULOMA VILOMA (ALTERNATE NOSTRIL BREATHING) Put your right thumb on the outside of your right nostril, and inhale through your left nostril while keeping your mouth closed. Close your left nostril with your ring finger, and hold momentarily. Lift your thumb, and exhale out of your right nostril. Switch nostrils. Anuloma viloma lowers the heart rate and relieves stress.

SITHALI (THE COOLING BREATH) Curl your tongue, and stick it slightly outside your mouth. Inhale through the divot of your tongue. Retain your breath, close your mouth, and exhale through your nose. Sithali cools the body.

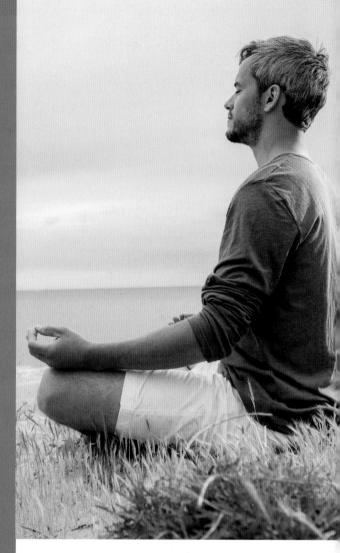

245 CHILL OUT

Getting fit is not always about the body. It often means changing or adjusting your mental attitude. What better way to approach fitness than with a discipline that teaches you how to focus your thoughts? Yoga meditation consists of "quieting a busy mind," a state you probably often wish for, but rarely achieve. In order to do this, yoga requires you to focus on one specific thing—like your breathing, a small statue, or a candle flame. It does not ask you to maintain a blank mind, only one that refuses to react to the thoughts that do intrude. Ideally, meditation should be practiced at a time of day when you are unlikely to be interrupted and in a place where you can sit comfortably on the floor. Some practitioners find it helps to repeat a resonating mantra, such as *"o-h-m-m-m ..."*

TO GET THE RIGHT VIBES

Many of the words used in yoga come from Sanskrit, the classical language of Greater India. It is called a "vibrational" language—merely hearing the words has value, even if their meaning is not understood.

ASANA Seat; yoga posture.

AYURVEDA The ancient Indian science of health.

BUDDHA An enlightened one. "The Buddha" refers to Siddhartha Gautama, an enlightened spiritual teacher who taught in India between the sixth and fourth century BC.

CHAKRA Energy center. The basic system has seven chakras (the root, sacrum, solar plexus, heart, throat, third eye, and crown). Each has its significance and is associated with a color, element, and syllable.

DRISHTI Gazing point used during asana practice.

GURU One who brings us from dark into light; a spiritual mentor.

KARMA Action; the law of karma is the law of cause and effect, based upon the complex web of conditions, individuals and relationships in the universe, not just a simple concept like "steal from someone, and you'll be robbed in return".

MANTRA A repeated sound, syllable, word or phrase; often used in chanting and meditation.

MUDRA A hand gesture; the most common mudras are anjali mudra (pressing palms together at the heart) and gyana mudra (with the index finger and thumb touching).

NAMASTE Greeting commonly translated as "the light within me bows to the light within you"; used at the beginning and end of a yoga class.

OM The original syllable; chanted "o-h-m" at the beginning and/or end of many yoga sessions.

PRANA Life energy; chi; qi.

PRANAYAMA Breath control; breathing exercises.

SAMADHI A state of complete self-actualization; enlightenment.

SAVASANA Corpse pose; final relaxation; typically performed at the end of hatha yoga classes.

SHAKTI Female energy.

SHIVA Male energy; a Hindu deity.

YOGI/YOGINI A male/female practitioner of yoga.

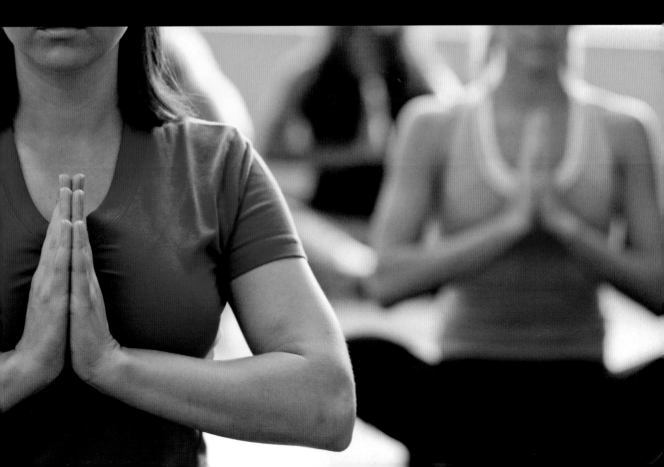

247 SALUTE THE SUN

This classic yoga flow will energize your body as it stretches and strengthens all your major muscle groups. Known as the sun salutation, or surya namaskar, it is a series of basic poses that appear in most yoga classes. On your first try, hold each of these poses for 10 to 15 seconds, and then flow into the next. Check the chart opposite for the muscle groups worked and the Sanskrit names for the poses, which many yoga instructors will refer to during class.

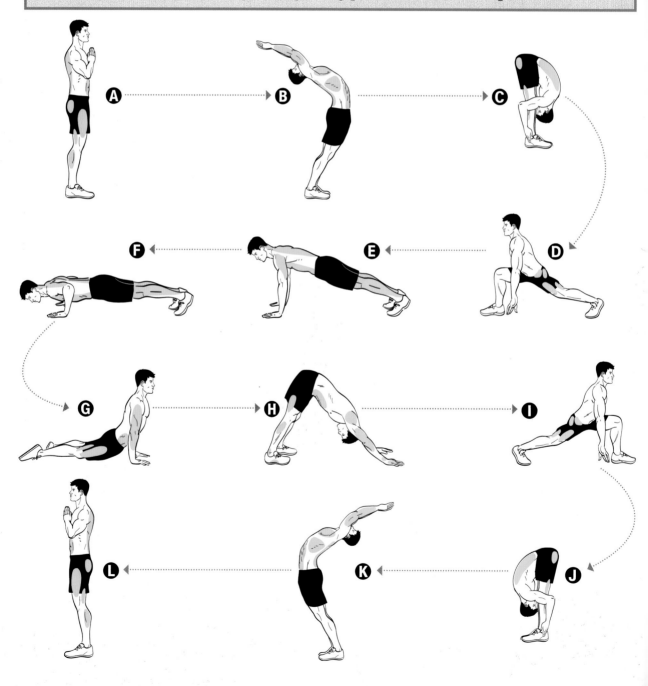

A **MOUNTAIN POSE** Stand with both feet touching, back straight, arms pressed against your sides, and your weight evenly distributed on both feet. Flex the muscles in your legs, stomach, and glutes. Bring your hands in front of you in a prayer position

B **STANDING BACKBEND** From their prayer position, lift your hands until your arms are straight over your head. Lift your chest toward the ceiling, and then bend your shoulders and upper back slowly backward. Stop bending if you experience any pain or discomfort. Hold for two breaths, and then return to mountain pose.

C **FORWARD FOLD** Bend forward from the hips. Keep your knees straight, and reach your fingertips to the floor. If you can't reach, put your hands on the back of your ankles, or cross your forearms and hold your elbows.

D **HIGH LUNGE** Bend your knees, then step your left foot back until your right knee forms a right angle. Rest your torso on the front of your thigh, and put your hands on either side of your right foot. Look forward with your neck straight and long.

E **PLANK** Step your right foot back to meet your left. Hold yourself up in a high push-up stance, your arms perpendicular to the floor, your back straight, and your hips up (not sagging toward the floor).

F **HALF-PLANK** From plank, lower your torso toward the floor, keeping your elbows tight against your sides until your body is a few inches off the mat. Keep your tailbone firm and your legs active and engaged.

G **UPWARD-FACING DOG** Lower your body to the floor, then stretch your legs back, pushing the tops of your feet into the floor. Spread your palms on the mat, then push your chest off the mat until your arms are straight. Tilt your head up so that your neck is straight.

H **DOWNWARD-FACING DOG** Flip from the tops of your toes onto the bottoms, while also pushing your hips up into the air. Your body should form an upside-down V with your palms on the mat and your fingers spread wide. Push your heels down toward the floor, then widen your shoulder blades, and pull them toward your buttocks.

I **HIGH LUNGE** See D, but step back with your right foot to reverse the movement of the pose.

J **FORWARD FOLD** See C.

K **STANDING BACKBEND** See B.

L **MOUNTAIN POSE** See A.

EXERCISE	TARGET	SANSKRIT NAME
MOUNTAIN POSE	Legs, glutes, and stomach	Tadasana
STANDING BACKBEND	Abdominals, rib cage, arms, chest, and back	Ardha anuvittasana
FORWARD FOLD	Glutes, back, hamstrings, and calves	Uttanasana
HIGH LUNGE	Hip flexors, quads, glutes, and hamstrings	Aekpaadprasarnaasana
PLANK	Abdominals, lower back, chest, neck, shoulders, upper trapezius, biceps, triceps, glutes, thighs, and calves	—
HALF-PLANK	Abdominals, lower back, chest, neck, shoulders, upper trapezius, biceps, triceps, glutes, thighs, and calves	Chaturanga
UPWARD-FACING DOG	Arms, legs, and core	Urdhva mukha svanasana
DOWNWARD-FACING DOG	Hamstrings, calves, ankles, arches, hands, wrists, arms, shoulders, and abdominals	Adhomukha svanasana

PLAY DEAD Most yoga classes end in savasana, or corpse pose. The name is an apt one—you lie still and completely relaxed. It may look easy, but it takes practice to learn how to release the tension in all your muscles, yet still remain conscious and alert.

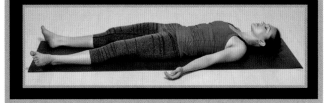

248 CONNECT MIND AND BODY WITH PILATES

Pilates aids the development of a balanced body by focusing on core strength, flexibility, body alignment, and stability, and by using your own body weight to create resistance. Joseph Pilates developed the system (originally called Contrology) in Germany in the early twentieth century. Inspired by his study of Asian philosophy and the Greek ideal of the perfect integrated human, he created a series of exercises based on the connection between the body and the mind. With its similarity to yoga and emphasis on resistance work, this versatile discipline exploded in popularity across the world in the 1980s—and has never lost its appeal.

Pilates, once the province of dancers and athletes, now benefits adults, seniors, and kids of all fitness levels, as well as those in rehab and women getting in shape after pregnancy. Advocates insist that Pilates not only makes them stronger, longer, and leaner, but also enables them to move with grace and coordination. They have better posture and feel more "aligned and together" as they handle the stress of their daily lives. The system can be practiced at any time and almost anywhere, and unlike fitness methods that require a lot of reps, Pilates asks only that, no matter how few you can perform, you should fully and precisely execute each movement.

249 PRACTICE THE PRINCIPLES

There are six principles of Pilates: concentration, centering, control, breathing, precision, and flow. When you integrate them during a workout, you can dramatically improve your fitness results.

CONCENTRATION Concentrate on the mind-body connection during an exercise, and picture the specific muscle pathways that will complete that movement. Then form a mental image of yourself performing the exercise correctly, in proper alignment.

CENTERING Pay special attention to the muscles of your core—the Pilates powerhouse—which include the abdomen, lower back, hips, and butt. They help all your body's muscles function more efficiently.

CONTROL Controlled exercises do not focus on intensity or reps, but on quality of movement. Control also develops strength, stamina, flexibility, equilibrium, and good posture—preventing stress on bones, muscles, and joints.

BREATHING Each Pilates exercise has a specific breathing pattern, so it takes practice in order to coordinate breathing and movement. Start by inhaling deeply through your nose during prep and return, and exhaling fully from your mouth during the rigorous phase.

PRECISION Pay attention to your form—in Pilates, quality matters more than quantity. Start and end correctly, tracing with your mind—and then your body—each step that composes the complete movement.

FLOW Exercise as though you were a dancer, with graceful connections and transitions from one position to the next as you lengthen your body.

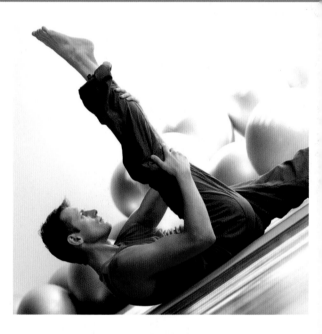

GYM
etiquette

250 TONE IT DOWN

The gym may not be a noise-free zone like a library, but it helps to keep the background noise down whenever possible, especially in classes like yoga and Pilates. It's best to keep your phone in the bag, but if you must have it, set it on vibrate while you exercise, so that incoming ringtones won't disturb others. If you must answer a call, go out to the lobby or parking lot. And try not to chat on the phone while using equipment that others are waiting for. You might appear more focused on your phone call than on your workout.

251 CHOOSE A PILATES CLASS

If your gym or studio has specialized Pilates equipment, take a few classes to familiarize yourself or, better yet, invest in some one-on-one time with a Pilates instructor who can help you apply the six principles. Exercising safely is a key aspect of this discipline, and you don't want to risk injury because you don't know how a certain apparatus works. Make sure to try out the reformer, a machine that utilizes pulleys and resistance from the participant's own body weight and with graduated levels of springs. Most of the Pilates exercises done on a mat can also be performed on the reformer.

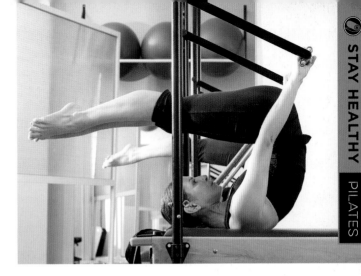

252 EQUIP YOURSELF

Pilates exercises can be done on a mat on the floor or by using the special exercise apparatuses developed by Joseph Pilates. There are also portable Pilates aids you can use in class or at home.

MAT Pilates mats are thicker than yoga mats and not sticky. Look for a supportive mat at least a half-inch thick (1.27 cm) and long enough and wide enough so that you can exercise without shifting off the edges.

PILATES BALL This small inflatable ball, which measures about 9 inches (23 cm) in diameter, can be grasped between the knees to work those stubborn inner-thigh muscles or placed behind your back for support during mat exercises.

FOAM ROLLER These tubular aids comes in a variety of sizes, colors, and densities; they provide cushioning and can also be used for stretching, strengthening, balance training, and self-massage (see #227–230).

MAGIC CIRCLE Also called a fitness circle, exercise ring, or fitness ring, this flexible rubber-encased metal ring with two pliable handles adds gentle resistance to Pilates movements when you squeeze the sides together or place tension on it from the inside.

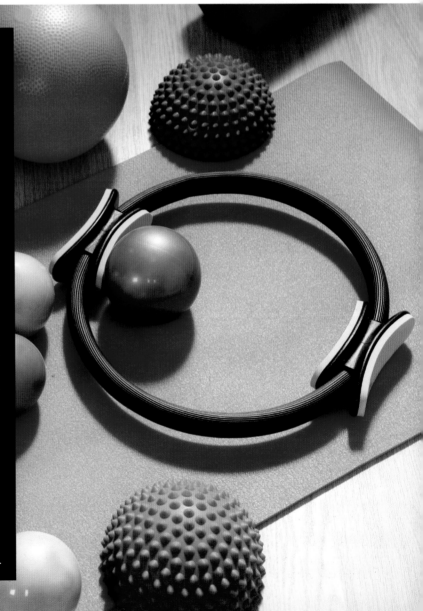

253 FLATTEN YOUR TUMMY

Pilates is known for its ability to help you achieve a toned and flat midsection. The following workout, known as the Stomach Series, Abdominal Series, or Belly Burner, lets you sample five of the classical Pilates mat exercises that really challenge your abdominal endurance. Your ultimate goal is to move seamlessly from one exercise to the next. If you are new to Pilates, begin by working on the first exercise, then when you feel comfortable performing it with precision and control, move onto the next in the series, gradually adding until you can perform all five in one rhythmic flow.

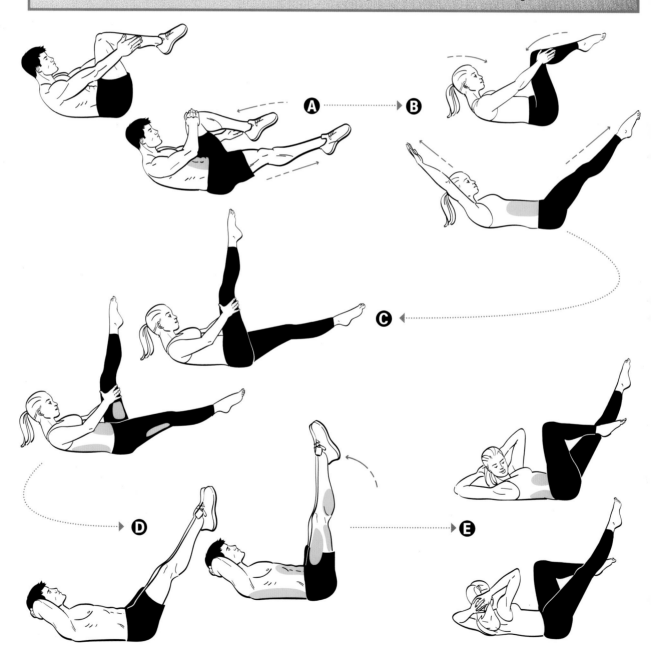

A SINGLE LEG STRETCH Lie faceup on the mat. Exhale, and curl your head and shoulders up off the mat, bend both knees into your chest, extending one leg straight out. Put your outside hand on the ankle of your bent leg and your inside hand on the knee of your bent leg. Inhale, switching legs two times in one inhalation and switching hand placement simultaneously. Exhale, switching legs two times in one exhalation, keeping hands in their proper placement.

B DOUBLE LEG STRETCH Lie faceup on your mat, and then curl your upper body into a half-curl position, pulling your knees to your chest with your hands on your ankles. Inhale, simultaneously extending your arms back and your legs forward. Exhale while hugging your knees back into the center. Make sure you are keeping your upper body lifted off the mat.

C SCISSORS Lie faceup on your mat with your arms by your side and your legs raised in the tabletop position. Inhale, drawing in your abdominals. Exhale, reaching your legs straight up and lifting your head and shoulders off the mat. Inhale, holding the position while lengthening your legs. Exhale, stretch your right leg away from your body, and raise your left leg toward your trunk. Hold onto your left leg with both hands, pulsing twice with a small, rhythmic back-and-forth motion while keeping your shoulders down. Inhale, switching your legs in the air, and then exhale, reaching for the opposite leg.

D DOUBLE STRAIGHT LEG LOWER/LIFT Lie faceup on your mat, and extend both legs up to the ceiling, squeezing your heels, sitting bones, and inner thighs together as you externally rotate the legs in the Pilates V-stance. With hands behind the head and elbows wide, lengthen the back of your neck, and curl up into a C-curve with your shoulder blades cresting the mat. Inhale, and lower both of your legs. Exhale, as you draw your legs up using lower abs, not your hip flexors.

E CRISS CROSS Lie faceup on the mat with your legs in tabletop position. Place your hands behind your head with shoulders down and elbows wide. Exhale, and curl your upper body off the mat. Inhale, then exhale, and extend your right leg as you rotate your ribcage to the right, keeping your elbows wide as you bring your left armpit toward the right knee. Turn your torso a little more with a small pulse as you continue to exhale. Inhale, and return to center. Exhale, extend your left leg, and rotate your torso to the left. Continue to alternate sides.

EXERCISE	REPS	BENEFITS
SINGLE LEG STRETCH	4 to 12 reps with each leg	Strengthens abs, promotes coordination, and stabilizes torso
DOUBLE LEG STRETCH	4 to 6 reps	Strengthens and builds abdominal endurance, promotes coordination, and stabilizes trunk
SCISSORS	4 to 12 reps with each leg	Strengthens abs, stretches hamstrings and hip flexors, and increases spine flexibility
DOUBLE STRAIGHT LEG LOWER/LIFT	4 to 6 reps	Strengthens abs, lengthens legs, and strengthens hips flexors
CRISS CROSS	4 to 12 reps	Strengthens abs and obliques and challenges trunk rotation

KEEP GOOD FORM Form is all-important in Pilates, and certain positions will often come up during a mat workout.

NEUTRAL POSITION You maintain the natural curve of your spine—typically when lying on your back.

IMPRINTED POSITION Press your navel toward your spine. This move flattens your abdominal wall and lengthens and strengthens your lower-back muscles.

C-CURVE C-curve describes the shape of your back and spine when you scoop in your stomach, stretching the muscles surrounding your spine in the process.

PILATES V-STANCE The legs are together, straight, and rotated outward from the top of the thigh, which brings the heels together with toes pointing slightly out, forming a V.

TABLETOP You lie faceup with legs raised, knees bent, and shins parallel to the mat. From this position, you will then lift your torso for many Pilates exercises.

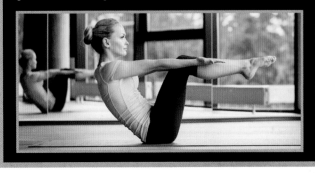

DIG DEEP The finish line may be in sight, but this moment is when many competitors feel they're starting to lose steam. Maybe it's been a tough, uphill battle, and you're unsure you can go all the way. Perhaps your daily obligations to your job and family are becoming too demanding, especially after you've been "otherwise engaged" for 11 weeks. Now is the time to really dig deep and find that extra grit to make fitness and health your priority for just one more week, and to make it to the end.

 GIVE YOURSELF A PEP TALK As you near the finish line, if your resolve falters, it can help to remind yourself that you are on a mission and to re-emphasize your specific goal: losing weight, shaping up, overcoming health risks, or other concerns. Some find it helpful to approach the Challenge just one gym visit at a time—especially if contemplating a 12-week haul seems daunting. If you feel that you haven't made it far as you'd like, remind yourself how far you've come. Look at your before picture and

remember why you are doing this. Focus on the ground that you *have* gained and the shape you're *now* in, an outcome you may have doubted you'd ever achieve. Ask yourself, "Is one more week really that far?"

STAY IN THE GAME FOR YOUR

 "FANS" Peer pressure can sometimes be a good thing at a time like this. Stop and think of all the people rooting for you, the ones who maintain faith in you and your goals—your family, friends, coworkers, gym buddies, and trainers.

FOLLOW A WINNER'S JOURNEY
Johnelle Burnett
Female Winner, Ages 18–29

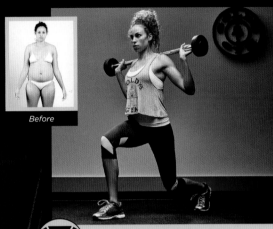

Before

LOST 49.5 pounds (22 kg), 21.5 inches (54.6 cm), and 14.7% body fat

In college, Johnelle played basketball and was in awesome shape. Then she got married and gained weight during each of her two pregnancies. After an unexpected cross-country move, she started using fast food as a crutch to avoid cooking. In spite of taking Zumba classes at Gold's Gym, her weight hardly budged. When she saw posters for a 12-week body transformation challenge at her gym, she thought, "I want to do this, and I want to win it by losing the most weight." She signed up that day.

Her trainer made a meal and exercise plan and cheered her on. She started working out six days a week, taking classes like interval training, weight lifting, cycling, and Pilates. She focused on eating unprocessed foods, whole grains, and lean protein. Twelve weeks later, she'd lost nearly 30 percent of her body weight and won the Gold's Gym challenge for her age and gender.

Now that she has her "dream body," Johnelle is setting new goals, like running a half marathon. She says, "This is beyond what I ever thought I could accomplish. Doing the Challenge has helped me learn to push myself to accomplish new things."

They've seen the many positive changes in your body and your attitude, and remarked on them. Let those encouraging comments be the inspiration that keeps you going. If you let your fans know you won't disappoint them, there's a good chance you won't let yourself down either. There is also a dedicated Gold's Gym Challenge community on Facebook, where you and others can work to support each other. Let everyone know you have just one more week to go, and you can rally each other to the finish line!

WINNER'S WORDS

"Set goals. ... It's important to find something that motivates you to push yourself."

~ Johnelle Burnett

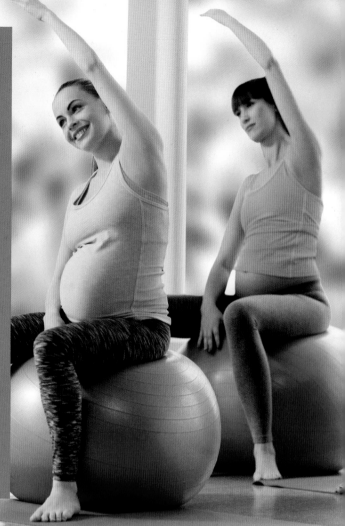

254 EASE INTO PREGNANCY

Fitness-conscious celebrities often take flak from the press for continuing their strenuous workouts well into pregnancy. So is exercise really safe while you are carrying a child? Medical research confirms that working out while pregnant provides a host of benefits. Exercise improves energy levels, posture, muscle tone, and endurance, and it decreases the risk of long-term obesity and gestational diabetes. It can also reduce backaches, swelling, and bloating, and it's even possible that being fit can result in a faster delivery. It definitely speeds up recovery time.

So, which exercises are safe? Yoga, Pilates, dance, cycling, and running are fine, but common sense dictates no martial arts or anything that might risk trauma or cause you to fall. Some Gold's Gyms have classes just for pregnant women (search your local area for "Mommy and Me" classes), often with stability balls or other low-impact aids.

Keep active with cardio and light lifting to combat first trimester fatigue. In the second trimester, use a stability ball to ease your back by raising your lower torso with your legs. In the third trimester, avoid twisting motions, or lying supine or prone; try walking, flexibility training, and light resistance training. If in doubt about the rigors of a routine or exercise, err on the side of caution. See your doctor if there are any symptoms of fetal distress.

255 EAT FOR TWO

In spite of that old expression, "She's eating for two now," which can be a license for indulgence, most pregnant women only require an additional 300 calories daily—the equivalent of one grilled cheese sandwich.

Pregnancy is not an excuse to load up a plate, but there are certain things that you should be adding to your diet to ensure good health for you and your baby. Eat a variety of foods that supply a range of nutrients. Include whole grains, low-fat dairy products, and lean meat, and fill up your plate with a cornucopia of colorful vegetables and fruits. To meet vitamin and nutrimental needs, take antenatal supplements during and after your pregnancy, especially those that contain folic acid, necessary for fetal bone development during the first 12 weeks, and iron, to build up your reserves. It's also important to take at least 1000 mg of calcium daily; augment that with dairy products and leafy green vegetables.

256 PREPARE FOR BIRTH

Many gyms offering classes for moms-to-be and their partners, recommend specific exercises to ready the body for childbirth. There are a few that can ease delivery. Simple pelvic tilts can also help relieve backaches and keep your abs strong. Just stand straight with your back to a wall, and relax your spine. Breathe in deeply, and press the small of your back against the wall. Exhale, and continue the exercise for about five minutes. You can also do this lying down (see #257).

Squat exercises (see #125) are a great addition to a pregnancy fitness plan because they open up the pelvic outlet by a quarter inch to a half inch. Sitting cross-legged will also strengthen and stretch your pelvic muscles (as well as the back and thighs). Sit on the floor with your back straight, your soles touching, and your knees dropped to opposite sides. As you gently press both of your knees toward the floor with your elbows, you'll feel the stretching in your inner thighs.

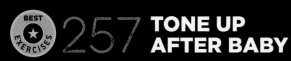

257 TONE UP AFTER BABY

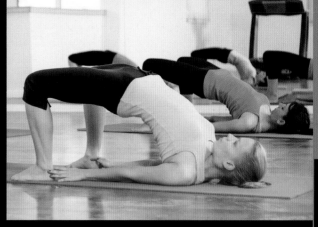

Most new moms would love to get their pre-baby body back as quickly as possible, but how soon is too soon? The rule of thumb has long been that is okay to begin exercising six weeks after birth. Many doctors are now revising that time frame: if you had an uncomplicated vaginal delivery, it's generally safe to begin exercising as soon as you feel ready. If you had a C-section or other complicated birth, work with your doctor to determine a proper exercise plan and schedule—and when you can start it.

When you are ready to begin getting back into shape, it may be hard to find the time—taking care of a newborn usually doesn't allow for hours spent at the gym. You may also feel you simply have no energy. But exercising after pregnancy offers benefits beyond helping you to lose weight and tone muscles. Exercising boosts both your mood and your energy levels, and it ups your stamina and endurance—things you certainly need to look after a newborn. Here are two easy exercises to get you started.

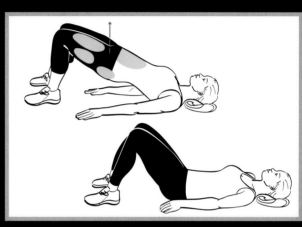

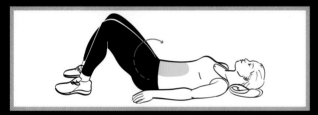

Ⓐ PELVIC TILT This is a gentle abdominal-strengthening move that many women can begin to perform as early as a week after birth. Try for 5 to 10 reps.

HOW Lie on your back with knees bent (you can place a pillow under your hips and another between your knees if you are uncomfortable at first). Flatten your back against the floor by tightening your abdominal muscles and bending your pelvis up slightly. Hold for up to 10 seconds. Repeat.

Ⓑ PELVIC BRIDGE Also known as the shoulder bridge, this exercise tones your legs and glutes while strengthening the abs, lower-back, and pelvic floor muscles. Try for 5 to 10 reps.

HOW Lie on your back with your knees bent and your feet flat, and about one hip-width apart. Press your feet into the mat and squeeze your glutes, raising your hips until your body makes a straight line from your shoulders to your knees. Hold for up to 10 seconds. Repeat.

258 GET IN SHAPE WITH YOUR KIDS

Many fitness centers, including Gold's Gym, offer "Mommy and Me" classes for new moms and their toddlers. Yet the parent-child fitness bond doesn't have to end once your baby grows out of this stage. Try exposing your young children to some of the same fitness classes or pursuits you love (and that many gyms offer for kids)—yoga, martial arts, sports conditioning, or dance. That way, you can pursue them together at home, at the beach, or in the park. You will enhance your relationship through these shared interests and also be guiding your child toward a fitness-based future.

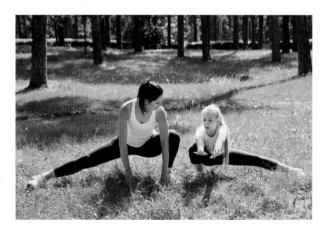

259 STAY MOBILE

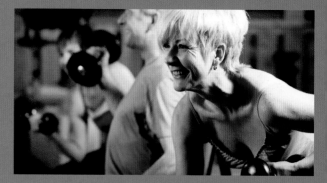

You tend to lose mobility as you age, but there is no reason you cannot stave off this trend by adding an exercise regimen to your weekly schedule. Remaining active can help seniors (and those still on their way there) combat bone loss, aids circulation, boosts energy, and bolsters memory and mood.

For many in the aging population, mobility also means independence—access to shopping facilities, as well as social, cultural, and medical outlets. The loss of mobility, even a marginal amount, can signal a turning point in vitality and interest in the outside world. It's therefore critical that aging baby boomers do whatever they can to foster it. Below are some suggestions for how to get in motion and stay in motion.

EXERCISE DAILY Even if you don't jog or bike, the simple act of walking integrates the functions of musculoskeletal, cardio-respiratory, sensory, and neural systems.

CHECK VISION AND HEARING Impaired vision or hearing can make the outdoors a dangerous place—especially if you don't see oncoming cars or hear their horns. Be sure your faculties are in good working order before you venture out.

MAINTAIN YOUR WEIGHT Extra weight is hard on an aging body. Consider small, nutritionally dense meals or snacks every three or four hours. Avoid flour, sugar, and rice.

FOCUS ON POSTURE AND BALANCE Standing up straight and long with your abdominal muscles tightened protects the spine. Maintaining good balance through exercise helps prevent falls and injuries.

LOSE THE STRESS Studies reveal that exercise can reduce the effects of stress-induced aging at the cellular level. It is noted that those who keep fit and feel young for their age also score better on cognitive tests.

260 AGE GRACEFULLY

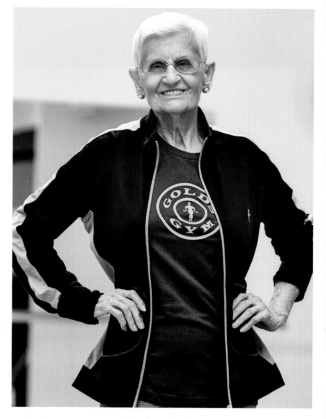

Many fitness centers, including Gold's Gym, offer low-impact classes geared for senior citizens, some of them under names like Silver Sneakers, Fabulous Fitness 50+, and Always Active. Low impact does not mean no impact, however. You'll definitely get a workout. Depending on location, seniors can choose from weight training, cardio, stretching, cycling, yoga, Pilates, aqua aerobics, Zumba, and dance classes, among many others. And if certain floor routines are too taxing for some individuals, most gyms even offer the option of performing them while seated in a chair. Check your local listings for health clubs in your area that offer senior classes. Remember, you're never too old to improve your health!

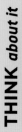

THINK *about it*

Your genetic makeup accounts for only about 25 percent of your longevity and health. Many of the potential health threats you face as you get older are ones you can work to prevent, or even reverse.

261 GO THROUGH THE MOTIONS

Each of your joints has a prescribed path that it follows, called its range of motion (ROM). In order for a joint to have full range of motion, it must have good flexibility, but as you age this flexibility is often compromised. Keeping your joints moving is therefore essential for maintaining easy movement. There are three kinds of exercises used to build, recover, and maintain ROM.

PASSIVE RANGE OF MOTION (PROM) Often used by older folk with severe movement limitations or anyone recovering from a sports injury or joint replacement, PROM calls for you do nothing as a therapist or equipment (such as a knee machine) moves the compromised joint through the range of motion.

ACTIVE ASSISTIVE RANGE OF MOTION (AAROM) Here, you use the muscles surrounding a joint in order to perform the exercise, relying on help from a therapist, trainer, or equipment.

ACTIVE RANGE OF MOTION (AROM) With AROM exercises, you use the muscles surrounding a joint to do the movements with no outside assistance.

262 EXTEND YOUR RANGE

To keep your muscles and joints healthy, include a few ROM exercises in your fitness plan. The following sample exercises focus on ankles, knees, and shoulders—three areas at which you might notice compromised range of motion. Definitely target problem areas, but look for exercises that also target joints that are working well to maintain your body's full range of motion throughout your life.

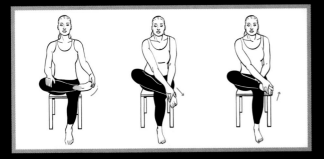

Ⓐ ANKLE FLEX-EVERT-INVERT This exercise combines three moves to take your ankles through their full ROM.

HOW Sit with your right leg crossed over your left knee. Use your left hand to pull the top of your foot and toes toward you until you feel a gentle stretch on the top of your foot and ankle. Next, place your thumb on the top of your foot and your fingers across the bottom. Gently push your foot downward with a slight rotation so that your littlest toes rise slightly toward the ceiling. You should feel a gentle stretch on the inside of your ankle. Move your thumb to the bottom of your foot, and place your fingers across the top. Gently pull your foot so your smallest toe comes toward you, and your thumb pushes the inside of the ball of your foot away from you until you feel a gentle stretch on the outside of your ankle. Repeat all steps with your left foot.

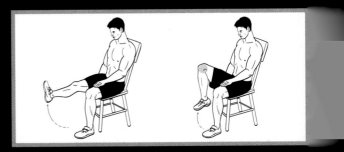

Ⓑ EXTEND AND MARCH This compound move can improve the range of motion of your knees.

HOW Sit with your back straight and feet planted firmly on the floor. Extend one leg straight out, holding the extended position for 5 to 10 seconds. Slowly lower, and then bend the knee of the same leg to lift your leg as if you were marching. Slowly lower, and alternate extending and marching for the desired reps before switching to the other side.

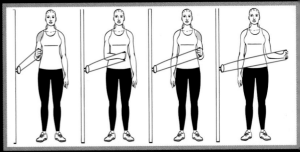

Ⓒ INTERNAL AND EXTERNAL SHOULDER ROTATION This simple move targets your deltoids and rotator cuff (see #090) to improve the range of motion of your shoulders.

HOW Attach a resistance band to a doorknob. Take hold of the handle, and, keeping your upper arm close to your side, bend your elbow to 90 degrees. Bring your hand across your body. Return to the start, switch hands, and bring your hand away from the middle of your body. Repeat in the opposite direction.

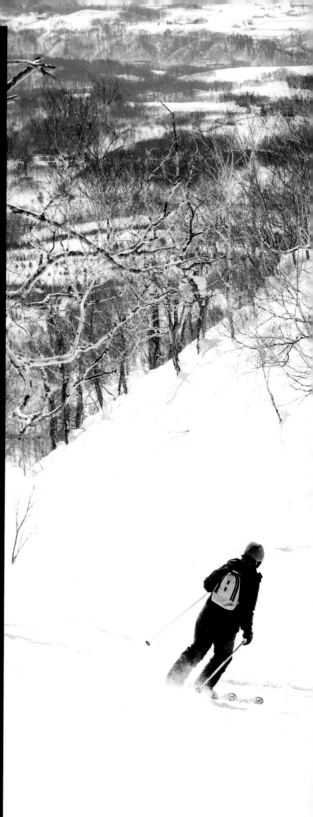

263 BOOK A FIT-CATION

If you are one of a growing number of individuals who now seek fitness-based destinations in lieu of relaxing vacation spots or family fun parks, here are some faraway locations that offer breathtaking scenery, along with lots of challenging physical activities. Be sure to check out a nearby Gold's Gym—they are part of the global community, after all—where you can put your travel pass to work.

PADDLE A BOARD Bohol in the Philippines, also known as God's Little Paradise, offers stand-up paddleboarding on the Loboc and Abatan Rivers, with miles of flat stretches for observing native wildlife, such as tarsiers, monitor lizards, and geckos. Paddleboarding provides a low-impact, full-body ° workout and improves balance. Also check out the multiple Gold's Gym locations in nearby Cebu City.

HIT THE SLOPES If the cardio exhilaration of skiing or snowboarding is your winter mania, try Japan's "powder paradise," Niseko. With nearly 50 feet of snow annually, Niseko's runs will definitely wow you. Try an afternoon of snowmobiling, and then have a soak in a volcanic hot spring. Tokyo has a multitude of Gold's Gyms, which you will pass through getting to and from Niseko.

CHALLENGE THE ROCKIES The United States has no shortage of fitness destinations, but mountain biking in Ogden, Utah, also offers spectacular scenery and famous national parks, along with a full-muscle workout and lung-bursting cardio. Ogden attracts world-class riders, but provides trails for cyclists of every level. There are at least four Gold's Gyms in the Salt Lake City area.

FIND YOUR INNER LIGHT Follow in the footsteps of the Beatles, and travel to Rishikesh, India, to study in the yoga capital of the world. Seek enlightenment at the Ganga Aarti ceremony at Triveni Ghat or find peace while rafting on the holy Ganges River. The less spiritual can mingle with Bollywood stars at the Gold's Gym in Dehradum—or more than 90 other locations in India.

HIKE SIBERIA Every year, nearly 4,500 volunteers hack hundreds of miles of trails around stunning Lake Baikel, the deepest lake in the world, known as the Pearl of Siberia. This rugged wilderness offers hiking and outdoor activities, including seal sightings. Check out the Moscow Gold's Gyms before you embark on the Trans-Siberian Railway. All aboard for adventure!

EXPLORE MACHU PICHU This ancient Inca city, one of the wonders of the New World, is located at an elevation of 8,000 feet (2,440 m)—so consider the cardio benefits of getting there during a four-day trek through three mountain passes. As you pass through Lima prior to embarking, check out one of the dozen Gold's Gyms in the area.

264 SURVIVE A LONG FLIGHT

If you're stuck on a long flight, it's important to keep moving. This not only helps you avoid cramping and stiffness, it can prevent deep-vein thrombosis, a serious condition that may occur during extended air travel. Once the seatbelt sign is off, move around the cabin every hour or so—stroll the aisles and give your legs a stretch. You may also require a glass of wine to maintain your sanity, but go easy on the alcohol, because it can dehydrate you; opt instead for water or juice.

265 STAY FIT ON THE ROAD

Whether you are traveling for pleasure or business, you probably want to work out the kinks of your journey before you sightsee or head for your conference. Most upscale hotels have complimentary health clubs and pools. You can also take advantage of fitness centers outside the hotel—ask the concierge about guest passes. And if you are a Gold's Gym member, search online for locations—there are more than 700 facilities in 42 states and 30 countries. Runners, hikers, and cyclists can find city trails by checking out mapmyfitness.com. Don't forget to use the stairs for a super cardio blast, and check your pedometer or wearable monitor to make sure you're meeting your step goals.

266 CREATE A HOTEL ROOM GYM

It's easy to set up a mini-gym in the privacy of your hotel room using portable fitness gear—and a towel or two.

TOWEL WARM-UP Hold a stretched towel overhead, and bend side to side for five reps, and then stretch it horizontally in front of you, swivel to the right, hold for five seconds, and then swivel to the left. Sit down on the floor with your legs outstretched, and loop a towel around your feet. Pull both ends toward you to stretch your back.

JUMP ROPE This lightweight fitness aid can furnish a taxing cardio workout.

AQUABELLS Before heading to the hotel pool, fill these collapsible dumbbells with tap water; when filled, they can weigh up to 16 pounds (7 kg) each. You're now ready to add some resistance training to your swim routine.

BODY WEIGHT Your body is the most important piece of exercise equipment. Using your own weight in exercises such as situps and pushups is a workout with no added gear.

267 STAY FIT ON THE JOB

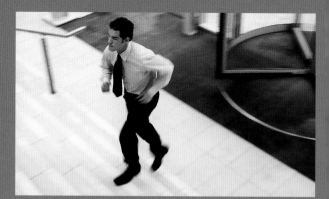

You'd be surprised at how many opportunities there are to incorporate fitness into the workplace—even if you are a sedentary desk jockey—as well as during your commute.

DON'T SKIP BREAKFAST Your body needs that early meal to boost post-sleep metabolism. Research also shows that skipping breakfast can increase your desire for fatty foods at lunchtime. If there's no time for breakfast before work, keep some instant oatmeal or low-fat yogurt in the office breakroom, and eat at your desk.

WALK WHENEVER Head outside during your lunch break to gain the many benefits of walking. If you drive to work, park at the far end of the lot. And, of course, walk to work if you can.

COMMUTE TO HEALTH If you carpool to work, you and your fellow passengers can make use of this downtime. Engage your core by contracting your abs and pressing hard on the roof of the car with both hands for 10 seconds. Or do an elbow squeeze: touch your elbows together and press as hard as you can for 10 to 20 seconds. You can do these and many other isometrics just about anywhere there is a seat—a car, plane, bus, train, or subway. If you commute via subway, choose to stand, and use the strap, pole, or bar to do some isometrics.

TAKE THE STAIRS Avoid the elevator, and use the stairs when moving from floor to floor. To get in some morning cardio, sprint up and down the stairs at the train station or at your building.

MEET FACE TO FACE Instead of phoning or texting co-workers so you can discuss something, get up from your desk and walk over to their cubicles. The same applies to meetings in nearby buildings—ditch the conference call, and discuss your agenda in person. This also combats the impersonality of so much technology-driven office contact.

PREPARE FOR SNACK ATTACKS Office workers can gain up to six pounds a year from just eating unhealthy vending machine snacks. Stay away from those tempting chips and candy bars and instead keep some fruit or nuts in your desk.

Ask the EXPERT

HOW CAN I KEEP FIT AT MY DESK?

Fitness-based office furniture (like treadmill, stationary bike, elliptical desks, and stability ball chairs) is meant to address a growing health threat to our computer-oriented workforce—physical inactivity, which the World Health Organization ranks as the fourth biggest killer on the planet, over obesity. The obvious benefit of these workout desks is that they keep you moving. The downside is that in recent studies, which compared treadmill-desk workers to seated workers, the former performed worse on all aspects of thinking, including math, comprehension and concentration, as well as typing. Perhaps a better option is an elevated workstation. Standing upright causes your body to shift, naturally, from side to side. You can also simply stretch at your desk, or get up from the computer, and get some isometrics exercises or stretch every 20 minutes. You can also try the exercises on the opposite page (#268).

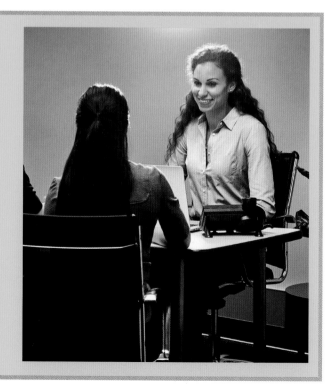

Don't let a busy schedule stop you from getting an effective workout. These four sweat-free exercises are just a sampling of the many that the fitness experts at Gold's Gym have designed for the workplace. You just need a resistance band and a few extra minutes throughout the day, so stop making excuses, and use that office downtime to up your fitness level.

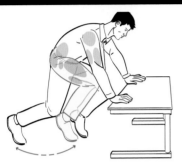

Ⓐ DESK MOUNTAIN CLIMBER When you perform this exercise, really focus on keeping your core tight—the more you use your abdominals, the less strain you feel in your back. Perform three sets of 15 to 20 reps.

HOW Stand facing a desk or counter an arm's length away. Rest your hands on the edge, palms down and slightly wider than shoulder-width apart. Lean in, then walk your feet out behind you. Lower your hips slightly so your body forms a diagonal. Balancing on your toes, bring your right knee toward your chest. Alternate legs continuously.

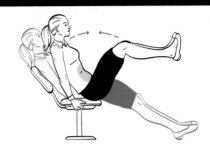

Ⓒ IN AND OUTS This move may seem tough at first, so beginners should start by keeping one leg on the floor and lifting the other knee up, then alternating. And be sure to take your time when you do these. Perform three sets of 10 reps.

HOW Sit on the front edge of a chair (without wheels). Place your hands along the sides of your body, holding the sides of the chair. Kick your legs straight out in front of you, toes flexed, and then lean back in the chair as far as you can while keeping your back straight. Then simultaneously bring your knees and chest toward each other as close as you can. Return to your starting position, and repeat.

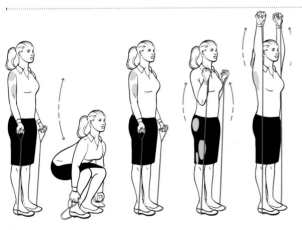

Ⓑ STAND-UP HANDS UP This exercise is great for a midday energy burst because it works more than three muscle groups. Perform three sets of 10 reps.

HOW Stand with your feet hip-width apart. Put a resistance band under your feet while gripping one end in each hand. Lower your hips to a squat position, and slowly stand up. Next, curl your hands up to your shoulders like you're doing a biceps curl, then raise your hands above your head. Lower your arms, and repeat all steps.

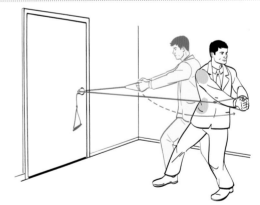

Ⓓ 3 O'CLOCK TO 9 O'CLOCK This exercise works your obliques and shoulders. You can increase the intensity of the move by walking farther from the door to pull the resistance band tighter. Perform three sets of 15 reps on each side.

HOW Tie a resistance band around a doorknob, and close the door. Stand with your feet shoulder-width apart and your body at a 90-degree angle from the door. Grab the band with both hands, and hold it at shoulder height. Pivot on your feet to turn away from the door while pulling the band across your body. Switch sides, and repeat.

269 ASSESS YOUR PAIN

It's no surprise that professional athletes dread sports-related injuries that can take them out of the game. But many gym-goers also share this fear—they know that their success in the gym is based on regularity and repetition, and that anything that jeopardizes their schedule can derail their fitness goals. So if you are feeling any level of pain, you need to determine if your muscles are fatigued, sore, or actually injured—and whether or not to seek treatment. Here are some guidelines.

FATIGUE Muscles that are fatigued by strenuous work undergo physiological changes, including buildup of lactic acid (the "burn"), increased tissue acidity, and chemical energy depletion, so you might feel mild pain at the end of an exercise. This discomfort is temporary and diminishes quickly.

SORENESS Muscle pain that occurs a day or two after working out is known as delayed onset muscle soreness, or DOMS. It is associated with eccentric muscle contractions (the nonworking phase of lifting) and can be the result of microscopic tears in the muscle or connective tissue. DOMS may be mild, moderate, or so severe that sitting down in a chair is painful. Avoid any resistance training until it eases, usually in a day or two, and treat it with warm baths, heating pads, stretching, range-of-motion body movements, and acetaminophen.

INJURY Any pain that begins during or directly after working out and lasts for several days or more is likely to be a strain, also called a muscle pull. Strains happen when small tears occur in muscles and tendons after stretching them beyond capacity—a popping sensation is often the first sign. Strains can also occur from excessive training or a fall. They are classified as mild, moderate, or severe, but if you suspect a strain, have a doctor examine you as soon as possible in order to avoid complications.

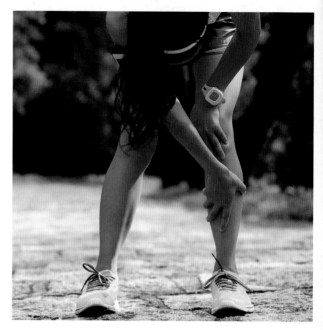

270 REST AND RECOVER

It's great to have that "gung ho!" attitude when it comes to getting in shape, but it's also important to know when you need to say "gung whoa!" Recovery is the term that fitness trainers use when describing the time it takes sore muscles to repair themselves. Ideally, you should wait for at least 48 hours before focusing on the same muscle group, so stagger your target areas—upper body followed by lower body, for example. As well as helping you physically recuperate, a period of rest also allows you to recover psychologically.

Ask the EXPERT

STRAIN OR SPRAIN?

This is a question that fitness trainers often hear, and there is a distinct difference. Strains and sprains both involve damage to the body's supporting framework: the bones, muscles, tendons, and ligaments.

When a muscle or tendon—a fibrous cord connecting muscles to bones—is stretched or torn, the injury is called a strain. Acute strains occur at the junction where the muscle is becoming a tendon, when the muscle is stretched and suddenly contracts, as during running or jumping. Chronic strains develop from overuse or repetitive stress, such as serving a tennis ball, which leads to an inflamed tendon—tendonitis. Strains can be accompanied by symptoms including sharp pain, swelling, bruising, or redness. They are treated by rest, cold packs, compression, and elevation.

Ligaments are the tissues that connect bones to each other. Sprains involve the stretching or tearing of a ligament or a joint capsule. Forcing a joint beyond its normal range of motion, such rolling your ankle, is the most common cause of sprains. You will experience pain and inflammation, and, because ligaments provide joint stability, you may temporarily lose the ability to move your limb properly.

Both strains and sprain require speedy medical intervention, but with due care, most of these injuries heal without long-term problems.

271 ICE IT OR APPLY HEAT

There are two accepted ways to ease muscle pain or injury (icing and heating) but most people have no clue which treatment to apply, and so they end up using the wrong one, or both … or neither. Here are some guidelines to make remembering less difficult.

ICING The application of cold packs (or bags of frozen peas) to an injury relieves pain by numbing the area as well as reducing swelling, inflammation, and bleeding. Always ice the site immediately (remember: **I**ce **I**mmediately) after the injury occurs and for the next two days. To make your own cold pack, freeze a wet, folded hand towel inside a plastic zip bag.

HEATING Applying a heating pad, warm compress, or other source of heat brings blood to an injured area and reduces joint stiffness and muscle spasms. Use these methods only after 48 hours of icing an injury. And don't apply a heating pad directly to the skin—wrap it in flannel or a towel.

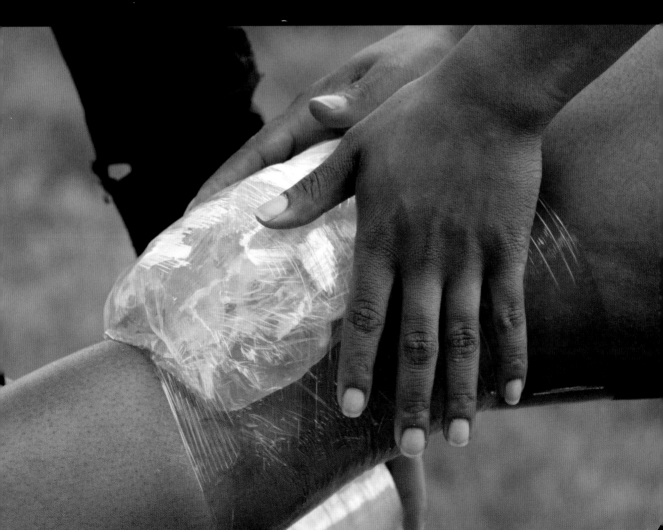

272 CALL THE DOCTOR!

If you are experiencing pain and suspect you have a strain, sprain, or other exercise-related injury—meaning the pain began while you were exercising and did not let up for a day or two—it's time to visit a health care professional to get an examination. After determining the type and severity of the injury, he or she will recommend a protocol to expedite healing, possibly including physical therapy. In the case of some more extreme strains, such as a ripped tendon, surgery might be in order. But even with more moderate injuries, proper and timely treatment is imperative—otherwise scar tissue could form around the tear and limit your range of motion, requiring visits to a physiotherapist or chiropractor.

In addition to strains and sprains, here are some injuries that might require a doctor's care.

BACKACHE Even though strength and flexibility exercises often ultimately relieve lower-back pain, you might initially experience lumbar aches when you begin to work out or perform repetitive motions. Make sure that you warm up properly, and treat any pain with stretching, strength work, and cold packs.

GROIN PULL Stressing groin muscles that are stiff, a bit weak, and prone to strains is frequently the cause of this painful condition. Always go slowly when exploring the range of motion of a new exercise. Treat by icing the inner thigh and with compression, ibuprofen, and stretching and strengthening exercises. Full recovery could take 12 weeks.

SHIN SPLINTS Those stabbing pains along the front of the lower legs are caused by intensifying your running or biking routine too quickly or not allowing enough recovery time. Shin splints occur from damage to one of two muscle groups along the shinbone. Treatment includes cessation of activity, stretching, strength work, cold packs, and ibuprofen, and adding arch supports or heel lift inserts to running shoes.

RUNNER'S KNEE The knee may be the most likely body part to be injured during exercise. Runner's knee, which can be caused by tight hamstrings, improper foot support, or weak thigh muscles, causes a dull pain around the front of the knee (patella) where it connects with bottom of the thighbone (femur). It is especially painful going up and down stairs. Treatment involves cessation of running, cold packs, compression, elevation, ibuprofen, stretching, and the addition of arch supports.

BLISTERS These tender fluid-filled bubbles can ruin a workout or run; if they become infected, they take a lot longer to heal and can adversely affect your routine. To reduce the friction that causes blisters, wear properly fitting shoes and moisture-wicking socks. A bit of petroleum jelly also helps lubricate blister-prone areas.

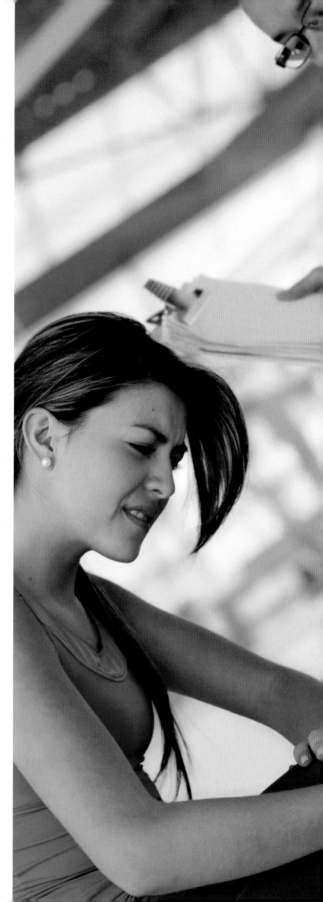

273 TAKE IT EASY

If you are diagnosed with a serious sports or fitness-related injury, it's important that you abide by your doctor's instructions regarding recuperation time. Muscles, tendons, and ligaments can sometimes take longer than bones to mend. Make sure that you don't skip or shorten any physical therapy sessions, and if home exercises are called for, do them for as long as prescribed.

Another part of recovery is understanding what happened to cause the injury and doing your best to ensure that it will not occur again. If you forgot warming up, overtrained, or tried a difficult move without guidance from a trainer, then those are situations you can avoid in future. If you took a misstep, got a cramp, or fell, then those are not circumstances you could have changed. Accepting that and moving on is important. Even the best and strongest athletes occasionally suffer a hard knock through no fault of their own.

274 COME BACK SLOWLY

Once your doctor or physical therapist clears you to go back to the gym, make sure to follow these suggestions for a seamless—and painless—re-entry.

MAKE A PLAN Work with your doctor, physiotherapist, and trainer to come up with an exercise-based rehab plan. Your physical therapist or trainer can also spot any faulty movements or muscle imbalances that might cause future injuries.

STAY FUELED During recovery and re-entry you need to eat right and maintain proper hydration. Avoid alcohol, refined sugar, or white flour; stick with lean protein, complex carbs, and lots of greens. You might also consider taking joint-building supplements like glutamine or MSM and chondroitin.

TAKE YOUR TIME Even after you start to feel like your old, pre-injury self, stick with your rehab plan for at least another two weeks. That way you continue to build strength. Once your rehab rules have relaxed, continue to focus on exercises that emphasize stability, flexibility and the core.

ROLL WITH IT It's critical to warm up your injured muscles before exercising, so consider massaging the vulnerable spots with a foam roller.

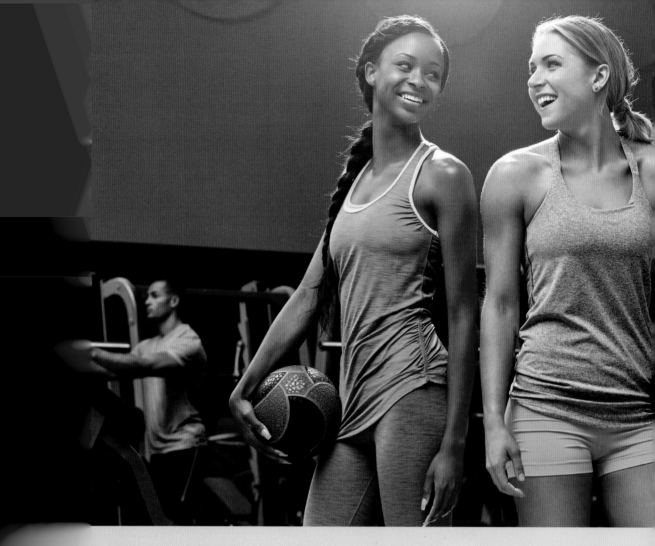

 LEARN FROM THE JOURNEY The end of the Challenge is only the beginning. A key part of any transformative experience is the journey from an unsatisfactory physical state to improved strength and increased flexibility, and greater confidence. You've honed the skills that are used use to maintain your healthy lifestyle—patience, discipline, determination, and the ability to dig deep and sometimes even surprise yourself. Take a moment to congratulate yourself on completing 12 weeks of rigorous training. Only you know the physical difficulties you faced and the personal battles you fought. Celebrate that success, and compare your "before" and "after" photos. Maybe your weakness was snacks, or lack of discipline. Whatever the struggles, you came out on the other side a winner. You shed pounds, and gained muscle and improved self-respect.

 AVOID BACKSLIDING Momentum is nearly as important after the Challenge as it is during the 12-week process. This time you're competing only with yourself. Still, you already know the drill: continue to schedule those gym hours each week, investigate new classes that pique your interest, keep your home or office fitness tools at hand, enjoy weekend rewards—a visit to the zoo or museum or a night out with friends—or treat yourself to new fitness gear, and stay in touch with those gym buddies. The end of the challenge is a time to schedule a session with your personal trainer and map out the route forward from here.

 WRITE A LETTER TO YOUR OLD SELF Remember that old you? A person who felt ancient before your time, and

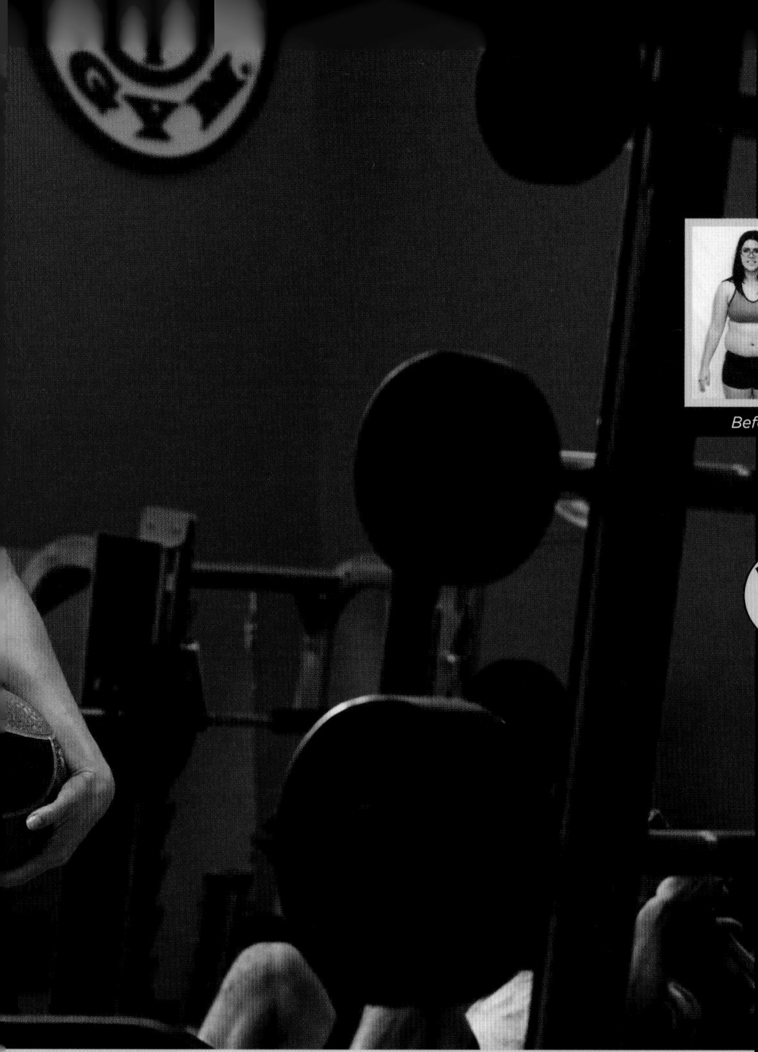

FOLLOW A WINNER'S JOURNEY
Chelsea Meza
Female Winner, Ages 18–29

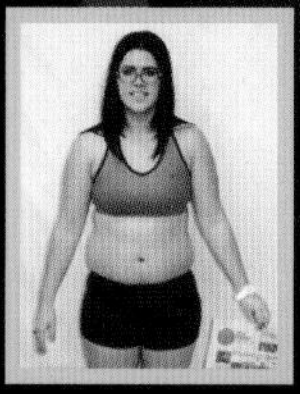

Before

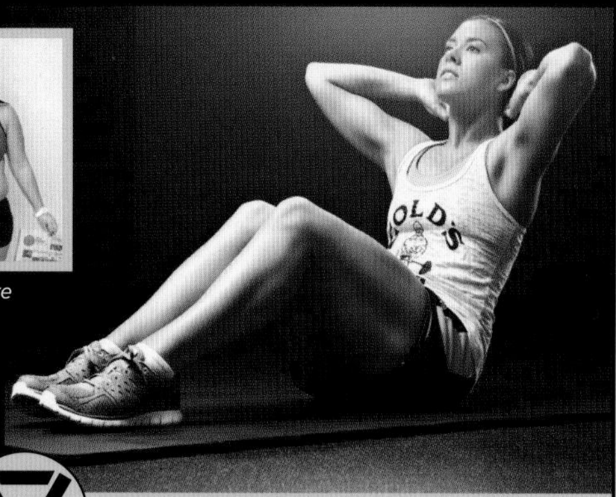

LOST 33 pounds (15 kg)

Chelsea knows how it feels to be stressed, tired, moody, and overweight. Chelsea was training to become a cosmetologist and was married young, but still felt unmotivated and uninspired by much of her life. It took competing in the 2013 Gold's Gym Challenge to change her attitude—and she ended up a state and national winner!

"I'm not saying this to brag," she explains, "I am saying it so you will trust me and listen to what I'm going to tell you. ... The Challenge was so many things to me—hard, awesome, tiring, cool, exhausting, and invigorating! I lost 33 pounds, and gained so much more—confidence, joy, a hot bod, and lots of muscle!"

Chelsea warns that during the Challenge, your family can negatively influence your eating habits. She had to learn to say a firm "No!" to well-meaning relatives. She also recommends printing out an unflattering "before" photo and then finding a favorite photo of a version of yourself that you want to recapture. Whenever you are frustrated, take out both photos to remind yourself where you are going and why. Get excited, re-energize, and re-commit. "Tell yourself you are a rock star," she adds, "and push forward. Twelve weeks are going to fly by!"

who couldn't keep up with your kids, younger coworkers, or even peers? It's time to write that person a letter from the other side. Tell that "before" version of yourself how much you appreciate the decision that brought you to this healthy new place, and how you promise to devote yourself to holding on to the gains you've made. Let that person know that you are now less likely to develop type 2 diabetes or high blood pressure. Your new clean diet also reduces your risk for some cancers and heart disease and may add years to your life.

WINNER'S WORDS

"Finish the Challenge strong, and prepare for everyone to be amazed and say to you, 'Are you kidding me!'"

~ Chelsea Meza

MAINTAIN YOUR MOJO

Even if you are seeing results, it can be hard to stay motivated at the gym week in and week out. You might also hit a slump and find you're making excuses to stay home. Gold's Gym (and the Mayo Clinic) offer some possible solutions that will raise your level of enthusiasm and beat the blahs.

SET SHORT-RANGE GOALS We're always told to look at the big picture, but sometimes dealing with things in smaller increments is a lot easier on our psyches. Break your fitness goals into doable segments—for instance focus on losing 2 pounds a week rather than 24 pounds in 12 weeks. And be sure to write down those goals.

KEEP IT FUN Who said working out had to be so serious? Break up your strength or cardio routines with some free-form dancing to your MP3 player or do a circuit around the track—while skipping.

MAKE A SWITCH It helps to vary your workouts. If you always head to the treadmill for cardio, give the elliptical a go. Try a new piece of equipment, such as an EZ bar or a new modality, such as TRX or battle rope training, or sign up for a lively class, like Zumba or PiYo. Trying something new helps keep boredom at bay.

FIND OTHER OUTLETS Make fitness part of your home life, not just a gym experience. Get off the couch, and get yourself moving. Weed the garden, mow the lawn, paint the guest room, rake the leaves, hand polish the stair rails, or de-clutter the closets—remember, if you're moving, your core's moving.

DON'T BE RIGID If you make yourself a hostage to your fitness goals, then the gym will start to feel like a prison. Take a day or two off if you need to chill. Forcing yourself to exercise can sour you and end up derailing your efforts a lot quicker than a few days of R&R.

GIVE YOURSELF A REWARD If you've met a tough goal or beaten a personal best, how about rewarding yourself with something special? You can upgrade your gear—such as buying yourself new running shoes or a tote-bag for your yoga mat—or you could treat yourself to a new activity—such as a fun dance class or yoga in the park.

MAKE FITNESS TIME FAMILY AND FRIEND TIME Maybe this message keeps getting repeated because it's true—it is always more entertaining to work out with a friend or loved one. Make gym time couple time or try organizing an informal game of soccer or street hockey with your kids or friends.

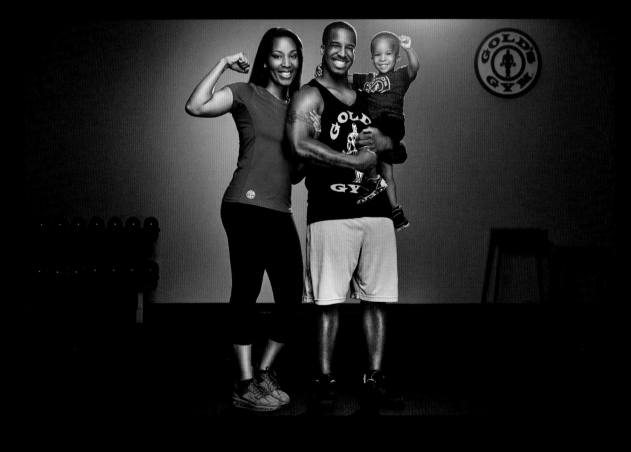

276 BRING ON THE SANDMAN

Adequate sleep is a key part of fitness—it is when the body and brain replenish. Lack of sleep won't just leave you foggy; chronic insomnia can also make you prone to diabetes, depression, cardiovascular disease, and weight gain. Still, you'd think that getting regular exercise would send you straight to dreamland at night, but even certain pro athletes find that sleep eludes them, resulting in a loss of aerobic endurance. Below are some triggers for sleep problems, along with how to avoid them so that you can wake up feeling fresh and alert.

KICK THE CAFFEINE Most people know enough not to drink caffeine in the evening, but even a cup of tea at 4:00 p.m. can affect your sleep patterns. If you are a restless sleeper, boycott any drinks with caffeine after 2:00 p.m.

SNOOZE WITH SEROTONIN Heavy meals should be avoided before bedtime, but some foods can actually help you sleep. An all-carbohydrate snack is beneficial for getting your body to make the most of its own store of sleep-inducing serotonin (as well as tryptophan, an amino acid that is converted to serotonin in the body). Try a late-night snack of graham crackers, or you can add serotonin or serotonin-precursor supplements, such as 5-HTP, to your nutrition plan.

SAY NO TO NIGHTCAPS It's true that alcohol will make you sleepy, but it is also true that it can disturb the second half of your sleep cycle and decrease deep sleep. Have wine or beer with dinner, not while watching the late news.

BATHE EARLY One traditional cure for insomnia—taking a hot bath before heading to bed—may actually keep you up. Anything that raises your body temperature near bedtime can stop you from falling asleep. The body likes to be cool as it slumbers, which is why we often wake up to find one foot outside the covers.

RELAX WITH YOGA Shedding mental and physical stress is an ideal way to invite sleep. At bedtime, try some gentle yoga moves, such as the reclined butterfly. Lie supine with your soles together, knees drooping. Then close your eyes, and inhale through your nose while slowly counting to four; exhale counting backwards to one. A 10-minute session should ease you into sleep.

BANISH LIGHT Exposure to bright lights or computer screens—which signal daytime to our brains—before bedtime can delay the onset of sleep. Dim the lights as you get ready for bed, and then turn off all technology, including your cell phone text alert.

277 PAT YOURSELF ON THE BACK

At some point in your fitness journey, you will realize that you got out of bed in the morning without any creakiness or pain. Perhaps you hefted your preschooler into your arms at the supermarket entrance and *ran* to the car in the rain. Or you slipped into that party dress or sports jacket from your college days, and it actually fit. "Wow," you think with a bit of shock. "It's really working."

This is where you congratulate yourself, when you comprehend that through dedication, application, and hard work, you have changed your physical appearance for the better. And that there are so many beneficial changes on the inside, ones you can't even see—like increased strength, greater stamina, a healthier heart and lungs, a boosted metabolism, and improved flexibility. Like being at a lower risk for high blood pressure and type 2 diabetes. Or that feeling you can conquer the world. So tell yourself "Well done!"—and eat a celebratory cupcake or plate of French fries. And then get right back on the gym floor, and start to work your butt off. *Again.*

278 KEEP UP THE GREAT WORK

For some people, reaching their goal is not the most difficult part of a fitness plan. Maybe you're one of them. You can apply yourself like gangbusters initially, but can't sustain the momentum to hold onto those gains afterward. If so, here are some suggestions to stop you from relapsing and losing the precious inroads you've made toward better health and fitness.

UPDATE YOUR GOALS Maintenance will require a different mindset than conditioning. Change your focus by giving yourself fitness goals outside the gym—joining a charity race, for example, or starting up a hiking group. Also engage in a physical activity you enjoy for its own sake, like horseback riding or softball.

SIDESTEP YOUR TRIGGERS Don't let personal drama or any negative emotions impact your health decisions during transition. If something is so upsetting that you vow to ditch the gym for the next month, take a yoga class instead to regain your centered self.

PASS IT ALONG Rather than spending your time obsessively recording miles or calories, become a message-bearer to keep yourself accountable. Share knowledge and experience with your friends, co-workers, or family members, and encourage them to find their own path to wellness.

BE PATIENT Remind yourself frequently that it takes time to shift gears into maintenance mode. For instance, ease up on high-intensity workouts and lower your caloric demand accordingly, but don't stop scheduling those gym visits or trainer sessions—and never lose that healthy desire to improve yourself. Remember that fitness is a lifelong journey, not a destination.

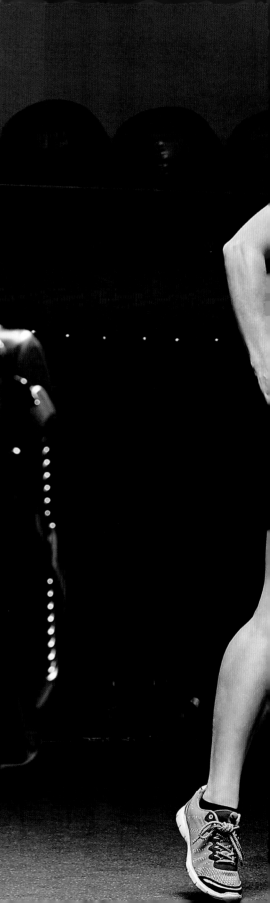

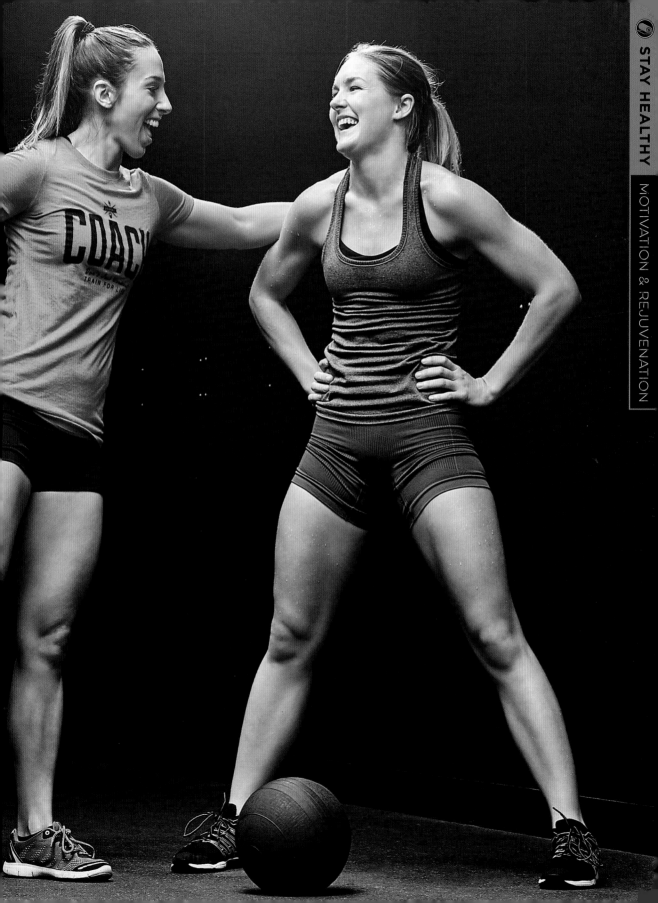

INDEX

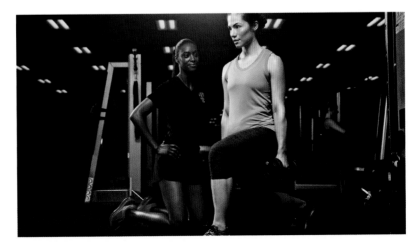

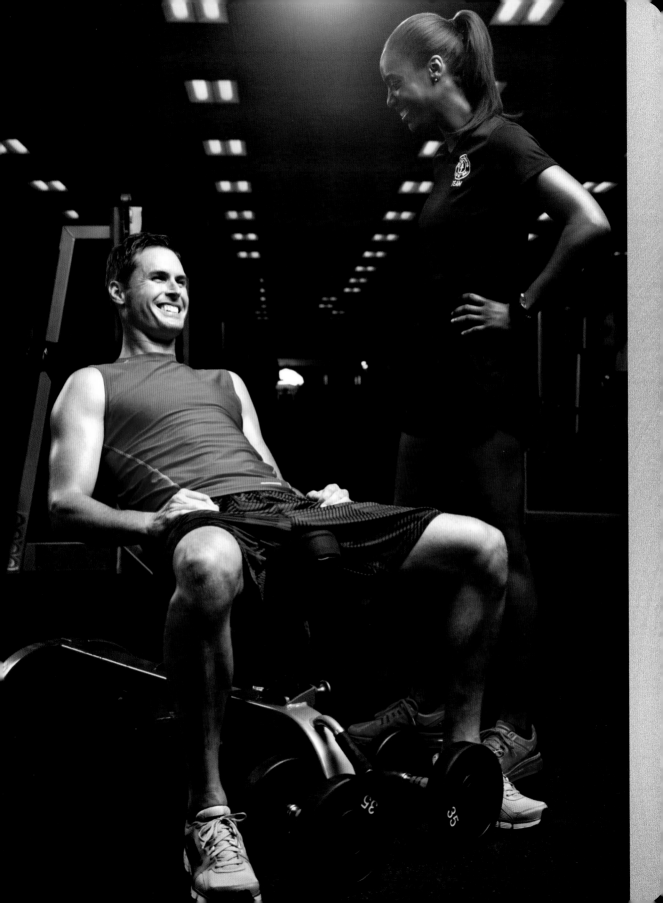

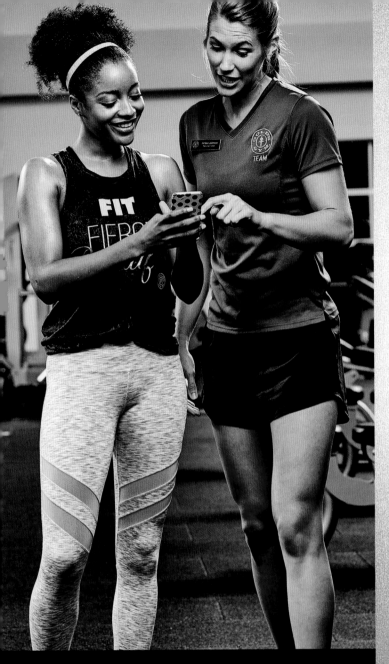

weldonowen

PRESIDENT & PUBLISHER Roger Shaw
ASSOCIATE PUBLISHER Mariah Bear
SVP, SALES & MARKETING Amy Kaneko
FINANCE & OPERATIONS DIRECTOR
Philip Paulick
ASSOCIATE EDITOR Ian Cannon
CREATIVE DIRECTOR Kelly Booth
ART DIRECTOR Allister Fein
ILLUSTRATION COORDINATOR
Conor Buckley
PRODUCTION DIRECTOR Chris Hemesath
ASSOCIATE PRODUCTION DIRECTOR
Michelle Duggan
IMAGING MANAGER Don Hill

© 2017 Weldon Owen Inc.
a division of Bonnier Publishing USA
1045 Sansome Street, Suite 100
San Francisco, CA 94111
weldonowen.com

Library of Congress Control Number
on file with the publisher.

ISBN 13: 978-1-68188-044-0
ISBN 10: 1-68188-044-X
10 9 8 7 6 5 4 3 2 1
2017 2018 2019 2020 2021
Printed in China by 1010 Printing International

MOSELEY ROAD INC

PRESIDENT Sean Moore
CONTRIBUTING WRITER/EDITOR
Nancy J. Hajeski
PROOFREADER Jessie Shiers
DESIGNER Lisa Purcell

**Special thanks to Hollis Liebman for
his fitness expertise and invaluable
contributions to the text.**

Thanks as well as to Brittany Bogan for
editorial assistance and to Kevin Broccoli
of BIM Creatives for creating the index.

CREDITS

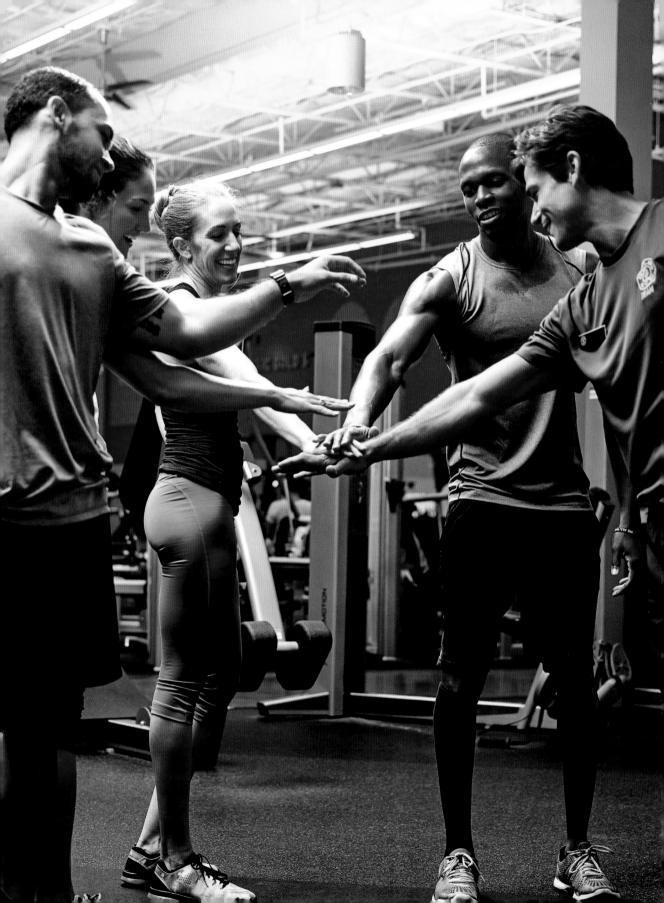